Surgery of Larynx and Trachea

Marc Remacle
Hans Edmund Eckel (Eds.)

Surgery of Larynx and Trachea

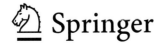 Springer

Prof. Marc Remacle
Dept. of ORL-Head & Neck Surgery
University Hospital of
Louvain at Mont-Godinne
Dr. G. Therasse avenue 1
5530 Yvoire, Belgium
marc.remacle@uclouvain.be

Prof. Dr. Hans Edmund Eckel
Landeskrankenhaus Klagenfurt
Hals-Nasen-Ohren-Abteilung
St. Veiter Str. 47
9026 Klagenfurt
Austria
hans.eckel@kabeg.at

ISBN: 978-3-540-79135-5   e-ISBN: 978-3-540-79136-2

DOI: 10.1007/978-3-540-79136-2

Springer Heidelberg Dordrecht London New York

Library of Congress Control Number: 2009926262

Cover design: eStudio Calamar, Figueres/Berlin

Printed on acid-free paper

Springer is part of Springer Science+Business Media (www.springer.com)

"To the memory of Prof. Dr. György Lichtenberger (1944–2009)"

Foreword

I have been honoured to write the foreword to this European Textbook on *Surgery of Larynx and Trachea.*

This multi-author textbook under the editorship of Professor Marc Remacle and Professor Hans Eckel is definitely a milestone in European laryngology and for the European Laryngological Society.

The editors and the chapter authors belong to the leading laryngologists in Europe. The book covers a broad field within larynx and trachea and represents the state of art within European laryngology today. The book covers physiology, phoniatrics, open, and endoscopic operative techniques in adults and in pediatrics. Even assisting drugs used in clinical practice as steroids, fibrin glue, mitomycin C, cidofovir, etc. have been covered.

The book is easy to read, but goes into depths of representative fields.

On the whole, the book is very well illustrated, not only with endoscopic photos, but also with a lot of illustrative drawings which complement and add to the quality of the chapters.

I am sure that this is a book that will be read, not only by laryngologists in Europe and outside, but also used in the teaching of residents and those superspecializing in laryngology.

As one of the founding members of ELS and President of EUFOS, I must congratulate all the authors and editors of this European Textbook on *Larynx and Trachea.* The book is an example of the standard and quality of European ORL-HNS and especially laryngology today. The book is definitely very promising for the future.

Jan Olofsson

Preface

Only 25 years ago, laryngology and laryngeal surgery mainly dealt with life-threatening conditions of the larynx, particularly those related to airway obstruction and laryngeal cancer. Endoscopic biopsies for diagnostic purposes, open laryngeal surgery to resect laryngeal tumours and tracheotomy for airway relief were the principal laryngeal procedures at most Ear, Nose and Throat departments throughout Europe and the world.

In the meanwhile, research into laryngeal anatomy and physiology, technical advances and pharmacological progress have provided us with an abundance of new insights into the basic laryngeal functions – protection of the lower airway during deglutition and voice production – and therapeutic options. During the same period, our attitude towards health and medical care has changed considerably. While cure was the only ambition of most medical and surgical interventions in the past, the preservation and improvement of physical function is now an equally important issue. Individuals in today's developed societies depend on communicative skills rather than on physical work, and laryngology has become a major medical subspecialty dealing with communication disorders.

Clinical pioneers, some of them are contributors to this textbook, have developed a wealth of new endoscopic and surgical techniques to improve the voice, to recover deglutition, to restore a laryngeal and tracheal airway and to treat cancer without sacrifice of laryngeal function. Refined diagnostic tools, to assess structural changes (endoscopy and imaging) or functional impairment (voice analysis) are available to identify both the origin and the consequences of laryngeal disease, and to direct symptom-related surgery. Different surgical traditions throughout the countries of Europe have developed into different solutions for clinical problems. This diversity of opinion and practice is part of this book. Each chapter reflects the personal experience and clinical skill of the contributing author. Differences in opinion may occur, and not all dilemmas in laryngology have been solved so far.

This textbook has been written to lay out the basic principles of contemporary laryngeal surgery from a European perspective. The description of these fundamentals of laryngeal surgery will not replace surgical atlases or detailed descriptions of individual laryngeal procedures. By providing context and perspective, the chapters of this textbook are meant to supply the reader with the fundamentals of laryngeal surgery.

The editors hope that this textbook may serve as a basis for future research, for discussion among laryngologists and as a source of inspiration to our readers.

We express our gratitude to Springer editors, who made this book possible, to the contributors to this project, and to our fellows, students and families.

September 2009   Mont Godinne and Klagenfurt
Marc Remacle and Hans Edmund Eckel
Editors

Contents

Contributors

Christoph Arens Universitätsklinikum Magdeburg A.ö.R.,
Universitätsklinik für Hals-, Nasen- und Ohrenheilkunde, Klinikdirektor,
Leipziger Str. 44, 39120 Magdeburg, Germany
e-mail: christoph.arens@med.ovgu.de

Alfons J. M. Balm Department of Head and Neck Oncology and Surgery,
The Netherlands Cancer Institute, Antoni van Leeuwenhoek Hospital,
Plesmanlaan 121, 1066 CX, Amsterdam, The Netherlands
e-mail: a.balm@nki.nl

Martin A. Birchall John Farndon Chair of Surgery, University of Bristol
e-mail: Martin.Birchall@bristol.ac.uk

Patrick J. Bradley Department ORL-NHS, Nottingham University Hospitals,
Queens Medical Centre Campus, Derby Road, Nottingham NG7 2UH England
e-mail: pjbradley@zoo.co.uk

Michiel W. M. van den Brekel Department of Head and Neck
Oncology and Surgery, The Netherlands Cancer Institute,
Antoni van Leeuwenhoek Hospital, Plesmanlaan 121, 1066 CX,
Amsterdam, The Netherlands

Dominique Chevalier Service ORL Hospital Huriez,
Centre Hospitalier et Universitairee de Lille, Rue Michel Polonovski,
59037 Lille Cedex, France
e-mail: d-chevalier@chru-lille.fr

Philippe H. Dejonckere The Institute of Phoniatrics & Logopedics,
University Medical Center Utrecht, AZU F.02.504,
P.O. Box 85500, 3508 GA Utrecht, The Netherlands
e-mail: Ph.deJonckere@umcutrecht.nl

Frederik G. Dikkers Department of Otorhinolaryngology,
University Medical Center Groningen, University of Groningen,
P.O. Box 30001, 9700 RB Groningen, The Netherlands
e-mails: f.g.dikkers@kno.azg.nl; f.g.dikkers@kno.umcg.nl

Suzy Duflo Equipe d'Audio-Phonologie Expérimentale et Clinique,
Laboratoire Parole et Langage, CNRS-Université de Provence,
Marseille, France
e-mail: sduflo@yahoo.com

Hans Edmund Eckel Department of Oto-Rhino-Laryngology,
A.ö. Landeskrankenhaus Klagenfurt, HNO, St. Veiter Str. 47,
A-9020 Klagenfurt, Austria
e-mail: hans.eckel@kabeg.at

Gerhard Friedrich Professor and Chairman,
Ear, nose and Throat University Hospital, Graz,
Head of Department of Phoniatrics, Speech and Swallowing,
Medical University of Graz, Auenbruggerplatz 26-28,
A-8036 Graz, Austria
e-mail: phoniatrie.hno@meduni-graz.at

Patrick Froehlich University Lyon 1 and Chair of Department of Pediatric
Otolarygnology, Head and Neck Surgery,
Hospital Femme Mère Enfant, 59 bd Pinel,
69677 Bron cedex, France
e-mail: patrick.froehlich@chu-lyon.fr

Antoine Giovanni Equipe d'Audio-Phonologie Expérimentale et Clinique,
Laboratoire Parole et Langage, CNRS-Université de Provence,
Marseille, France
e-mail: antoine.giovanni@ap-hm.fr

David G. Grant Specialist Registrar, Bristol Royal Infirmary,
Upper Maudin Street, Bristol BS2 8HW, UK
e-mail: mail@davisgrant.com

Orlando Guntinas-Lichius Department of Otolaryngology,
Friedrich-Schiller-University Jena, D-07740 Jena, Germany
e-mail: orlando.guntinas@med.uni-jena.de

Anastasios G. Hantzakos First Department of Otorhinolaryngology,
Head & Neck Surgery of the University of Athens Medical School,
Hippocrateion General Hospital, Athens, Greece
e-mail: ahantza@gmail.com

Frans J. M. Hilgers Department of Head and Neck Oncology and Surgery,
The Netherlands Cancer Institute, Antoni van Leeuwenhoek Hospital,
Plesmanlaan 121, 1066 CX Amsterdam, The Netherlands
e-mail: f.hilgers@nki.nl

Barış Karakullukçu Head and Neck Surgeon, The Netherlands Cancer Institute,
Antoni van Leeuwenhoek Academic Hospital, Plesmanlaan 121,
1066 CX Amsterdam, The Netherlands
e-mail: b.karakullukcu@nki.nl

Georges Lawson Department of ORL Head & Neck Surgery,
Cliniques Universitaires UCL de Mont-Godinne, Therasse avenue 1,
5530 Yvoir, Belgium
e-mail: george.lawson@uclouvain.be

György Lichtenberger[†] ORL-HNS, Szent Rokus Hospital & Institutions,
Gyulai P.u. 2, 1085 Budapest, Hungary

Jean-Paul Marie Service d'ORL & Chirurgie Cervico faciale,
Hopital Ch Nicolle, CHU Rouen, F-76031, Laboratoire de Chirurgie
Expérimentale UPRES EA 3830 GRHV, IFRMP 23,
Université de Rouen, France
e-mails: Jean-Paul.Marie@chu-rouen.fr; jean-paul.marie4@wanadoo.fr

Philippe Monnier Professor and Chairman, Otolaryngology, Head & Neck
Surgery Department, Centre Hospitalier Universitaire Vaudois,
Rue du Bugnon 46, CH-1011 Lausanne, Switzerland
e-mail: philippe.monnier@chuv.ch

Ferhan Öz Valikonagi cad.No:161/12 Nisantasi, 80200 Istanbul, Turkey
e-mail: ferhanoz@tkbbv.org.tr

Giorgio Perretti Department University of Brescia,
P.zzale Spedali Civili Brescia, 25100 Brescia, Italy
e-mail: g.peretti@tin.it

Miquel Quer Professor of Otorhinolaryngology, Head of the Department
of Otorhinolaryngology and Head and Neck Surgery, Hospital de la Santa Creu
i Sant Pau, Universitat Autonoma de Barcelona, Barcelona, Spain
e-mail: mquer@santpau.cat

Niels Rasmussen Department of Otolaryngology,
2100 Copenhagen, Rigshospitalet, Denmark
e-mail: niels.rasmussen@rh.regionh.dk

Marc Remacle Department of Otorhinolaryngology and Head & Neck surgery,
University Hospital of Louvain at Mont-Godinne, Dr. G. Therasse avenue 1,
5530 Yvoir, Belgium
e-mail: Marc.remacle@uclouvain.be

Christian Sittel Klinik für Hals-, Nasen-, Ohrenkrankheiten,
Plastische Operationen, Klinikum Stuttgart, Katharinenhospital,
Kriegsbergstraße 60, 70174 Stuttgart, Germany
e-mail: c.sittel@klinikum-stuttgart.de

I. Bing Tan Department of Head and Neck Oncology and Surgery,
The Netherlands Cancer Institute, Antoni van Leeuwenhoek Hospital,
Plesmanlaan 121, 1066 CX, Amsterdam, The Netherlands

Jochen Werner Department of Otolaryngology,
Head and Neck Surgery, Philipps-University of Marburg,
Deutschhausstr. 3, 35037 Marburg, Germany
e-mails: wernerj@med.uni-marburg.de; zapf@med.uni-marburg.de

Physiology of Voice Production

1

Antoine Giovanni and Suzy Duflo

Core Messages

> During phonation the respiratory cycle changes.
> The vocal fold is composed of the thyroarytenoid muscle, its fibrous tissue cover, and the facing mucosa.
> Cyclic repetition of closing and opening movements of the vocal cords results in vibration.
> Voice production depends on neuromotor coordination of all muscles involved in phonation.

Voice production corresponds to the physiological and physical processes by which vibration of the vocal fold is transformed into speech. The primary driving force for vocal fold vibration and voice production depends on conversion of aerodynamic energy to acoustical energy when the vocal folds are closed in the midline. The sound produced by vocal fold vibration is immediately modified and filtered in the cavities located between the vocal folds and the lips (buccopharyngeal resonator). Because a number of factors can affect phonation, voice production is a highly variable process, not only from person to person but also within the same person [24, 30].

A. Giovanni (✉)
Equipe d'Audio-Phonologie Expérimentale et Clinique,
Laboratoire Parole et Langage, CNRS-Université de Provence,
Marseille, France
e-mail: antoine.giovanni@ap-hm.fr

1.1 Breath Stream

The diaphragmatic muscle, innervated by the phrenic nerve, is the most important inspiratory muscle. Contraction increases airway capacity, allowing a larger volume of air to be inhaled. During its relaxation, the air is exhaled from the lungs, which can go back to their initial volume owing to their elastic properties. During quiet breathing, inhalation is shorter than exhalation. Under some conditions (e.g., during phonation), accessory respiratory muscles may also be used. The accessory inspiratory muscles are the external intercostal muscles, scalene muscle, and sternocleidomastoid muscle. The expiratory muscles are the internal intercostal muscles and abdominal muscles, including the three oblique muscles and the right and dorsal large muscles [25, 27, 32].

During phonation, the respiratory cycle changes with shortening of inhalation and lengthening of exhalation. After closure of the vocal folds, blocking the airflow, and increasing subglottal air pressure, the speaker strives to maintain a constantly higher-than-normal expiratory pressure in the lungs and trachea (see reference to phonatory threshold pressure, below). After taking a deep breath during the prephonatory phase, the forces of elastic recoil are called into play. The diaphragm is not relaxed until the recoil forces diminish. The second phase corresponds to involvement of the internal intercostal muscles, which tend to decrease the size of the thorax and thus increase air pressure. The third phase corresponds to activation of the abdominal muscles, which constitute the most important active component. When singing, expiratory pressure, in the best case scenario, is controlled by contraction of the oblique abdominal muscles rather than by contraction

M. Remacle, H. E. Eckel (eds.), *Surgery of Larynx and Trachea,*
DOI: 10.1007/978-3-540-79136-2_1, © Springer-Verlag Berlin Heidelberg 2010

of the right large abdominal muscles. Back muscles can also be used to stiffen the thorax.

1.2 Laryngeal Vibrator

The larynx sits on top of the trachea. The thyroid and cricoid cartilages, which are part of the larynx, provide reinforcement and prevent collapse of the airway. The other components of the larynx are mobile and form a closing mechanism that protects the trachea during deglutition. They include the arytenoid cartilage, epiglottis, and endolaryngeal muscles. For more information about the osteocartilaginous elements and the intrinsic and extrinsic muscles of the larynx, the reader is referred to classic anatomical descriptions [8, 33].

The vocal fold is a "multilayered" structure that exists only at the level of the anterior two-thirds of the fold (known as the "ligamentary" portion of the fold as opposed to the posterior cartilaginous portion, which corresponds to the vocal process). The vocal fold is composed of the thyroarytenoid muscle, its fibrous tissue cover, and the facing mucosa [7, 17, 18, 20] (Fig. 1.1).

The vocal fold features are specifically designed for vibration. The vibrating free edge is covered with squamous epithelium, which is more resistant to the mechanical constraints produced by vibration and contact than the pseudostratified respiratory mucosa that lines the rest of the larynx. In addition, the epithelium is covered with a mucus layer whose outer layer has a mucin film to prevent dehydration of the underlying

serous layer, cilia, and cells. The free edge of the vocal fold is glaborous (i.e., totally devoid of glands that might hinder mucosal wave formation); and most blood vessels as well as elastin and collagen fibers run parallel to the free edge of the vocal fold. The basement membrane is attached to the underlying lamina propria by interlacing fibers whose density appears to depend on genetic factors. Thus, genetics could predispose patients to develop certain lesions, such as nodules. The lamina propria has traditionally been divided into three layers according to the histological composition regarding elastin and collagen fibers (i.e., the superficial layer that corresponds to Reinke's space in the classic description and the middle and deep layers that correspond to the vocal ligament). Interstitial proteins regulate vocal fold viscosity, which is an essential physical factor in vibration. Proteins also contribute to absorption of mechanical shocks caused by vibration. Hyaluronic acid is especially important for both viscosity regulation and shock absorption. The distribution of fibrous and interstitial proteins probably depends on the mechanical stress to which the vocal folds are subjected and may be genetically determined.

Two of the most important cells of the lamina propria are fibroblasts and myofibroblasts. Fibroblasts play a key role in maintaining the integrity of the lamina propria. They allow replacement of proteins. Myofibroblasts are present only after trauma or damage requiring regeneration or repair of the extracellular matrix. This suggests that vocal folds are competent in repairing microscopic trauma within 36–48 hours. It has been reported that vocal rest is useful to give myofibroblasts time to act.

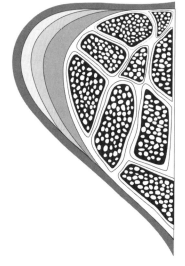 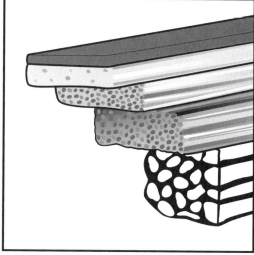

Fig. 1.1. Frontal section showing the multilayered structure of the vocal fold. (From Hirano [18], with permission)

1.3 Vocal Fold Vibration

All current theories and models of vocal fold vibration are based to some extent on the myoelastic-aerodynamic theory formulated by Van Den Berg. When the vocal folds are closed with appropriate tension on either side of the midline of the glottis (prephonatory attack position), airflow from the trachea is blocked and subglottic pressure increases. Vibration begins when subglottic pressure below the vocal folds exceeds fold resistance (phonation threshold pressure) and some air is released into the supraglottic region. As soon as the vocal folds separate, allowing some air to rush out, subglottic pressure decreases and the folds close back as a result of elastic recoil and the Bernouilli effect. Cyclic repetition of these closing and opening movements results in vibration [2, 6, 13, 16, 20, 23] (Fig. 1.2).

The mechanism underlying vocal fold vibration is comparable to that of a violin string. When the bow drags the string off the equilibrium point, countervailing elastic forces gradually build until they exceed the force of adhesion to the bow. At this point, the string "unhooks" and is free to oscillate (vibrate). When sufficient energy has been dissipated, the string adheres again to the bow. This is known as the stick–slip friction model involving alternation between a stick phase in which the string is dragged by the bow ("driving force") and a slip phase in which the string is free to oscillate at a frequency determined by the mass of the string and the amount of tension applied. In the larynx, airflow over the free edge of the vocal fold serves as the driving force (instead of a bow) [6, 13, 15] (Fig. 1.3).

According to Titze, phonation threshold pressure (i.e., the minimum air pressure required to sustain vocal fold oscillation) is the "missing link" in understanding vocal fold physiology [31]. The phonatory threshold pressure depends on several parameters.

- Stiffness of the vibrating portion of the vocal fold
- Viscosity of the vocal fold
- Thickness of the free edge of the vocal fold
- Width of the glottal opening prior to phonation
- Transglottic pressure gradient

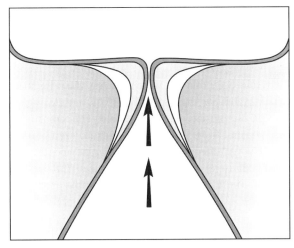

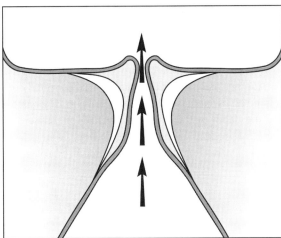

Fig. 1.2. Frontal section of the vocal folds shows resolution of the elastic conflict between subglottic air (*opening force*) and muscle and the elastic fold (closing force)

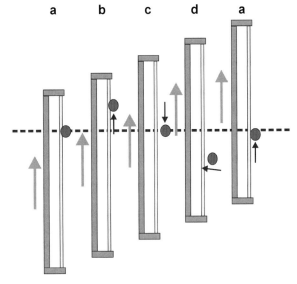

Fig. 1.3. Stick–slip friction model of fold vibration. (**a**, **b**) Stick phase. (**c**, **d**) Slip phase

Under normal conditions the phonatory threshold pressure is between 2 and 4 hPa and the subglottic pressure is around 7 hPa; however, higher pressures may be necessary when a louder voice is required. It has been shown that the increase of pitch has a relation with vocal fold tension, leading to higher phonatory threshold pressure. In disease states involving vocal fold lesions, mucosal stiffness leads to an increase in phonatory threshold pressure. In the case of unilateral laryngeal paralysis, the prephonatory glottic gap is too wide and the speaker must compensate by increasing the subglottic pressure. Increased phonatory threshold pressure is a fairly accurate indicator of voice strain in disease states.

There are numerous ways to decrease phonation threshold pressure. In general, decreasing the velocity of the tissues can be achieved by improving hydration, thereby decreasing tissue viscosity. Another way to decrease phonation threshold pressure is to decrease the mucosal wave velocity. This can be achieved by lowering surface tension (low-pitched voice) or by hydrating the surface mucus. The prephonatory glottic gap can be narrowed by tightening the muscles slightly. The goal of laryngoplasty in patients with laryngeal paralysis is to decrease the width of the prephonatory glottic opening. It can also be useful to increase the thickness of the vocal fold (e.g., by speaking in a lower-pitched voice or in some cases by changing the register: chest vs. head).

During a cycle of vibration, the vocal folds are not similar. This difference can be heard; but the coupling and adduction of the vocal folds has the effect of synchronizing the vibrating masses. This process is effective so long as differences between the two vocal folds stay within a certain range. Beyond the effective range, however, various abnormalities can appear, including biphonation, which corresponds to synchronization every other cycle. Another, more complex phenomenon is reciprocal modulation of the folds characterized by the presence of subharmonics and bifurcations (i.e., sudden state changes). This problem is frequently observed in patients with unilateral laryngeal paralysis, which is often associated with sudden voice shifts (bitonal voice) [4, 15, 22].

1.4 Pitch Control

The pitch of the human voice is related to the fundamental frequency (F_0) of vocal fold vibration. As shown in Table 1.1, pitch depends on the length of the vocal folds and the sex, age, and weight of the person. Vocal fold thickness has also been shown to affect pitch, which increases with thickness in both men and women [3, 9, 10, 14, 29] (Table 1.1).

Pitch control depends on adjusting the F_0 of vibration. This adjustment can involve regulation of mass or tension, which can be done actively by contracting the intralaryngeal muscles or passively by contraction of the perilaryngeal muscles. Basically, pitch control involves the combined actions of two muscles: the cricothyroid (CT) muscle, which acts on vocal ligament tension, and the thyroarytenoid (TA) muscle, which acts on the muscle mass of the fold. This adjustment mechanism can be viewed as bipolar, according to the "body-cover" theory described by Hirano and Titze. If the TA muscle is contracted and the CT muscle is relaxed, the total length of the vocal fold increases; moreover, the overall stiffness of all layers increases, so the F_0 increases. Conversely, if the TA muscle is contracted and the CT muscle is relaxed, the stiffness of the muscle mass and the F_0 increase. Accordingly, these two muscles with different sources of innervation—superior laryngeal nerve (SLN) (for the CT) and recurrent laryngeal nerve (RLN) (for the TA)—can be seen as exercising differential control over the F_0 (Fig. 1.4).

Another mechanism that can be used for pitch control involves increasing the cover tension by decreasing the depth of the vibrating tissue. This strategy is used to produce higher pitches, such as a falsetto sound. Decreasing the effective depth can lead to

Table 1.1. Voice pitch as a function of age and sex [1]

Subject	Weight (kg)	Height (m)	Fold length (mm)	Arytenoid length (mm)	F_0 (Hz)
Newborn	3.5	0.50	2	2	500
Eight-year-old	30	1.20	6	3	300
Adult woman	60	1.60	10	4	200
Adult man	75	1.80	16	4	125

F_0, fundamental frequency

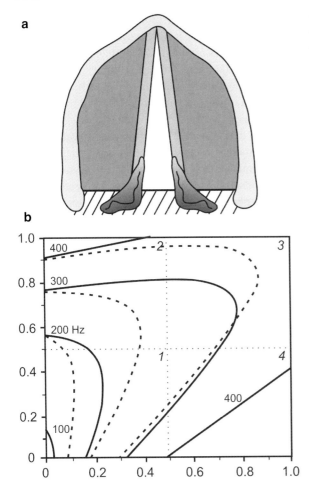

Fig. 1.4. Differential control of the fundamental frequency (F_0) by contracting the cricothyroid (CT) and thyroarytenoid (TA) muscles. (**a**) Action of the muscles. (**b**) Map of muscle activation. (From Titze [32], with permission)

changes in F_0 in the same way as changes in fold tension or length. The depth of the vibrating tissue can be regulated using the TA muscle. Although no accurate quantitative data are currently available, it can be speculated that the vocal fold ligament absorbs most of the elongation at high frequency so the remaining mucosa stays fairly loose. A taunt vocal ligament with a "free," loose tissue edge appears to represent the optimal condition for high-pitched phonation. For lower and middle-range frequencies, the muscle portion of the body can be used for elongation and tensioning. The vocal ligament can remain loose, providing a greater depth of vibration in the modal register [5, 26, 28].

The complex action of the TA on the F_0 is related to differences in tension and biomechanical properties of the tissue layers. According to Hirano, contraction of the TA muscle should be associated with an increase in body tension and a decrease in cover tension. If the vibrating tissue is composed only of mucosa, contraction of the TA muscle leads to lowering of the F_0. Conversely, if the vibrating tissue is composed mainly of muscle, contraction of the TA muscle leads to a rise in the F_0. Correlation between the F_0 and TA activity becomes more and more positive as the depth of vibration increases.

Each layer of the vocal fold has distinct biomechanical properties, depending on what is known as the length–tension ratio (i.e., tension induced in the material by changes in length, known as the stress–strain curve). In this regard, it has been shown that collagen fibers are more resistant to elongation than elastin fibers. Variations in the concentration of collagen and elastin in each layer of the lamina propria explain differences in behavior during elongation. A stress–strain curve can be obtained for the whole vocal fold. Total fold strain (tensile strain) corresponds to a combination of various active and passive actions that occur during tensioning.

1.5 Intensity Control

Current research indicates that the optimal glottic configuration for phonation is achieved when the vocal folds are in virtual contact and the vocal muscles are fairly relaxed. A slight gap should be established between posterior ends of the two vocal folds by balancing the activity of the adductor (interarytenoids and lateral cricoarytenoids) and abductor muscles. Under these conditions a quasi-sinusoidal signal with low harmonic content can produce a "pure voice" [11, 26, 28].

Intensity is controlled by combined regulation of subglottic pressure and glottic configuration. Higher intensity is achieved by simultaneously increasing vocal fold adduction and subglottic pressure. Because increased vocal fold adduction leads to longer contact time between the vocal folds, higher intensity is accompanied by a shortened open phase of the vocal folds cycle [19]. This raises the issue of the optimal adduction configuration. If the vocal folds do not touch, the voice is weak and of poor quality. Conversely, excessive contact leads to vocal straining, resulting in a tight, pressed voice quality. The ideal configuration appears to occur when the vocal folds are almost in contact before phonation (decreased prephonatory glottic width). In this configuration, the vocal folds are almost completely free and can express the full range of vibration modes. The signal produced is practically sinusoidal. This mode of functioning corresponds to what some singing teachers refer to as a "free-floating voice." According to this analogy, glottic resistance is adjusted to ensure the best possible yield from the conversion of aerodynamic to acoustical energy with minimal effect on vocal fold vibration. To increase the intensity, the glottis operates on a more "open–shut" than "wave" basis. However, glottal efficiency decreases, and a large amount of energy is dissipated at the vocal fold level in the form of friction, which can cause local inflammation and even fold lesions. These lesions, called dysfunctional lesions, are preferentially in the zone where contact of the vocal folds is the strongest (i.e., the middle third).

Increased tension in the voice apparatus can leads to "voice straining" on the part of the speaker. In the English-language literature, voice straining is often referred to as vocal misuse or abuse. In fact, the straining concept goes beyond vocal fold function and applies to all physiological components involved in communication. When striving to attract attention, the speaker increases muscle tension to produce a stronger, more effective ("projected") voice. This behavior, characterized by stiffening of the body, has been shown to result in increased muscle activity throughout the body. The breathing pattern changes in association with voice straining. Inhalation is deeper to increase subglottic pressure (prephonatory attack phase). Some subjects have trouble relaxing muscles sufficiently to inhale deeply and may need to use their accessory inspiratory muscles ("thoracic breathing" in place of the normal "abdominal breathing"). Stiffening is also observed in all posturing muscles including not only those of the neck and larynx but also those of the calves and back. Increased muscle activity in relation to increased vocal intensity requires more energy. If subjects do not or cannot rest sufficiently to offset the excess energy expenditure, they may develop complications such as dysfunctional laryngopathy (vocal overuse). Because voice straining affects all these components, rehabilitation should not be limited to changing the glottic configuration. Management must include a wide range of aspects, including general muscle tension, stress level, posture, and prephonatory respiration.

A number of factors promote synchronization of the vocal folds [12]. The first is symmetry of shape and tension of the vocal folds in the normal resting state. In this regard, unilateral laryngeal paralysis represents the worst possible condition. It should be noted that acceptable fold vibration can be obtained if contact is reestablished between the vocal folds, as can be observed during speech therapy or laryngeal manipulation. Another factor promoting synchronization is the Bernoulli effect, which applies equally to the two vocal folds and so tends to have the same effects as a function of glottic configuration. The most important synchronizing factor is the tissue mass-combining effect of direct contact between the vocal folds. The quality of contact is highly dependent on the vocal fold cover mucosa, with viscosity playing a major role. In vitro experiments on excised larynx models in our laboratory showed that the frequency of the vibration directly correlated with the viscosity of the artificial lubricant applied. The higher the viscosity of the lubricant used, the more the vibration frequency decreased when the vocal fold "closure" time increased. It has also been shown that more viscous mucosa increases the phonation threshold. Conversely, the greater the degree of asymmetry and freedom tend to be, the greater is the need for "forced" synchronization. It can thus be understood that the mechanism underlying "voice straining," used to increase loudness, is similar to the mechanism used to compensate for abnormalities in laryngeal vibration.

1.6 Vowel Production in the Vocal Tract

Human speech production depends on sound transformation in the vocal tract. According to the source-filter theory, the source sound is a pulsed airstream from the glottis containing numerous frequencies. Filtration consists of selecting certain frequencies for transmission through the mouth. The vocal tract acts as a resonator by suppressing the transfer of some frequencies. The concept of resonance in a tube is based on interference between waves submitted to multiple reflections. Like a wind instrument used to make music, the human vocal tract resonates at various source frequencies depending on the anatomical features that determine production of speech sounds (phonemes) [21, 30].

The resonance frequencies (formants) of the vocal tract are commonly numbered consecutively upward from the lowest frequency (F1–F5). Low-pitched formants correspond to the pharynx and high-pitched formants to the oral cavity. Vowels' formants are the lowest-pitched formants at F1 and F2. Thus, for vowel perception, the filtering process simplifies the code presented to the listener. In traditional phonetics, vowels are classified in regard to how the tongue is positioned in the mouth from top to bottom and from front to back. The tongue is placed at the bottom and back for the French /a/ vowel sound, at top and front for the French /i/ vowel sound, and top and back for the French /u/ vowel sound. These three vowels determine the vowel triangle on a F1 and F2 orthonormal representation.

To produce the French /eu/ vowel sound, the vocal tract is almost tubular with an almost constant cross section due to the neutral position of the tongue. The frequencies are about 500 Hz for F1 and 1500 Hz for F2. On the same diagram we can see the position of F1 and F2 with the tongue in different positions. For the French /a/ vowel sound, the vocal tract can be modeled as a narrow tube for the pharynx and a larger tube for the oral cavity.

Formants can be modified by articulatory movements. In general, the frequencies of all formants decrease evenly as the length of the tube increases. The length of the vocal tract can be changed by lowering the larynx or by projecting or retracting the lips. Because these movements cause frequency sliding without changing the interval between formants, there is no change in vowel identification. The sound of vowels can be modified by rounding the lips to reduce the mouth opening. Horn players sometimes cover the ends of their instruments to achieve this effect. The acoustical effect of obturation is the same as that of lengthening the tube (i.e., frequency sliding to a lower register). With the combination of adjusting the height of the larynx and the position and shape of the lips, it possible to enhance or muffle the pitch of the voice. Singers use several techniques to adjust pitch. Some sopranos can lower pitch by dropping the jaw. Using this technique, F1 can be brought into contact with F0; and acoustical power can be increased. By increasing acoustical power, contraction of the mouth lowers F1 and increases F2 to produce vowels with a wider spectrum (e.g., for the French /i/ vowel sound). Conversely, contracting the pharynx increases F1 and decreases F2 to produce a more compact vowel (e.g., for the French /a/ vowel sound).

Singers frequently talk about voice placement and claim that some vowels have exact locations in the vocal tract. The sensation that some vowels have precise locations could be related to the localization of pressure maxima of the standing waves in the vocal tract. Thus, there would be places where the sensations must be maximum (e.g., high pressure at the palate level for the French /i/ vowel sound, high pressure in the velar region for the French /u/ vowel sound, and high pressure in the pharyngeal region forthe French /a/ vowel sound). It is likely that some singers are able to use this sensation to customize vowel production. Other singing techniques based on sensations such as singing in a mask, using the jaw as a resonator, or directing the note at the level of the palate just behind the upper incisors may also be related to pressure maxima at precise locations in the vocal tract.

1.7 Nervous System Control

Voice production depends on neuromotor coordination of all muscles involved in phonation, ranging from posture and respiratory muscles to the muscles of the larynx, pharynx, and buccolabial articulatory apparatus [34].

1.7.1 Sensory Innervation of the Larynx

Sensory innervation of the larynx is provided mainly by the SLN, which receives fibers from the laryngeal vestibule and the laryngeal margin. These fibers merge with the vagus nerve at the level of the inferior vagus ganglion. Innervation of the vocal fold and subglottic region is also provided by fibers that merge with the RLN. There are sensory mucosal receptors in contact (mechanoreceptors) that induce the cough reflex when stimulated. They are mainly located at the vestibular level. In addition, intrinsic and extrinsic muscles present several types of articular and intramuscular mechanoreceptors (corpuscular, neuromuscular bundles, spiral) that supply nerve centers with proprioceptive information concerning vocal fold tension and elongation. The fibers penetrate the bulb of the vagus nerve and run in the direction of the nucleus of the solitary bundle.

1.7.2 Nerve Centers

The brain areas responsible for motor control of the pharynx and larynx are located in the lower part of the ascending frontal convolution (or precentral gyrus) of both hemispheres. When all or parts of these areas are stimulated, an overall laryeal response is observed with vocalization, inhibition of the posterior cricoarytenoid muscle, and bilateral activation of one or several adductor muscles. Cerebral damage in this area leads to unilateral paralysis.

There are many connections in the brain, particularly with language-related centers (e.g., the gyrus supramarginalis). The associative pathways between pharyngolaryngeal motor regions and cortical and subcortical auditory zones are especially noteworthy.

1.7.3 Reflex Control

Articulatory adjustment during phonation takes place during the prephonatory period and during sound production. Prephonatory adjustment is independent of audiophonatory control. This explains how singers produce sounds at a predetermined pitch and intensity. Prephonatory regulation in the cortex depends on input supplied by laryngeal mechanoreceptors concerning tension and position of the various muscles and articulations. During phonation, this input allows the adjustments necessary to maintain the glottic configuration to be made instantaneously. It is likely that other reflex arcs involving the abdomen thorax, neck, and tongue, among others, provide the feedback needed for continuous adjustment of the larynx during phonation.

1.7.4 Audiophonatory Control

Auditory feedback is a necessary component of voice control. This is demonstrated by the disordered, unmodulated voice produced by people with congenital deafness. Audiophonatory control probably depends on voluntary commands produced by corticobulbar pathways in response to acoustic input arriving in the auditory cortex as well as a range of acousticolaryngeal reflexes. However, these control mechanisms act in synergy with proprioceptive control, allowing prephonatory tuning.

During the first months after deafness, the proprioception input explains the almost normal voice of people who became deaf.

References

1. Baken RJ (1987) Clinical Measurement of Speech and Voice. Taylor and Francis, London
2. Berke GS, Moore DM, Hantke DR, Hanson DG, Gerrat BR, Burnstein F (1987) Laryngeal modeling: theoretical, in vitro, in vivo. Laryngoscope;97:871–888
3. Buck JM (1997) Organic variation in the vocal apparatus. In: Hardcastle WJ, Laver J (Eds). The Handbook of Phonetic Sciences. Blackwell, Cambridge, pp. 256–297
4. Davis PJ, Fletcher NH (1996) Vocal Fold Physiology: Controlling Complexity and Chaos. Singular Publishing, San Diego
5. Dejonckere PH, Hirano M, Sundberg J (Eds) (1995) Vibrato. Singular Publishing, San Diego
6. Dejonckere PH (1985) Le concept oscillo-impédantiel de la vibration laryngée. Rev Laryng (Bordeaux);106:275–282
7. Duflo S, Thibeault SL (2007) Anatomy of the larynx and physiology of phonation. In: Mesati AL, Bielamowicz SA (Eds). Textbook of laryngology, Chapter 3. Plural, San Diego
8. Fink BR, Demarest RJ (1978) Laryngeal Biomechanics. Harvard University Press, Cambridge
9. Fujimura O (1988) Vocal Physiology. Voice Production, Mechanisms and Functions. Raven Press, New York)
10. Fujimura O, Erickson D (1997) Acoustic phonetics. In: Hardcastle WJ, Laver J (Eds). The Handbook of Phonetic Sciences. Blackwell, Cambridge, pp. 256–297
11. Gauffin J, Hammarberg B (1991) Vocal Fold Physiology. Singular Publishing, San Diego
12. Giovanni A, Ouaknine M, Guelfucci B, Yu P, Zanaret M, Triglia JM (1999) Non-linear behavior of vocal fold vibration: role of coupling between the vocal folds. J Voice;13:341–354
13. Giovanni A, Ouaknine M, Garrel R, Ayache S, Robert D (2002) Un modèle non-linéaire de la vibration glottique. Implications cliniques potentielles. Rev Laryng (Bordeaux);123:273–277
14. Glaze LE, Bless DM, Milenkovic P (1988) Acoustic characteristics of children's voice. J Voice;2:312–319
15. Herzel H, Berry D, Titze I, Saleh M (1994) Analysis of vocal disorders with methods from nonlinear dynamics. J Speech Hear Res;37:1008–1019
16. Hirano M, Kakita Y (1985) Cover-body theory of vocal fold vibration. In: Daniloff R (Ed). Speech Science. College-Hill Press, San Diego
17. Hirano M, Sato K (1993) Histological Color Atlas of the Human Larynx. Singular Publishing Group, San Diego
18. Hirano M (1974) Morphological structure of the vocal fold as a vibrator and its variation. Folia Phoniatr;26:89–94
19. Ishizaka K, Isshiki N (1976) Computer simulation of pathological vocal-fold vibration. J Acoust Soc Am;60:1193–1198
20. Kahane JC (1988) Histologic structure and properties of the human vocal folds. Ear Nose Throat;67:322–330

21. Kent RD (1997) The Speech Sciences. Singular Publishing Group, San Diego
22. Matsuhita H (1975) The vibratory mode of the vocal folds in the excised larynx. Folia Phoniatr;27:7–18
23. Orlikoff RF, Kahane JC (1996) Structure and function of the larynx. In: Lass NJ (Ed). Principles of Experimental Phonetic. Mosby, St Louis
24. Rossing TD, Fletcher NH (1995) Principles of Vibration and Sound. Springer, New York
25. Sataloff RT (1997) Professional Voice: The Art and Science of Clinical Care. Singular Publishing Group, San Diego
26. Scotto Di Carlo N (1991) La voix chantée. La Recherche; 22:1016–1024
27. Seikel JA, King DW, Drumright DG (1997) Anatomy and Physiology for Speech and Language. Singular Publishing Group, San Diego
28. Sundberg J (1987) The Science of Singing Voice. Northern Illinois Press, De Kalb, IL
29. Titze IR, Jiang J, Drucker DG (1988) Preliminaries to the body-cover theory of pitch control. J Voice;1:314–319
30. Titze IR, Scherer RC (Eds) (1983) Vocal Fold Physiology: Biomechanics, Acoustics and Phonatory Control. The Denver Center for the Performing Arts, Denver
31. Titze IR, Schmidt SS (1995) Phonation threshold pressure in a physical model of the vocal fold mucosa. J Acoust Soc Am;97:3080–3084
32. Titze IR (1994) Principles of Voice Production. Prentice Hall, Englewood Cliffs
33. Tucker HM (1987) The Larynx. Thieme, New York
34. Webster DB (1995) Neuroscience of Communication. Singular Publishing, San Diego

Assessment of Voice and Respiratory Function

2

Philippe H. Dejonckere

Core Messages

> Voice is multidimensional.

> Audio recording is the most important basic requisite for voice quality assessment.

> Once a high-quality complete recording has been attained, it can be stored and remains available.

> Existing research does not support the complete substitution of instrumental measures for auditory perceptual assessment.

> To be valuable, however, perceptual assessment should follow a standard procedure, as does the voice recording. A currently used scale for making perceptual judgments is the GRBAS scale.

> Videolaryngostroboscopy is the main clinical tool for diagnosing the etiology of voice disorders, but it can also be used to assess the quality of vocal fold vibration and thus evaluate the effectiveness of a treatment.

> The simplest aerodynamic parameter of voicing is the maximum phonation time (MPT), in seconds. It consists of the prolongation of an /a:/ for as long as possible after maximal inspiration and at a spontaneous, comfortable pitch and loudness. A reduction of possible bias (e.g., supportive respiratory capabilities compensating for poor membranous vocal fold closure) is possible by computing the ratio or quotient : Averaged phonation airflow or PQ = VC (ml)/MPT (s).

> Accurate estimation of subglottal pressure can be achieved by measuring the intraoral air pressure produced during the repeated pronunciation of /pVp/ syllables (i.e., a vowel between two plosive consonants).

> Among Voice Range Profile parameters, the highest and lowest frequencies and the softest intensity (decibels, or dBA, at 30 cm) seem most sensitive for changes in voice quality.

> Although subjective by definition, self-evaluation is of great importance in clinical practice. Careful quantification is needed for self-evaluation to be compared and correlated with the objective assessment provided by the voice, an important adjuvant technique, laboratory. The Voice Handicap Index is a largely diffused, validated protocol.

> Electromyography (EMG), an important adjuvant technique, is an electrophysiological investigation of neuromuscular function.

2.1 Introduction

The voice laboratory is considered an essential tool for the assessment and treatment evaluation of voice patients and for clinical research on voice disorders. Several specific questions may be answered from the information obtained in the voice laboratory.

1. Is a given voice or voice function measurement considered normal (within normal limits) or pathological?
2. If the voice or voice function is considered pathological, how severe is the alteration?

P. H. Dejonckere
The Institute of Phoniatrics and Logopedics,
University Medical Center Utrecht, AZU F.02.504,
PO Box 85500, Nl-3508 GA Utrecht, The Netherlands
e-mail: Ph.deJonckere@umcutrecht.nl

M. Remacle, H. E. Eckel (eds.), *Surgery of Larynx and Trachea*,
DOI: 10.1007/978-3-540-79136-2_2, © Springer-Verlag Berlin Heidelberg 2010

3. Which aspects or mechanisms of voice production are involved with the voice disorder? How does the primary (medical) etiology or lesion explain the components of voice production that are perceived or analyzed as deviant (e.g., by limiting vocal fold closure or by eliciting irregular vibrations related to vocal fold asymmetry)? How do they account for the patient's complaints (e.g., voice fatigue or compensation mechanisms)?

4. What is the result of a comparison of voice production two or more times (e.g., before and after therapy), in two or several situations or voicing conditions (spontaneously vs. louder, when doing an Isshiki maneuver, or when applying a defined therapeutic technique)? Have the changes returned the voice to normal function as indicated by voice measurement [1]?

2.2 Prerequisite: Recording a Voice Sample

Audio recording is the most important basic requisite for voice quality assessment. Once a high-quality recording has been performed, it can be stored and remains available—as a document—for performing additional investigations at a later time (e.g., blind perceptual evaluation by a panel or sophisticated acoustical analyses) [2]. A sampling frequency of at least 20,000 Hz is recommended. Ideally, the recordings are made in a sound-treated room, although a quiet room with ambient noise permanently < 45 dB is acceptable. The mouth-to-microphone distance needs to be held constant at 10 cm. A (miniature) head-mounted microphone offers a clear advantage. Off-axis positioning (45°–90° from the mouth axis) reduces aerodynamic noise from the mouth during speech [3, 4].

In regard to voice/speech material, examples of protocol for standard recording are as follows.

- /a:/ at (spontaneous) comfortable pitch/loudness, recorded three times to evaluate variability of quality [5]
- /a:/ slightly louder to evaluate the possible change in quality (plasticity) and the slope of the regression line frequency/sound pressure level [6, 7]
- A single sentence or a short standard passage

Phonetic selection can be useful, such as a short sentence with constant voicing (no voiceless sounds and

spoken without interruption) and no fricatives. Such a sentence (e.g., "We mow our lawn all year") can be analyzed by a computer program for sustained vowels; and because it contains no articulation noise, there is no biasing of harmonics-to-noise computations. Computation of the percent voiceless (normal in this case is 100%) is useful for neurological voices or spasmodic dysphonia [9]. Furthermore, it allows easy determination of the mean habitual fundamental speaking frequency.

Another example of a criterion for phonetic selection is a multiplication of voice onsets, as they are critical in disturbed voices [10]. Such criteria are not language-linked.

A standard reading passage should also be recorded whenever possible. Two classic, often used reading passages for English-speaking persons are "The Rainbow Passage" (a phonetically selected passage including all the speech sounds of English) and "Marvin Williams" (an all-voiced passage) [3].

2.2.1 Perception

Existing research does not support the complete substitution of instrumental measures for auditory perceptual assessment. To be valuable, however, perceptual assessment must follow a standard procedure, as does voice recording. A currently used scale for making perceptual judgments is the GRBAS scale, which rates grade, roughness, breathiness, asthenicity, and strain on a scale of 0–3 [11]. The rating is made by assessing current conversational speech or when reading a passage. The severity of hoarseness is quantified under the parameter "grade" (G), which relates to the overall voice quality, integrating all deviant components. There are two main components of hoarseness, as shown by principal component analysis [12].

1. Breathiness (B): an auditive impression of turbulent air leakage through an insufficient glottic closure, including short aphonic moments (unvoiced segments)
2. Roughness or harshness (R): an impression of irregular glottic pulses, abnormal fluctuations in fundamental frequency, and separately perceived acoustic impulses (as in vocal fry), including diplophonia and register breaks. When present, diplophonia can also be noted as "d."

These parameters have shown sufficient reliability (inter- and intrarater reproducibility) [13, 14]. A reliability analysis provided further evidence to support the GRBAS scale as a simple, reliable measure for clinical use [15]. The behavioral parameters asthenicity (A) and strain (S) appear to be less reliable. The remaining simplified scale, GRB, then becomes similar to the RBH scale used in German-speaking countries [16].

For reporting purposes, a four point grading scale is convenient (0 = normal or absence of deviance; 1 = slight deviance; 2 = moderate deviance; 3 = severe deviance). However, it is also possible to score on a visual analogue scale (VAS) of 10 cm, possibly with anchoring points [14, 17].

It is proposed that the term "dysphonia" be used for any kind of perceived voice pathology. The deviation may concern pitch or loudness as well as timbre or rhythmic and prosodic features. "Hoarseness" is limited to deviant voice "quality" (or timbre) and excludes pitch, loudness, and rhythm factors. A limited number of voice pathology categories—such as those related to mutation or transsexuality—are specifically concerned with pitch and register. Rhinophonia is a specific abnormality of resonance and if present needs to be reported separately. Tremor is a characteristic temporal feature and when present must also be reported separately. A special protocol is required for substitution voices [19, 77].

Perceptual evaluation—if averaged among several blinded raters—is very well suited to demonstrate treatment efficacy in voice pathology [21].

2.2.2 Vocal Fold Imaging

2.2.2.1 Videolaryngostroboscopy

Videolaryngostroboscopy is the main clinical tool for diagnosing the etiology of voice disorders, but it can also be used to assess the quality of vocal fold vibration and thus evaluate the effectiveness of a treatment. Stroboscopy involves a video-perceptual series of judgments and ratings (e.g., glottic closure, regularity, symmetry, mucosal wave). The pertinence of stroboscopic parameters is based on a combination of reliability (inter- and intraobserver reproducibility), no redundancy (from the factor analysis), and clinical sense (relation to physiological concepts) [23].

The basic parameters are the following:

1. Glottal closure. It is recommended that the type of insufficient closure also be recorded and categorized.

   - Longitudinal. It is important to consider that a slight dorsal insufficiency—even reaching into the membranous portion of the glottis—occurs in about 60% of middle-aged healthy women during normal voice effort. Fifty percent of the women close the glottis completely during loud voice.
   - Ventral.
   - Irregular.
   - Oval. It is over the whole length of the glottis but with a dorsal closure.
   - Hour-glass shaped.

Rating glottal closure has been found highly reliable [24, 25]. Objective quantitative measurements are also possible [26]

2. Regularity: quantitative rating of the degree of irregular slow motion, as perceived with stroboscopy [27].
3. Mucosal wave: quantitative rating of the quality of the mucosal wave, accounting for the physiology of the layered structure of the vocal folds [11].
4. Symmetry: quantitative rating of the "mirror" motion of both vocal folds. Usually asymmetry is caused by the limited vibratory quality of a lesion (e.g., diffuse scar, localized cyst, leukoplakia) [28].

For each stroboscopic parameter, a four-point grading scale can be used (0 = no deviance; … 3 = severe deviance), but a VAS may also be useful [23, 28]. Videostroboscopy can be documented on hard copy and thus be archived. Rating *a posteriori* is possible.

It is classically recommended to observe and record videostroboscopic pictures under various voicing conditions. For example, the degree of glottal closure usually increases with increased loudness [24, 25]. However, this basic rating concerns a comfortable pitch and loudness. Laryngostroboscopic ratings and measurements have been found relevant for documenting therapeutic effects [20–22, 29].

2.2.2.2 Digital High-Speed Pictures

With modern technology, it has become possible to capture and store digital vocal fold images at a rate of 2000 (and more) per second with sufficient definition (several hundred pixels) and to display the image sequence at a rate of, for example, 20/s immediately after capture. This procedure does not seem to be appropriate for routine use in the diagnosis of voice problems as a long review time is needed for a short sequence without simultaneous sound. A specific indication for digital high-speed cinematography is to analyze and understand the vibratory characteristics in aperiodic voices, during voice onsets or accidents (breaks), or in case of diplo- or triplophonia [30, 31].

2.2.2.3 High-Speed Single-Line Scanning (Video-Kymography)

High-speed single-line scanning (video-kymography) is an imaging technique for investigating vocal fold vibration, especially when the vibration is irregular and

when the focus is on accidents or short events in this vibration, making conventional stroboscopy unsuitable. A modified video-camera selects a single horizontal line from the whole image and monitors it at high speed (8000/s). The displayed image shows successive high-speed line images below each other, thereby demonstrating the vibration of the selected ventrodorsal level of the vocal folds over time. An important practical advantage is that the display is in real time. This type of imaging provides relevant, timely information e.g., for comparing the vibration amplitude of both folds or for understanding diplophonia [32, 33]. It also clearly demonstrates the mucosal wave phenomenon and its absence or asymmetry.

Single-line scanning can also be performed on a high-speed video recording (Fig. 2.1). If several lines are displayed, phase shifts between different ventrodorsal segments of one or both vocal folds—as

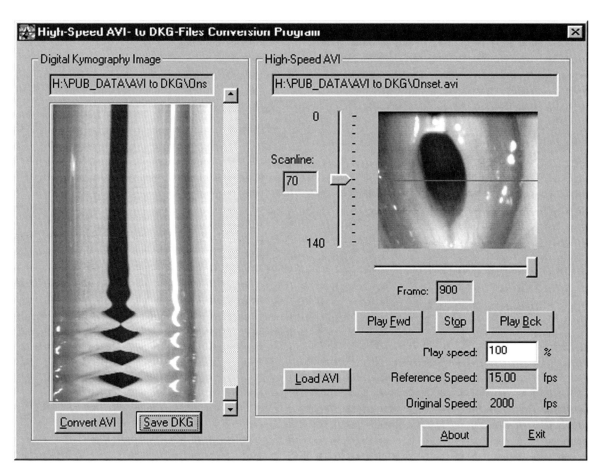

Fig. 2.1. Single-line scan (video-kymography) obtained from a high-speed video recording in a normal subject (Kay System; Kaypentax, Lincoln Park, NJ, USA). *Right* Vibrating vocal folds and the *single line* that was selected. *Left* Oscillation pattern at that specific level during a voice onset

frequently occurs in case of a vocal fold cyst—can be demonstrated [34].

2.2.3 Aerodynamics

Aerodynamic analysis of voice production includes measurement of airflow and air pressure, and their relation during phonation. Using appropriate instrumentation, a number of derived measurements can provide information regarding vocal efficiency, although for certain measurements only a stopwatch is needed.

2.2.3.1 Phonation Airflow

The simplest aerodynamic parameter of voicing is the MPT (in seconds). It consists of the prolongation of an /a:/ for as long as possible after maximum inspiration and at a spontaneous, comfortable pitch and loudness. It is one of the most widely used clinical measures in voice assessment worldwide [35]. A prior demonstration is necessary, and three trials are required, the longest being selected for comparison to the norm [36]. As it concerns an "extreme" performance, it has been shown to be extremely sensitive to learning and fatigue effects. Furthermore, in good voices the duration of "apnea" can become the limiting factor, rather than the available air. Children show significant lower MPT values as their lung volume is smaller [37]. A reduction of possible bias (e.g., supportive respiratory capabilities compensating for poor membranous vocal fold closure) is possible by computing the following ratio: (Phonation Quotient).

Averaged phonation airflow or PQ = VC (ml)/MPT (s)

Vital capacity (VC) is defined as "the volume change at the mouth between the position of full inspiration and complete expiration." It can be measured in a reliable way using a hand-held spirometer [38]. In normal subjects, the VC depends on anthropometric factors and is quite strongly correlated, for example, with height [39]. It is also sensitive to lung disease. As the VC is not directly related to voice quality, it is meaningful to take it into account, especially if a child is being investigated.

The mean airflow rate can also be measured using pneumotachography. This technique directly measures the mean airflow rate (ml/s) for sustained phonation over a comfortable duration, usually 2–3 s, at the habitual pitch and intensity level and following habitual inspiration. Pathophysiological backgrounds and normative values have been reported [11, 35, 40–43].

The variation of averaged phonation airflow varies considerably among normal subjects, and there is a large overlapping range of values in normal and dysphonic subjects, which limits its value for diagnostic purposes [44]. Nevertheless, when comparing glottal function before and after surgical intervention or nonsurgical voice training techniques, airflow measurement may be useful for monitoring therapeutic effects [45] (e.g., in the case of paralytic dysphonia [46–48] or when microlaryngeal phonosurgery is performed) [42]. The method is especially useful for demonstrating changes in a single test subject over time. For comparisons (pretreatment/posttreatment), it is recommended that the same technique (PQ or mean airflow rate measured by pneumotachography) be used for each measurement.

Flow glottography (FLOG) consists of inverse filtering of the oral airflow waveform. The basic tool is a high-frequency pressure transducer incorporated into an airtight Rothenberg mask [49]. The inverse filtering procedure removes the resonant effects of the vocal tract and produces an estimate of the waveform produced at the vocal folds. The special advantage of this technique is that it differentiates, and after calibration quantifies, leakage airflow (the DC component of the air flow) and pulsated airflow (AC component). Leakage airflow is an important concept: It assumes that there is an opening somewhere along the total length of the vocal folds through which air escapes. Calibration is critical for reliable measurements. FLOG can also be used to analyze voice onset.

2.2.3.2 Subglottal Air Pressure

Measurements of subglottal air pressure using esophageal balloons or pressure transducers, transglottal catheters, or tracheal puncture are semi-invasive or invasive and are limited to research situations. Subglottal pressure can be accurately estimated by measuring the intraoral air pressure produced during the repeated pronunciation of /pVp/ syllables (i.e., a vowel between two plosive consonants). A thin catheter is introduced into the mouth through the labial commissure, is sealed by the lips, and is not occluded by the tongue. If there is no closure of the vocal folds, the intraoral air pressure should be similar to the pressure elsewhere in the respiratory tract. During production of a voiceless consonant, the vocal folds are abducted and should not impose any significant obstruction to airflow from the lungs. Thus, the pressure behind the lips is the same everywhere and reflects the pressure available to drive the vocal folds if they were to vibrate [50, 51]. This technique also allows measurement of the phonation threshold pressure (PTP), the minimum pressure required to initiate phonation [52]. Pressure is usually reported in pascal units: $1 Pa = 1 N/m^2$; and $1 kPa = 10 cm H_2O$.

2.2.3.3 Efficiency of Phonation

Together with airflow and vocal intensity, subglottal air pressure can be used to estimate the efficiency of phonation. Obviously, reduced efficiency is expected to induce voice fatigue. Vocal efficiency—defined as the ratio of acoustical power to aerodynamic power—can be estimated by dividing the acoustical intensity of the utterance by the product of the air pressure and the airflow used to produce the utterance [54].

2.2.3.4 Flow Versus Volume Loops

Spirometry is important for investigating cases in which voice problems are associated with laryngeal obstruction, such as bilateral abduction paralysis, stenosis caused by extensive webs and scars, cancer, or even severe Reinke's edema. The flow–volume loop is generated when measurements of maximum forced expiration and maximum forced inspiration are plotted on a graph, with the flow rate on the ordinate and lung volume on the abscissa (Fig. 2.2). Lack of effort is easy to detect because there is reduced flow at the beginning of the expiratory curve, and the inspiratory curve is abnormal (Fig. 2.2b). Obstructive lesions of the larynx are easily detected and quantified because the morphology of the flow–volume loop is altered. Variable extrathoracic obstruction (as with bilateral vocal fold paralysis) manifests as a decrease in inspiratory flow only (Fig. 2.2c), whereas a fixed obstruction of the upper airway (e.g., extensive laryngeal cancer) is demonstrated and quantified by a symmetrical

reduction of inspiratory and expiratory flow (Fig. 2.2d) [55–57].

2.2.4 Acoustics

Acoustical measures provide, in an objective and noninvasive way, a great deal of information about vocal function. Increasingly, these measures have become available at affordable cost and appear to have succeeded well in monitoring changes in voice quality across time (e.g., before and after treatment). Acoustical measures reflect the status of vocal function and do not relate specifically to certain voice disorders because basic biomechanical changes resulting in acoustical differences can be induced by various lesions and dysfunctions.

2.2.4.1 Visible Speech

Acoustical analysis can be used to make the voice and speech visible (e.g., in spectrograms) [50]. This visual representation may be a considerable aid to the perception and description of voice characteristics. Spectrograms are also useful for comparing normal phonation with phonation characterized by excessive noise. Commercially available software packages provide synchronized displays of the microphone signal and the spectrogram, showing the frequency distribution of acoustical energy over time. A choice can be made between narrowband filtering (frequency resolution, mainly demonstrating fundamental frequency, harmonics, interharmonic and high-frequency noise, subharmonics) and broadband filtering (temporal resolution, mainly demonstrating periodicity but also formant location). Voice characteristics such as the sound pressure level (SPL), fundamental frequency, and formant central frequency can also be displayed over time for analysis of the singing voice. Visualizing fast Fourier transform (FFT) graphics (power spectrum) and long-time average spectra (LTAS) is usually possible (Fig. 2.3). When visible speech is provided simultaneously with voice sound, the interrater consistency of the perceptual quality evaluation significantly increases [8, 9]. Martens WMAF, Versnel H, Dejonckere PH (2007) The effect of visible speech on the parceptual rating of pathological voices. Arch Otolaryngol Head Neck Surg 133 : 178–185.

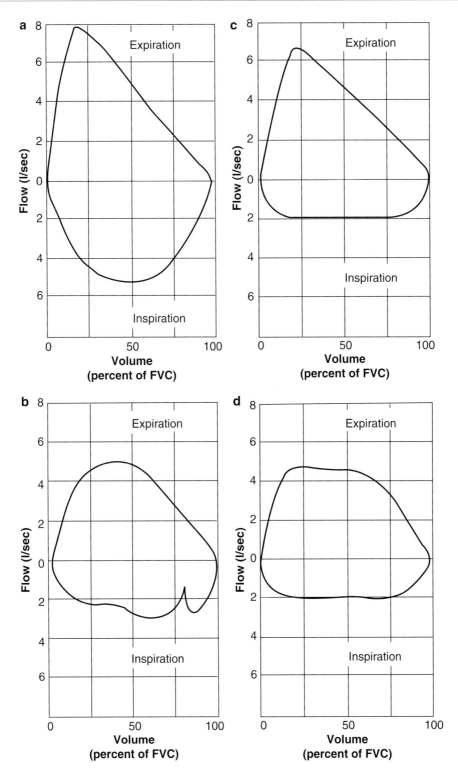

Fig. 2.2. Flow-volume curves. Measurements of a maximum forced expiration and a maximum forced inspiration are plotted on a graph with flow rates on the ordinate and lung volume on the abscissa. (**a**) During normal respiration the expiratory flow curve decays linearly. (**b**) When effort is poor, the initial slope of part of the expiratory curve is decreased, and the inspiratory curve is also abnormal. (**c**) A variable extrathoracic obstruction decreases only the inspiratory flow rate. (**d**) In case of fixed obstruction of the upper airway, inspiratory and expiratory flow rates are both reduced

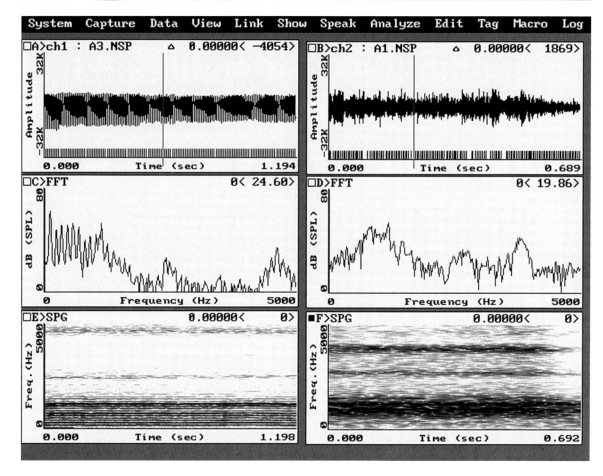

Fig. 2.3. Visible speech or sonagraphy, as displayed by the Computerized Speech Laboratory (Kay Elemetrics, Lincoln Park, NJ, USA). Sustained /a/: on the left by a normal voice and on the *right* by a breathy voice. *From top to bottom* : microphone signal), power spectrum (0–5000 Hz), and spectrogram (sonogram), frequency display 0–5000 Hz over time: about 1.2 s *left* and 0.7 s *right* , narrowband fi ltering 25 Hz with frequency (resolution). *Left panels*: in Power spectrum and spectrogram the harmonics are easy to identify, whereas they are lacking on the *right panels* . Here the power spectrum and spectrogram are replaced by aperiodic acoustical energy (noise). This kind of display also provides information about formant location

2.2.4.2 Acoustical Parameters

Acoustical analysis can also provide precise numerical values for many voice parameters, from averaged fundamental frequency to sophisticated calculations for noise components or tremor features.

Factor analysis allows the large number of acoustical parameters to be reduced to a limited number of clusters [14].

• Short-term fundamental frequency perturbation
• Short- or medium-term amplitude perturbation and voiceless segments
• Harmonics-to-noise ratio
• Long-term frequency and amplitude modulation
• Very long-term amplitude variation

• Subharmonics
• Tremor

Perturbation measures (in period and amplitude) and harmonics-to-noise computations on a sustained vowel (/a:/) at comfortable frequency and intensity appear to be the most robust measures and seem to determine the basic perceptual elements of voice quality: grade, roughness, and breathiness. Nevertheless, correlations with perceptual data remain usually moderate [14, 58]. *Jitter* is computed as the mean difference between the periods of adjacent cycles divided by the mean period. It is thus a fundamental frequency (F_0)-related measurement (Fig. 2.4). For *shimmer*, a similar computation is made on peak-to-peak amplitudes. Voice breaks must always be excluded. For pathological voices, the coefficients of

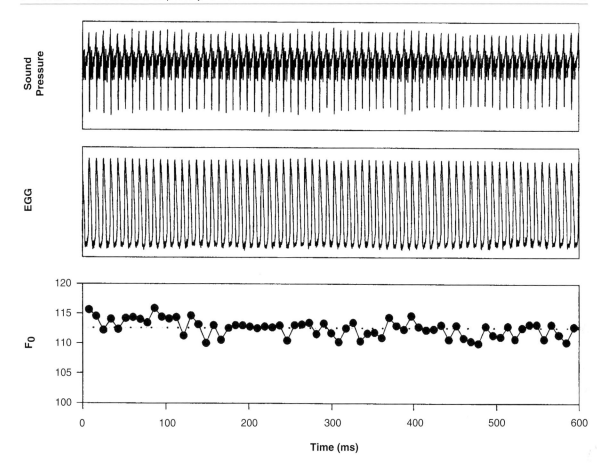

Fig. 2.4. Normal male voice, sustained /a:/. Microphone signal, electroglottogram, and F₀ plot across time. Normal voice is characterized by slight (< 1%) random variation of the fundamental frequency. In most cases of pathology, this aperiodicity (jitter) increases

variation of jitter and shimmer for a sustained /a/ are in the order of 20–30% for successive single trials as well as trials on different days [20–22]. A general limitation is that the systems employed for acoustical analysis cannot (or not in a reliable way) analyze strongly aperiodical acoustical signals. Perturbation measures of less than about 5% have been found to be reliable [59]. Only "quasi-periodic" voices are suited for perturbation analysis. Therefore, visual control of the period definition on the microphone signal is always necessary: Even in regular voices, a strong harmonic or subharmonic may account for erratic values. Alternatives from the field of nonlinear dynamics, such as the coefficient of Lyapunov, have been proposed for analyzing "chaotic" or "bifurcated" signals [60]. Also for substitution voices, special acoustical approaches of frequency perturbation have been proposed [18, 19].

For signal-to-noise ratio computations—e.g., normalized noise energy (NNE), harmonics to noise ratio (HNR), cepstral peak prominence (CPP)—there is currently insufficient standardization of the optimal algorithm(s) and insufficient knowledge about normative values for widespread clinical use. The harmonics-to-noise ratio was also found to be less well suited for demonstrating the effects of therapy [20–22].

Rhinophonia is a particular resonance characteristic of the voice. It may be present without a concomitant articulation disorder. Acoustical nasometry provides objective measurements by (schematically) computing the ratio between nasal and whole voice (nasal + oral) sound pressure levels [61].

2.2.4.3 Phonetography/Voice Range Profile

The phonetogram plots the dynamic range (dBA) as a function of the fundamental frequency range (Hz), thereby documenting the extreme possibilities of voice.

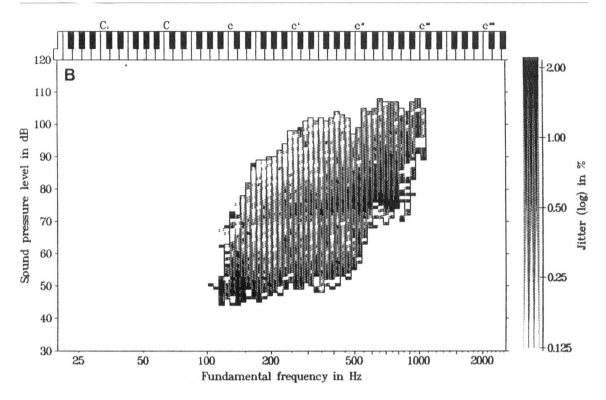

Fig. 2.5. Computerized phonetogram (voice range profile), with a gray scale indicating the amount of jitter (normal female voice). The more jitter, the darker the area. *Horizontal axis*: fundamental frequency in Hz (or musical tones on a keyboard). *Vertical axis*: sound pressure level, measured at 30 cm (dBA). This plot combines information about extreme possibilities of voice as well as an aspect of voice quality

These extremes are of importance for professional voice users, especially singers [62], but they must be interpreted with care [52, 53] because the acoustical energy is related to spectral distribution. Normative values for children and teachers have been defined [63].

Computerized systems make possible real-time measurement and display of fundamental frequency versus SPL and also of quality parameters such as jitter. Jitter results in various color gradations within the voice area, showing specific altered zones, or register boundaries (Fig. 2.5). Such computerized systems can also provide range profiles of current speech, possibly coupled with provocation tests, such as the task of reading at a controlled, louder intensity. These profiles are expected to be relevant for occupational voice users.

The highest and lowest frequencies and the softest intensity (dBA at 30 cm) seem most sensitive for changes in voice quality [5, 64–66], the latter being related to the phonation threshold pressure (PTP) [52, 53]. Measuring the lowest frequency allows one to compute the fundamental frequency range. Such a "three points range profile" can be obtained without completing a (time-consuming) whole voice range profile. However, as these three points represent "extreme" performances, they are (as are the MPT and CV) highly sensitive to learning and fatigue effects.

2.2.5 Self-Evaluation by Patient

Although subjective by definition, self-evaluation is of great importance in clinical practice. Careful quantification is needed for self-evaluation to be compared and correlated with the objective assessment provided by the voice laboratory. The purpose of subjective self-evaluation is to determine the deviance of voice quality and the severity of disability or handicap in daily professional and social life and the possible emotional repercussions of the dysphonia.

The basic aim is to differentiate the deviance of voice quality *stricto sensu* and the severity of the disability/handicap in daily social and/or professional life. A Voice Handicap Index can be computed on the base

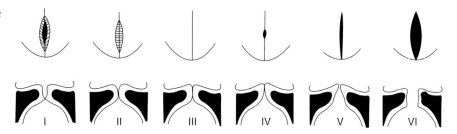

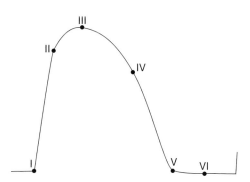

Fig. 2.6. Electroglottographic waveform with the corresponding laryngoscopic view and a frontal section through the midportion of the glottis. Point *III* corresponds to minimum impedance, which is at maximum closure of the glottis

of the patient's responses to a carefully selected list of questions [67]. It also investigates the possible emotional repercussion of the dysphonia. Rosen et al. [68] proposed a validated shortened version of the Voice Handicap Index: the VHI–10. However, for a basic protocol, a minimal subjective evaluation can be provided by patients themselves on a double VAS of 100 mm: their impressions about voice quality *stricto sensu* and about the repercussion of the voice problem regarding every-day social and, if relevant, professional life and activities. A score of "0" (maximum left) means a normal voice on the first scale and no handicap (related to voice) in daily life on the second scale. A score of "100" (maximum right) means extreme voice deviance on the first scale and extreme disability or handicap in daily social (and, when relevant, professional) activities, as rated by the patients themselves. A comparative study does not suggest that the exhaustive questionnaire is more reliable than the simple scales [20–22].

2.2.6 Adjuvant Techniques

2.2.6.1 Electroglottography

Electroglottography (or electrolaryngography) (EGG) is a method for monitoring vocal fold contact, rate of

vibration, and perturbation of regularity during voice production (Fig. 2.6). The major advantage of EGG is that it does not interfere with the physiologic processes of speaking or singing. The signal originates from two electrodes lightly placed on the speaker's neck at the level of the thyroid cartilage. Pitch extraction from the EGG waveform is particularly reliable—so long as there is at least partial vocal fold contact during the vibration cycle—because the waveform is unaffected by vocal tract resonances and environment noise [69, 70].

The main applications of EGG are as follows:

- Fundamental frequency computations (e.g., range, regularity, distribution, display across time, cross plots) so long as there is vocal fold contact
- Voice onset time
- Prephonatory and postphonatory laryngeal gestures
- Closed phase information (hyperkinetic vs. hypokinetic adduction)
- Voice range profile of spontaneous speech (falsetto excluded)
- Triggering of a stroboscopic light source

2.2.6.2 Electromyography

Electromyography is an electrophysiological investigation of neuromuscular function. The main indications are mobility disorders (especially reduced mobility). Neuromuscular pathological conditions in laryngeal muscles do not basically differ from neuromuscular pathological conditions in other muscles, so it is recommended that these investigations be performed in cooperation with a general myography specialist [71–74]. With the patient supine and the neck extended, a concentric needle electrode is inserted through the cricothyroid ligament to approach the thyroid muscle. The needle electrode is then angled cranially 45° and laterally 20° to an approximate depth of 1.5–2.0 cm. The cricothyroid muscle is reached by inserting the electrode off the midline close to the inferior border of the thyroid cartilage. EMG is also used for monitoring *Botulinum* injections in vocal muscles. An evidence-based review has been provided by Sataloff et al. [75].

2.2.7 Specific Techniques for Substitution Voices and Spasmodic Dysphonia

A special protocol for perceptual evaluation is required for substitution voices (i.e., voices in which the sound is not generated by two vocal folds) [18, 19]. Substitution voicing cannot be evaluated accurately by the GRBAS perceptual rating scale as most substitution voices are G_2 or G_3 and because an optimal substitution voice is never G_0. Therefore, the IINFVo scale was proposed as an alternative (and was found reliable). It has the following parameters [76, 77].

- I—overall impression of voice quality, acceptability and adequacy for daily communication
- I—impression of intelligibility
- N—unintended additive noise, a parameter that reflects the amount of annoyance caused by the audibility of all sorts of uncontrolled noises (e.g., bubbly noise, air turbulence, clicks) produced during speech
- F—fluency, which reflects the perceived smoothness of the sound production and accounts for all kinds of undesirable interruptions
- Vo—voicing, which means that utterances are heard as voiced or voiceless when they need to be voiced or voiceless

Scoring is similar to the GRBAS scale, with a four-point scale (from no deviance to severe deviance), or using a VAS. Spasmodic dysphonias can also be rated in this way.

Classic acoustical parameters, such as perturbation measures, are not suited for substitution voices or spasmodic dysphonias, as they are not "quasi-periodic" signals but usually show chaotic "bifurcations," such as breaks or diplophonic moments. Nonlinear approaches are promising in this field.

Using a program based on a peripheral auditory model, Moerman et al. [18, 19] analyzed 10-ms frames of the signal and confirmed by objective acoustical analysis that the quality of tracheoesophageal speech is superior to that of esophageal speech but inferior to that of normal speech or speech with the preservation of one vocal fold.

In cases of spasmodic dysphonia (AD type), simple acoustical measures for fluency, such as the total duration of the sentence (ms) and the ratio of the total duration of voiced segments to the total duration of the sentence—both parameters measured in a short 100% voiced sentence for normal speakers—appear to be valuable objective criteria for effectiveness of treatment. They are useful for monitoring the evolution and timing of a new *Botulinum* injection [8, 9].

For patients with substitution voices, a slightly corrected version of the Voice Handicap Index has been proposed [18, 19].

2.2.8 Basic Protocol for Functional Assessment of Voice Pathology Recommended by the European Laryngological Society, Especially for Investigating Efficacy of (Phonosurgical) Treatments and Evaluating New Assessment Techniques

The basic protocol for functional assessment of voice pathology proposed by the European Laryngological Society was an attempt to reach better agreement and uniformity concerning the basic methodology for functional assessment of pathological voices. The purpose was to allow relevant comparisons with the literature when presenting/publishing the results of any kind of voice treatment (e.g., a phonosurgical technique or a new/improved instrument or procedure for investigating the pathological voice) [78]. A few basic principles served as guidelines.

1. Voice function is multidimensional [35].
2. A (minimum) set of basic requirements for presenting (publishing) results of voice treatments is necessary to make comparisons and meta-analyses possible.
3. New and more sophisticated measurement or evaluation techniques and procedures are to be encouraged, but the basic set must be performed in all cases for comparison.
4. The recommendations must be suited to all "common" dysphonias, but a few specific categories of voice pathology need a specific protocol for increasing sensitivity (e.g., substitution voices and spasmodic dysphonia) [8, 9, 18, 19].
5. In the basic set, or "truncus communis," for the assessment of common dysphonias, the following components need to be considered. Each provides quantitative data.

    a. Perception
    b. Videostroboscopy
    c. Acoustics
    d. Aerodynamics/efficiency
    e. Subjective rating by patient

When investigating substitution voices and spasmodic dysphonias, elements such as intelligibility and fluency should be added. Furthermore, scales and algorithms should be adjusted for the dimensions "perception," "videostroboscopy" and "acoustics."

6. Each of the above items has its own specific relevance when reporting results or statistics, as it provides a particular insight (multidimensionality). Combined scores or indexes [66] integrating these or other data into a single value may be useful, but optimal evaluation and understanding of the treatment effect also requires intrinsic comparison of the scores for the different components [79]. An example of such an Index is the Dysphonia Severity Index (DSI): it was constructed by logistic regression (Fisher discriminant analysis) and combines the highest fundamental frequency (F_0) (Hz), softest intensity, MPT, and jitter (%) according to the formula $DSI = 0.13 \times MPT + 0.0053 \times$ highest $F_0 - 0.26 \times$ lowest intensity $- 1.18 \times$ jitter (%) + 12.4. For normal voices the DSI is +5, and for severely dysphonic voices it is −5. The first implementation studies pointed out that for some patients treatment effects can vary considerably from one dimension to another [80].

7. When assessing treatment outcomes, maximum objectivity must be constant. However, even objective data, such as audio recordings or videolaryngostroboscopic pictures, may be subjectively rated and interpreted. Nevertheless, for research purposes, it remains possible to improve the validity considerably by (1) averaging the ratings of a panel and (2) rating blindly, which means without knowing the conditions (e.g., before and after treatment).
8. Although the present guideline concerns only basic, nonsophisticated approaches, it is not to be considered as the ultimate way to conduct a basic assessment of voice function. Further implementation studies and more research are necessary and are warmly encouraged [81].
9. Instrumentation is kept to a minimum although considered essential for professionals performing phonosurgery. The ENT surgeon can be assisted in performing this basic set of measurements by a qualified, trained speech therapist.
10. In summary, two of the dimensions are considered objective (so long as the subject is cooperating normally): aerodynamics and acoustics. Although these two dimensions are considered objective, they are rated subjectively by the examiner (ratings can be made blindly by a panel!) via recording a voice sample and videostroboscopy. Finally, one dimension remains totally subjective (self-rating by the patient).

Implementation of this protocol demonstrates the clinical relevance of each item, and the low redundance. When investigating treatment effects, the correlations between the pre-post changes for the different parameters are weak [20–22, 82]. Multidimensional information about changes induced by therapy helps clinicians better understand the way in which a treatment works.

2.2.8.1 Example of a report using the proposed basic protocol

The patient was a 26-year-old woman who was diagnosed with vocal fold nodules. These results were obtained before treatment.

Perception	G34 B52 R18d
Stroboscopy	Clo 40hs Reg10 MW25 Sym0
Aerodynamics	PQ 285 ml/s (MPT 13 s)
Acoustics	Ji 1.2%; Shi 6.1%; F_0 – range c–g1; softest intensity 5 dBA 30 cm
Subjective evaluation	Vo30 Dis50

Explanation

Perception was rated on three VASs of 100 mm: grade, roughness, breathiness. Grade is scored 34/100, 52/100, and 18/100, where 0 = normal (no deviance) and 100 = extremely deviant. Diplophonia is present (d).

Stroboscopy was rated on four VASs of 100 mm: closure, regularity, quality of mucosal wave, symmetry. For closure, if abnormal, a categorical choice is also recommended; in this case, there was an hourglass-shaped pattern. Symmetry was normal.

Aerodynamics: phonation quotient (ml/s) and maximum phonation time (s). VC was 3705 ml.

Acoustics: jitter% and shimmer% on a sustained /a:/, at comfortable pitch and loudness. The "c" corresponds to 131 Hz and "g1" to 392 Hz. As for phonetography, the distance of the microphone must be 30 cm.

Subjective evaluation: provided by the patient himself on a double VAS of 100 mm. The first scale concerns the impression about voice quality *stricto sensu* (i.c. 30/100 = slight to moderate), and the second scale concerns the impression about repercussions of the voice problem during everyday social and, if relevant, professional life and activities (i.c. 50/100 = moderate to severe).

References

1. Dejonckere PH (2000) Perceptual and laboratory assessment of dysphonia. Otolaryngol Clin North Am;33:731–750
2. Titze I (1995) Workshop on Acoustic Voice Analysis: Summary Statement. National Center for Voice and Speech. The University of Iowa, Denver Co, 36 pp
3. Sataloff RT (1997) Professional Voice. Singular Publishing Group, San Diego
4. Watson C (1994) Database management of the voice clinic and laboratory. J Voice;3:99–106
5. Speyer R, Wieneke GH, van Wijck-Warnaar I, Dejonckere PH (2003) Effects of voice therapy on the voice range profiles of dysphonic patients. J Voice;17:544–556
6. Dejonckere PH (1998) Effect of louder voicing on acoustical measurements in dysphonic patients. Logoped Phoniatr Vocol;23:79–84
7. Dejonckere PH, Lebacq J (2001) Plasticity of voice quality: a prognostic factor for outcome of voice therapy? J Voice;15:251–256
8. Dejonckere PH (2007) Améliorer la fiabilité de l'analyse perceptive de la voix pathologique par un support visuel sonagraphique. In: Klein-Dallant C (Éd). Voix parlée et chantée. Editions Ortho, Paris, pp. 35–45
9. Dejonckere PH (2007) Critères acoustiques de fluence pour l'évaluation des dysphonies spasmodiques. In: Klein-Dallant C (Éd). Voix parlée et chantée. Editions Ortho, Paris, pp. 63–73
10. Revis J, Barberis S,Giovanni A (2000) Definition of a new temporal voice onset measurement. Rev Laryngol Otol Rhinol (Bord);121:291–296
11. Hirano M (1981) Clinical Examination of Voice. Springer, New York
12. Dejonckere PH, Lebacq J (1996) Acoustic, perceptual, aerodynamic and anatomical correlations in voice pathology. ORL J Otorhinolaryngol Relat Spec;58:326–332
13. De Bodt, M, Wuyts, F,Van de Heyning, P, Croeckx, C (1997) Test - re-test Study of GRBAS-Scale. J Voice;11:74–80
14. Dejonckere PH, Remacle M, Fresnel-Elbaz E, Woisard V, Crevier Buchman L, Millet B (1996) Differentiated perceptual evaluation of pathological voice quality: reliability and correlations with acoustic measurements. Rev Laryngol Otol Rhinol;117:219–224
15. Webb AL, Carding PN, Deary IJ, MacKenzie K, Steen N, Wilson JA (2004) The reliability of three perceptual evaluation scales for dysphonia. Eur Arch Otorhinolaryngol;261: 429–434
16. Nawka T, Anders LC, Wendler J (1994) Die auditive Beurteilung heiserer Stimmen nach dem RBH-System. Sprache Stimme Gehör;18:130–133
17. Wuyts F, De Bodt M, Van de Heyning PH (1999) Is the reliability of a visual analog scale higher than of an ordinal scale ? An experiment with the GRBAS-scale for the perceptual evaluation of dysphonia. J Voice;13:508–517
18. Moerman M, Martens JP, Dejonckere PH (2004) Application of the voice handicap index in 45 patients with substitution voicing after total laryngectomy. Eur Arch Otolaryngol;261: 423–428
19. Moerman M, Pieters G, Martens JP, Van Der Borgt MJ, Dejonckere PH (2004) Objective evaluation of the quality of substitution voices. Eur Arch Otorhinolaryngol;261: 541–547
20. Speyer R, Wieneke GH, Dejonckere PH (2004) The use of acoustic parameters for the evaluation of voice therapy for dysphonic patients. Acta Acustica United Acustica;90:520–527
21. Speyer R, Wieneke GH, Dejonckere PH (2004) Documentation of progress in voice therapy: perceptual, acoustic and laryngostroboscopic findings pretherapy and postterapy. J Voice;18: 325–339
22. Speyer R, Wieneke GH, Dejonckere PH (2004) Self-assessment of voice therapy for chronic dysphonia. Clin Otolaryngol;29:66–74
23. Dejonckere PH, Crevier L, Elbaz E, Marraco M, Millet B, Remacle M, Woisard V (1999) Quantitative rating of videolaryngostroboscopy: factor analysis of the vibratory characteristics. In: Dejonckere PH, Peters H (Eds). Communication and its Disorders: A Science in Progress. Nijmegen University Press, Nijmegen, pp. 170–171

24. Södersten M, Hertegard S, Hammarberg B (1995) Glottal closure, transglottal air flow and voice quality in healthy middle-aged women. J Voice;9:182–197

25. Sulter AM, Schutte HK, Miller DG (1996) Standardized laryngeal videostroboscopic rating: differences between untrained and trained male and female subjects, and effects of varying sound intensity, fundamental frequency, and age. J Voice;10:175–189

26. Speyer R, Wieneke GH, Hosseini EG, Kempen PA, Kersing W, Dejonckere PH (2002) Effects of voice therapy as objectively evaluated by digitized laryngeal stroboscopic imaging. Ann Otol Rhinol Laryngol;111:902–908

27. Dejonckere PH, Wieneke GH, Lebacq J (1989) Laryngostroboscopy and glottic dysrhythmia's. Acta Otorhinolaryngol Belg;43:19–29

28. Hirano M, Bless DM (1993) Videostroboscopic Examination of the Larynx. Singular Publishing, San Diego

29. Speyer R, Wieneke GH, Kersing W, Dejonckere PH (2005) Accuracy of measurements on videostroboscopic images of the vocal folds. Ann Otol Rhinol Laryngol;114:443–450

30. Eysholdt U, Rosanowski F, Hoppe U (2003) Measurement and interpretation of irregular vocal fold vibrations. HNO;51: 710–716

31. Imagawa H, Kiritani S, Hirose H (1987) High speed digital image recording system for observing vocal fold vibration using an image sensor. J Med Electron Biol Eng;25: 284–290

32. Neubauer, J, Mergell P, Eysholdt U, Herzl, H (2001) Spatiotemporal analysis of irregular vocal fold oscillations: biphonation due to desynchronization of spatial modes. J Acoust Soc Am;110:3179–3192

33. Svec JG, Schutte HK (1996) Videokymography: high-speed linescanning of vocal fold vibration. J Voice;10:201–205

34. Dejonckere PH, Versnel H (2005) High speed imaging of vocal fold vibration: analysis by 4 synchronous line-scans of onset, offset and register breaks. Proceedings IFOS Congress, Rome, 9pp*

35. Hirano M (1989) Objective evaluation of the human voice: clinical aspects. Folia Phoniatr;41:89–144

36. Neiman GS, Edeson B (1981) Procedural aspects of eliciting maximum phonation time. Folia Phoniatr;33:285–293

37. Kent RD, Kent JF, Rosenbek JC (1987) Maximum performance tests of speech production. J Speech Hear Res;52: 367–387

38. Rau D, Beckett RL (1984) Aerodynamic assessment of vocal function using hand-held spirometers. J Speech Hear Dis;49: 183–188

39. Morris S, Jawad MSM, Eccles R (1992) Relationships between vital capacity, height and nasal airway resistance in asymptomatic volunteers. Rhinology;30:259–264

40. Colton RH, Casper JK (1996) Understanding Voice Problems. Williams & Wilkins, Baltimore

41. Verdolini K (1994) Voice disorders. In: Tomblin JB, Morris HL, Spriesterbach OC (Eds). Diagnosis in Speech-Language Pathology. Singular Publishing Group, San Diego, pp. 247–306

42. Woo P, Casper J, Colton R, Brewer D (1994) Aerodynamic and stroboscopic findings before and after microlaryngeal phonosurgery. J Voice;8:186–194

43. Woo P, Colton RH, Shangold L (1987) Phonatory air flow analysis in patients with laryngeal disease. Ann Otol Rhinol Laryngol;96:549–555

44. Schutte HK (1980) The efficiency of voice production, Thesis. University of Groningen. Kemper, Groningen

45. Schutte HK (1992) Integrated aerodynamic measurements. J Voice;6:127–134

46. Fritzell B, Hallen O, Sundberg J (1974) Evaluation of teflon injection procedures for paralytic dysphonia. Folia Phoniatr; 26:414–421

47. Hirano M, Koike Y, von Leden H (1968) Maximum phonation time and air usage during phonation. Folia Phoniatr; 20:185–201

48. Murry T, Bone RC (1978) Aerodynamic relationships associated with normal phonation and paralytic dysphonia. Laryngoscope;88:100–109

49. Rothenberg M (1973) A new inverse filtering technique for deriving the glottal airflow during voicing. J Acoust Soc Am;53:1632–1645

50. Baken RJ, Orlikoff R (2000) Clinical Measurement of Speech and Voice. Singular Thomson Learning, San Diego

51. Rothenberg M (1982) Interpolating subglottal pressure from oral pressure. J Speech Hear Disord;47:218–224

52. Titze IR (1992) Phonation threshold pressure – a missing link in glottal aerodynamics. J Acoust Soc;91:2926–2935

53. Titze IR (1992) Acoustic interpretation of the voice profile (phonetogram). J Speech Hear Res;35:21–34

54. Colton RH, Woo P (1995) Measuring vocal fold function. In: Rubin JS, Sataloff RT, Korovin GS, et al (Eds). Diagnosis and Treatment of Voice Disorders. Igaku - Shoin, New York, pp. 290–315

55. Hyatt RE, Black LF (1973) The flow-volume curve: a current perspective. Am Rev Respir Dis;107:191

56. Robin ED (1982) Respiratory Medicine. In Medicine, Scientific American, New York, 14;III:1–7**

57. Slavit DH (1995) Role of the pulmonary junction in voice assessment. In: Rubin JS, Sataloff RT, Korovin GS, Gould WJ (Eds). Diagnosis and Treatment of Voice Disorders. Igaku - Shoin, New York, pp. 327–340

58. Wolfe V, Fitch J, Martin D (1997) Acoustic measures of dysphonic severity across and within voice types. Folia Phoniatr Logop;49:292–299

59. Titze I, Liang H (1993) Comparison of Fo extraction models for high precision voice perturbation measurements. J Speech Hear Res;36:1120–1133

60. Yu P, Ouaknine M, Giovanni A (2000) Clinical significance of calculating the coefficients of Lyapunov in the objective assessment of dysphonia. Rev Laryngol Otol Rhinol (Bord); 5:301–305

61. Dejonckere PH, van Wijngaarden HA (2001) Retropharyngeal autologous fat transplantation for congenital short palate: a nasometric assessment of functional results. Ann Otol Rhinol Laryngol;110:168–172

62. Schultz-Coulon HJ (1990) Stimmfeldmessung. Berlin, Springer

63. Heylen L, Wuyts FL, Mertens F, De Bodt M, Dan de Heyning PH (2002) Normative voice range profiles of male and female professional voice users. J Voice;16:1–7

64. Heylen L, Wuyts F, Mertens F, De Bodt M, Pattyn J, Croeckx C, Van de Heyning P (1998) Evaluation of the vocal performance of children using a voice range profile index. J Speech Lang Hear Res;41:232–238

65. Van de Heyning PH, et al (1996) Research work of the Belgian study group on voice disorders. Acta Otorhinolaryngol Belg;50:321–386

66. Wuyts F, De Bodt M, Molenberghs G, Remacle M, Heylen L, Millet B, Van Lierde K, Raes J, Van de Heyning PH (2000) The Dysphonia Severity Index: an objective measure of quality based on a multiparameter approach. J Speech Lang Hear Res;43:796–809

67. Jacobson BH, Johnson A, Grywalski C, Silbergleit A, Jacobson G, Benninger MS, Newman CW (1997) The Voice Handicap Index (VHI): development and validation. Am J Speech Lang Pathol;6:66–70

68. Rosen CA, Lee AS, Osborne J, Zullo T, Murry T (2004) Development and validation of the voice handicap index – 10. Laryngoscope;114:1549–1556

69. Dejonckere PH (1996) Electroglottography: a useful method in voice investigation. In: Pais-Clemente M (Ed). Voice Update. Excerpta Medica. Elsevier, Amsterdam, pp. 29–33

70. Fourcin A, Abberton E, Miller D, et al (1995) Laryngography. Eur J Disord Commun;30:101–115

71. Blitzer A (1995) Laryngeal electromyography. In: Rubin JS, Sataloff RT, Korovin GS, Gould WJ (Eds). Diagnosis and Treatment of Voice Disorders. Igaku - Shoin, New York, pp. 316–326

72. Dejonckere PH (1987) EMG of the Larynx. Press Productions, Liège

73. Dejonckere PH, Knoops P, Lebacq J (1988) Evoked muscular potentials in laryngeal muscles. Acta Otolaryngol Belg;42:494–501

74. Munin MC, Murry T, Rosen CA (2000) Laryngeal electromyography. Otolaryngol clin North Am;33:759–770

75. Sataloff RT, Mandel S, Mann EA, Ludlow CL (2004) Practice parameter: laryngeal electromyography (an evidence-based review). J Voice;18:261–274

76. Moerman M, Martens JP, Crevier-Buchman L, de Haan E, Grand S, Tessier C, Woisard V, Dejonckere PH (2006) The INFVo perceptual rating scale for substitution voicing: development and reliability. Eur Arch Otorhinolaryngol; 263(5):435–439

77. Moerman M, Martens, JP, Van Der Borgt MJ, Pelemans M, Gillis M, Dejonckere PH (2006) Perceptual evaluation of substitution voices: development and evaluation of the (I)INFVo rating scale. Eur Arch Otorhinolaryngol;263:183–187

78. Dejonckere PH, Bradley P, Clemente P, Cornut G, Crevier-Buchmann L, Friedrich G, Van De Heyning P, Remacle M, Woisard V (2001) A basic protocol for functional assessment of voice pathology. Eur Arch Otorhinolaryngol;258:77–82

79. Verdonck-de Leeuw IM, Mahieu HF (2000) Multidimensional assessment of voice characteristics following radiotherapy for early glottic cancer and the DSI. Eur Arch Otolaryngol; 257(Suppl 1):S20

80. Dejonckere PH, Crevier L, Elbaz E, Marraco M, Millet B, Remacle M, Woisard V (2000) Clinical implementation of a multidimensional basic protocol for assessing functional results of voice therapy. In: Jahnke K, Fischer M (Eds). Proceedings EUFOS Congress. Monduzzi editore, Berlin, pp. 561–565

81. Friedrich G, Dejonckere PH (2005) The voice evaluation protocol of the European Laryngological Society. First results of a multicenter study. Laryngorhinootologie;84:744–752

82. Dejonckere PH, Crevier-Buchman L, Marie JP, Moerman M, Remacle M, Woisard V (2003) Implementation of the European Laryngological Society (ELS) - basic protocol for assessing voice treatment effect. Rev Laryngol Otol Rhinol; 124:279–283

Fundamentals of Laryngeal Surgery: Approaches, Instrumentation, and Basic Microlaryngoscopic Techniques

3

Hans Edmund Eckel and Marc Remacle

Core Messages

> Most laryngeal lesions are located in the mucosa or submucosal space, making them easily accessible to endoscopic surgery.

> Advantages of the endoscopic approach include the avoidance of skin incisions, division of the thyroid cartilage, and tracheotomy.

> Open laryngeal surgery is required for the cartilaginous structures of the larynx, if the position of the larynx is to be altered, or if the anatomical situation prevents adequate endoscopic visualization.

> Endolaryngeal surgery is done using Kleinsasser's microlaryngoscopy technique.

> CO_2 laser systems are frequently used for laryngeal surgery, particularly phonosurgery, stenosis surgery, and resection of most laryngeal tumors.

Laryngeal endoscopy and surgery aims are a refined diagnosis of laryngeal, tracheal, and hypopharyngeal disease; improvement or restoration of laryngeal function (i.e., phonation, airway protection during deglutition, airway patency); and removal of neoplastic alterations of a benign or malignant nature. In recent years, transoral endoscopic surgery has seen enormous progress, whereas open surgery is now usually restricted to ablative or reconstructive surgery at the cartilaginous framework of the larynx.

3.1 Historical Background

Modern endoscopic laryngeal surgery traces its origins to the second half of the 19th century. Turck and Czermak of Vienna first used angled mirrors for clinical examination of the larynx in 1857, and 2 years later Stoerk used these mirrors for endolaryngeal cauterization of the larynx. As a result of these efforts, endolaryngeal surgery became more widely practiced, and techniques were advanced by McKenzie, Fränkel, Kirstein, Killian, and Jackson. Thus, the development of endolaryngeal surgery was contemporaneous with, but essentially separate from, that of open laryngeal surgery. The decisive breakthrough for endolaryngeal surgery as a universal approach for laryngeal operations occurred when Oskar Kleinsasser of Cologne, Germany, introduced microlaryngoscopy during the early 1960s [1]. This method provides access to most of the mucosal lesions of the larynx and a number of submucosal lesions. At the same time, it requires a specialized set of microinstruments that are controlled with both hands, requiring a high degree of manual skills.

The rich vascular supply of the tissues in the larynx, however, makes it difficult to carry out more extensive procedures, tending to cause troublesome bleeding from the cut tissues that obscures the operative field and makes precision microsurgery difficult or impossible. An early solution to this problem involved using monopolar electrocautery probes in endolaryngeal surgery to improve hemostasis during operations involving the relatively extensive division of submucosal tissues

H. E. Eckel (✉)
Department of Oto-Rhino-Laryngology,
A.ö. Landeskrankenhaus Klagenfurt, HNO, St. Veiter Str. 47,
A-9020 Klagenfurt, Austria
e-mail: hans.eckel@kabeg.at

(e.g., cordectomy, arytenoidectomy). In light of the above situation, the introduction of laser systems into laryngeal surgery marks an important milestone in the development of this operative approach [2]. By coupling a CO_2 laser to the operating microscope and controlling the invisible treatment beam with a micromanipulator, guided by a visible-wavelength coaxial aiming beam, a relatively stationary, noncontact technique was achieved for dividing endolaryngeal tissues while simultaneously coagulating small blood vessels. This approach overcame several basic problems in endolaryngeal surgery: The laser beam does not obstruct the surgeon's view of the confined operating field, it provides adequate tissue hemostasis for greater visibility, and it facilitates the surgical dissection.

The obvious advantages of endolaryngeal laser surgery were not generally appreciated at first. A major objection was that laser incisions always caused thermal tissue damage (burns) and therefore did not meet the requirement of clean, atraumatic tissue division with margins that could be evaluated histologically. Over time, technical refinements eliminated most of these objections, and laser use not only made it easier to carry out known surgical procedures but also laid the foundation for developing new therapeutic concepts, especially in the field of oncological surgery. Remarkably, these concepts were not developed in the United States, where lasers were first used in laryngology. It was left to clinical pioneers in Europe to research, describe, apply, and publicize the clinical potential of endolaryngeal laser surgery. In addition, endoscopic laser surgery has led to a modification of numerous operative procedures for benign lesions of the larynx. Van Overbeek pioneered the CO_2 laser-assisted endoscopic treatment of Zenker's diverticulum. Carruth in the United Kingdom and Freche in France advocated the use of CO_2 laser for benign lesions and bilateral vocal fold immobility. These techniques are briefly reviewed in this chapter.

In France, Marc Bouchayer, one of the best phonosurgeons of his time, improved the cold steel instruments especially for microphonosurgery. The new lines developed more recently on the Unites States, such as the Sataloff's or Benninger's sets, are directly inspired from Bouchayer's tools.

Until Kleinsasser, endolaryngeal surgery was frequently performed as indirect laryngoscopy under general anaesthesia. Afterward, It was much less popular even it was still practiced mainly in Japan or Eastern European countries.

The development of the "chip tip fiberscope" including a camera in the distal tip and an operating channel, the recent financial incentives for office-based procedures, and new injectable substances and laser wavelength have induced a shift for procedures performed transcutaneously or transnasally. A good balance between these two approaches, however, has still not been found.

In the United States, the gap between endolaryngeal surgery and open laryngeal surgery is still evident; although head and neck surgeons in the United States are skilled in open laryngeal surgery, they often take a skeptical view toward endoscopic laryngeal surgery, which is the domain of "laryngologists." This "overdivision" into subspecialties helps explain the long delay in acceptance of endolaryngeal laser surgery in the United States.

3.2 Endolaryngeal Versus Extralaryngeal Approach to the Larynx

Most benign laryngeal lesions are located in the mucosa or submucosal space of the larynx, making them easily accessible to endoscopic inspection. Advantages of the endoscopic approach include avoidance of skin incisions, division of the thyroid cartilage, and tracheotomy. Therefore, it causes less surgical trauma and its related morbidity. As a consequence, open operations on the larynx are now considered obsolete unless surgery is required for the cartilaginous structures of the larynx, if the position of the larynx is to be altered, or if there are particular problems that prevent adequate endoscopic visualization of the anatomicical structures. In most cases, surgical resection of benign laryngeal pathology is the only reasonable therapeutic option in cases where treatment is warranted. Except for oncological surgery, which aims to remove diseased structures, laryngeal surgery is driven by functional considerations, aiming at improving voice, deglutition, or airway patency. If doubt exists as to the nature of a given lesion, it may be prudent to leave some of the pathology behind and resect it at a later time if it better preserves the functional integrity of the larynx.

3.3 Surgical Endoscopy

Direct laryngoscopy under general anesthesia is indicated for all laryngeal diseases in which the larynx cannot be examined in the conscious patient (children) or in which mirror laryngoscopy, telescopic laryngoscopy, or flexible endoscopy has revealed findings in the larynx, hypopharynx, or trachea that require further investigation. Suspension laryngoscopy uses an identical approach but fixes the laryngoscope by means of a chest support. The surgeon's hands are free for bimanual manipulation. It provides ideal access for many diagnostic and therapeutic procedures in the trachea, in which the laryngoscope can serve as a "sheath" for introduction of tracheoscopes and operating instruments (Fig. 3.1). Using an operating microscope additionally provides a three-dimensional view of the endolaryngeal anatomy. In addition to inspection of the mucosal surface with the operating microscope and introduction of rigid endoscopes, this technique allows selective excisional biopsies, even enabling the surgeon to take large samples if required. In additional, visual inspection can be supplemented by tactile examination (e.g., to assess the mobility of an ankylosed arytenoid cartilage). Currently, CO_2 laser can be used for excisional biopsies, completely resecting small mucosal lesions of indeterminate nature in a procedure that is both diagnostic and therapeutic.

3.4 Fundamentals of Endolaryngeal Surgery and Equipment

Endolaryngeal surgery is done using Kleinsasser's microlaryngoscopy technique. The patient is positioned in a supine position. A rigid laryngoscope of appropriate size is inserted through the oral cavity, and the oropharynx and held in place using a chest support. The use of an operating microscope allows three-dimensional visualization of the endolaryngeal structures and bimanual surgical handling of instruments inside the larynx. The basic setup is shown in Figure 3.2 [3, 4].

In Figure 3.2, red lines indicate the patient's head positioning. The operating table has been adjusted in a way that allows the surgeon to sit comfortably on an operating chair, with arms supported by armrests, footswitches for steering the operating microscope, laser, and electrocautery; a red line indicates the viewing axis from the microscope to the larynx. Proper positioning of the patient is usually achieved with the patient's neck in

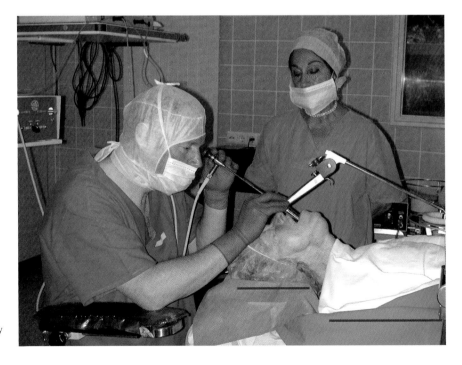

Fig. 3.1. Basic setup for direct laryngoscopy. A rigid endoscope is used to visualize the anatomical structures of the larynx and trachea. Positioning of the head and body is indicated by *red lines*

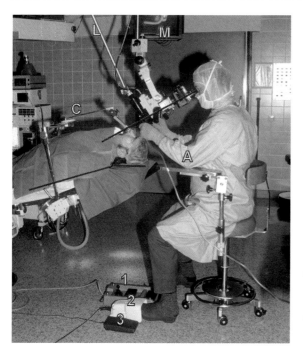

Fig. 3.2. Basic setup for microlaryngoscopic surgery. *C*, chest support; *L*, laser arm; *M*, monitor; *A*, arm rest; *1*, foot switch for microscope; *2*, foot switch for laser; *3*, foot switch for electrocautery

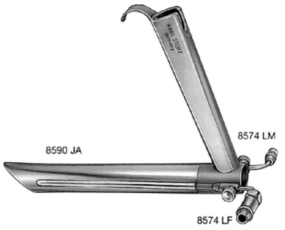

Fig. 3.3. Kleinsasser laryngoscope. (Courtesy of Karl Storz Company, Tuttlingen, Germany)

flexion and the head in slight hyperextension (Fig. 3.3). Other important prerequisites are preoperative assessment of dental status, adequate mouth protection during the procedure to prevent dental injuries, and a trained, proficient surgeon. Suitable options for anesthesia–ventilation include general endotracheal anesthesia (using a laser-safe ventilation tube), jet ventilation, and mask ventilation with intermittent apnea. The necessary equipment includes an assortment of laryngoscopes and stands, an operating microscope, microinstruments, CO_2 laser, monopolar cautery probes, rigid telescopes, and suction. Some procedures also require implants and their corresponding application instruments (collagen, fat, cartilage, dispersed silicone) and photographic or video equipment. The essential problems in any minimally invasive procedure, regardless of whether it is in the abdominal cavity, knee joint, or larynx, are obtaining an adequate view of the operative field and the ability to use the necessary instruments at the surgical site. For laryngeal surgery, operating laryngoscopes are employed. Because no laryngoscope can satisfy all requirements, the laryngeal surgeon should have an assortment of models on hand. The most important are listed below.

- Kleinsasser laryngoscopes (sizes A–C, DN, J, JL) (Fig. 3.3) are still valid for microsurgery of benign laryngeal lesions. Recent modifications have been proposed by major companies for better exposition of the anterior commissure or for laser-assisted microsurgery. Laryngoscopes are now equipped with wall-integrated channels for smoke evacuation and a light guide. The inner part of the scopes should be ebonized or sandblasted to prevent laser beam reflection and to favor maximum dispersion of the beam.
- The Bouchayer laryngoscope remains a gold standard for cold steel microphonosurgery for many phonosurgeons, particularly in France.
- Bivalved laryngoscopes in various sizes (Rudert, Steiner, Weerda) are necessary for approaching the supraglottic larynx and the hypopharynx (Fig. 3.4).
- The Lindholm laryngoscope, when inserted into the vallecula epiglottica, affords an excellent view of supraglottic structures (ideally of the whole larynx) (Fig. 3.5).
- Diverticuloscope for endoscopic cricopharyngeal myotomy.
- Pediatric laryngoscopes (various models).

Optimal instrumentation is just as important when treating benign laryngeal lesions as it is for surgery of malignant tumors. It may be even more so inasmuch as tumor surgery is basically a destructive process whereas surgery for benign laryngeal lesions is often a tailoring procedure. The goal of this type of surgery is not just to remove abnormalities but rather to modify

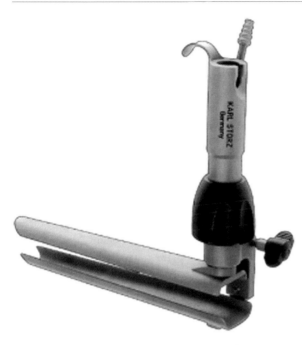

Fig. 3.4. Bivalved laryngoscope. (Courtesy of Karl Storz Company, Tuttlingen, Germany)

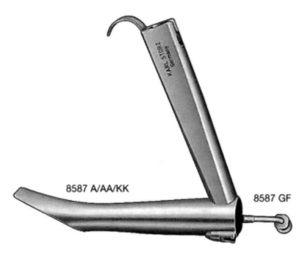

Fig. 3.5. Lindholm laryngoscope. (Courtesy of Karl Storz Company, Tuttlingen, Germany)

and adapt (tailor) anatomical changes to allow optimum functional rehabilitation of the voice, swallowing, and respiration.

No single company provides the ideal tool box so far. Surgeons, according to their own practice, experience, and professional surroundings, may prefer one instrument to another. Moreover, many companies provide similar instruments. Personal relations with these companies and their local representatives have, de facto, a major influence.

These instruments were originally designed for cold steel microsurgery. Many of them have been adapted for laser-assisted surgery with a channel for smoke evacuation.

The microinstruments are usually 22 cm in length, and most are paired symmetrical sets with a right and a left directed working end. The basic box should have the instruments designed originally by Kleinsasser: thin, curved forceps that have serrated teeth and cup forceps for biopsies. The Bouchayer "heart-shaped" forceps are ideal for microsurgery of the vocal fold. The head of the forceps is directed 45° to the left or right sides and 45° to the top, allowing perfect, gentle holding of the vocal fold. Microscissors, sickle knives, flap elevators, straight or curved, are of course mandatory for cold steel surgery. Three to four suction tubes with various diameters are also necessary.

Monopolar electrocautery is also necessary for bleeding control. Electrocautery connected to a suction tube or a forceps is available and can be recommended. Many surgeons achieve coagulation simply by contact between a basic electrocautery blade and the suction tube or forceps.

Stronger, larger forceps are available for endoscopic cancer surgery when large specimens have to be handled. The table is completed with wet towels for protecting the patient's face in case of laser-assisted surgery, swabs soaked in epinephrine solution (1:100,000) for controlling oozing and for protecting the cuff of the ventilation tube in case of laser surgery, and a silicone tooth guard or folded gauze sponge for protecting the teeth.

Other instruments may be necessary according to the specific surgery, such as Brünings syringe or the Ford injection device for injecting fat, collagen, or other substances. These choices are also related to the surgeon's own preferences and experience. They are discussed in the following chapters.

3.5 Laser Systems Used for Endoscopic Surgery of Benign Laryngeal and Tracheal Lesions

The CO_2 laser is the undisputed workhorse of laser surgery in laryngology. Owing to its frequent use in tumor surgery, nowadays it is available in the ear/nose/throat

(ENT) departments of most large hospitals. Designed for surgery, its wavelength is 10,600 nm, with absorption by water inducing minor peripheral thermal effects in the surrounding tissues. CO_2 laser meets the requirements for use for most benign laryngeal lesions, particularly during phonosurgery, stenosis surgery, swallowing rehabilitation, and resection of most benign laryngeal tumors.

The initial CO_2 laser microwave was a continuous wave. At a given power, it provided continuous output. The continuous exposure resulted in much heating of collateral, nontarget tissue by conduction. To minimize the thermal effect; a pulsed mode was developed for the CO_2 laser (Sharpulse). The thermal reduction is even more important with Superpulse or Ultrapulse waves. SuperPulse and UltraPulse are pulsed waves with the high peak of power delivered in millisecond pulses or less. The resultant average pulse power, preset during programming, usually ranges between 1 and 10 W. The interpulse pause of approximately 1 ms, called thermal relaxing time, permits the tissue to cool. This significantly reduces the thermal effect and consequent coagulation of the area surrounding the impact. SuperPulse has higher peak power (400–500 W) than UltraPulse (200 W) but less energy because its delivering time is shorter (Fig. 3.1). This pulse energy determines tissue impact and must reach the necessary threshold for ablation. Energy below ablation threshold leads to stronger thermal impact. UltraPulse adjusts its pulse energy automatically such that it is always above ablation threshold. This is not the case with SuperPulse (Fig. 3.2). The SuperPulse is cone-shaped, which means that some part (the rising and falling parts) is below ablation threshold, which in turn means this part of the energy goes into tissue and heats it more. UltraPulse is rectangular. Hence, there may be slightly more thermal damage with SuperPulse than with UltraPulse.

In addition to the laser unit itself, accessories are available for optimal delivery of laser energy to the operative site.

In terms of laser light delivery from the laser arm to the target, currently available are the Acuspot micromanipulator and scanner. The micromanipulator, which is attached to the operating microscope and connected to the laser arm, yields the smallest possible beam diameter presently available (i.e., 250 µm for a focal length of 400 mm). This micromanipulator makes possible the accurate tissue incision and dissection required for phonosurgery. By means of a computer-guided system of rotating mirrors, the scanner allows the beam to sweep a given surface with extreme rapidity. This feature makes it a highly effective tool when macroscopic vaporization is required. A "shaving" effect a few microns deep is achieved during each beam sweep, with little in-depth thermal penetration. The usual shape chosen for the surface is the circle. This mode of laser use is suitable for selective, superficial removal of mucosal lesions in cases where histological examination is not required and the main aim is to achieve uniform tissue ablation with the least possible collateral injury. An example is the removal of papillomas or patchy areas of leukoplakia, which can be histologically confirmed prior to laser ablation. The result of this procedure is a superficial mucosal wound with no thermal alteration of the underlying tissue. This type of wound undergoes rapid secondary epithelialization and can heal with an excellent functional result.

The Acublade is a scanner software modification that allows the beam to travel across the target as a straight or curved incision line instead of "shaving" a given surface (Fig. 3.3). Various lengths (0.5–3.5 mm) and penetration depths (0.2–2.0 mm) are programmable. The operator can, at all times, modify the parameters proposed by the laser-controlling software. This incision line can be rotated to the left or right thanks to a driving belt articulated with the scanner. The belt is moved with a joystick-controlled electrical motor (Fig. 3.4a).

The software-calculated penetration depth is based on average absorption of the CO_2 laser by living soft tissues. Depending on the desired length and penetration, the software calculates the required power and pulse duration for the single pulse mode. The Acublade was designed for SuperPulse and continuous modes that can originate from the same optical cavity. The Acublade is now available with UltraPulse technology. The guiding system of the incision line is fully electronic and integrated in the scanner (Fig. 3.4b).

Incisions are sharper with UltraPulse, making the dissection more comfortable, mainly when approaching a major vocal fold structure, such as the vocal ligament. This difference in efficiency is of interest for delicate phonosurgery of the vocal fold in single-pulse mode, but it is not an advantage for other procedures, such as cordectomy, when the shooting is usually in continuous mode. On the other hand, there may be more coagulation along the incision line.

The differences between SuperPulse and UltraPulse when used with Acublade are only perceptible during surgery. The differences do not affect the postoperative period or the functional results. For the selection of suitable laser parameters (e.g., pulse shape and duration, power output), the reader is referred to selected publications and to Chapters 1, 2, and 6 of this volume.

When treating laryngeal hemangiomas, especially when they are large, the neodymium:yttrium aluminum garnet (Nd:YAG) laser or other fiber-guided lasers with good absorption in the red spectrum, such as potassium titanyl phosphate (KTP) and diode lasers, have the advantage of greater penetration depth in tissue than other lasers, producing deeper coagulation of the hemangioma. Nd:YAG laser emits at 1064 nm. Its frequency is doubled by passing the light through KTP to produce KTP laser, which then emits at 532 nm. The diode laser, made from arsenium and gallium, has a wavelength of 805 nm, which situates it between the CO_2 and Nd:YAG lasers. As a result, the tissue effects of the KTP and diode lasers are altogether different from those of the Nd:YAG laser, mainly regarding the thermal effects. It must be remembered that the thermal diffusion of Nd:YAG is more than 4 mm into the surrounding tissues.

When approached carefully, however, circumscribed hemangiomas can be successfully shrunken by coagulation or excised locally with the CO_2 laser.

Argon lasers can also be used to treat vascular neoplasms owing to the absorption of the light by the red blood pigment. A special laser treatment modality is photodynamic therapy (PDT) (tissue lasing following selective uptake of a photosensitizing agent). The efficacy of PDT has been documented for a number of benign, preneoplastic, and neoplastic mucosal lesions. However, the cost of the procedure and concerns about unpredictable mucosal scarring limit its application in the treatment of benign lesions of the larynx and trachea. PDT is more frequently used for palliative treatment of head and neck cancer no longer treatable by surgery, radiotherapy, and/or chemotherapy. Foscan is presently one of the most used photosensitizing agents.

New wavelengths such as those of thulium or holmium-YAG which are fiber-guided, are presently on trial and are promising for office-based surgery. A hollow fiber transmitting the CO_2 laser is also commercially available. So far only rough ablations or incisions are possible.

Pulse-dye laser (PDL), originally developed to treat skin conditions that involve blood vessels, such as birthmarks, have been used transnasally in the office for treating angiectatic polyps or Reinke's edema. Long-term results are pending.

3.6 Alternatives to Surgical Laser Use

Surgical lasers, particularly CO_2 laser, can be used in various ways to treat benign laryngeal and tracheal lesions.

- Tissue ablation (precise cutting with minimum coagulation for resecting abnormal tissue)
- Coagulation (of blood vessels or highly vascular neoplasms)
- Vaporization (of tissues, as for papilloma removal)
- Induction of photochemical processes (in photodynamic therapy)

Alternative techniques are available for all of these applications and are briefly described below.

3.6.1 Tissue Cutting

Tissue incision and cutting can be accomplished with sharp cutting instruments (knives, scissors)—the essential tools for selective tissue ablation in every surgical discipline. Special small knives and microscissors are available for traditional tissue ablation in the larynx and trachea, but these instruments require expert manual skill and rigorous practice. They are designed to have a long shaft that must be passed down the operating laryngoscope, making them less effective than the scalpels and scissors used during open operations. At the same time, the division of tissues with cutting instruments always involves capillaries and small arterial or venous vessels, leading to diffuse bleeding at the surgical site. Although blood loss in the larynx is not quantitatively significant in itself, the bleeding nevertheless obscures the operative field and makes it difficult to assess the progress of the operation. This type of bleeding is particularly troublesome in the situation of maximum precision microsurgery. Not infrequently, it prevents the surgical precision that is desired from a functional standpoint and prolongs the operating time. The bleeding and the associated obstacles created during the surgery can result in functional failures and persistent, undesired anatomical changes (scars, synechiae). On the other hand, "cold" instruments offer the significant advantage of precise cutting with no thermal damage to surrounding tissues. This makes it easier for the pathologist to evaluate the margins of the excised tissues and eliminates the deleterious effects of collateral thermal damage on wound healing. Moreover, the use of cutting microinstruments in laryngeal surgery does not require the elaborate technical precautions necessitated by laser use. In summary, there is no question that the ability of cold instruments to remove small lesions confined to the mucosa, especially with phonosurgery, is the equal of surgical lasers and is even superior to lasers in some situations. CO_2 laser should be used for phonosurgical ablation of mucosal lesions only by a highly skilled surgeon and only in settings where optimal technical facilities are available.

In addition to conventional instruments, powered instruments (microdebriders, shavers) for use in laryngeal and tracheal surgery have been described recently. These instruments have been widely used in paranasal sinus surgery. Basically, they consist of a motorized blade rotating in a sheath with suction at the tip. Tissue is excised superficially by the rotating blade and simultaneously aspirated out of the sheath. Those advocating this type of instrument for endolaryngeal surgery (especially papilloma removal) have noted that shaver systems require less time for tissue ablation and do not generate a smoke plume. This argument is worth mentioning because human papillomavirus (HPV) DNA has been identified in the plume produced during the CO_2 laser vaporization of respiratory tract papillomas. Its clinical significance is uncertain, however. The difficult healing of "tissue burns" caused by endolaryngeal laser surgery has been cited as another argument for the use of microdebriders. However, bleeding is possible, which can be a factor in the dissemination of HPV.

One fact should be emphasised at this point: Surgical lasers cause burns in the larynx and trachea only if the surgeon is using an outdated device or is not well trained in laser surgery. In other words, burns following laser surgery are the fault of the operator, not of the method. Modern, fully equipped CO_2 laser systems enable the surgeon to divide tissue with absolute precision with a focused beam, without causing clinically significant thermal damage to normal surrounding tissue. Thus, the concern voiced by many authors that lasers cause "burns" is based on observations either from the early days of laser surgery or

improper laser use. When all facts are considered, the argument of thermal tissue damage and its implications for wound healing can no longer be taken seriously. Moreover, it is unclear whether motorized instruments used on the fine structures of the vocal cord mucosa pose an equal or even greater risk of inadvertent tissue damage than present-day laser technology. Let us consider an analogy with middle ear surgery: CO_2 lasers have gained an established place in stapes surgery, and today no ear surgeon would think of using shaver systems on the auditory ossicles. At the same time, microdebriders are probably an effective supplement to the surgical armamentarium for the rapid removal of large neoplasms that do not require further histological evaluation.

3.6.2 Coagulation

In addition to surgical lasers (CO_2, KTP, Nd:YAG), electrocautery probes are commonly used to coagulate blood vessels and tissues having a rich blood supply. Before the advent of surgical lasers, electrocautery probes were widely used in endolaryngeal surgery. They were used for cutting (e.g., arytenoidectomy), tissue ablation (suction–coagulation during papilloma removal), and selective cauterization of small blood vessels. Today, classic electrosurgery is more of an adjunct to endolaryngeal laser surgery than a competing modality. It is no longer considered an acceptable tool for most procedures because it causes far more extensive thermal damage and cauterization of specimen margins than the CO_2 laser and cannot be manipulated as precisely as the laser beam. When used as an adjunct to CO_2 laser, electrosurgery is indispensable in all major endolaryngeal procedures because CO_2 laser can only coagulate blood vessels no larger than 0.5 mm. It is unable to coagulate large bleeders, such as those encountered during an arytenoidectomy or endolaryngeal partial laryngectomy, even when applied in the continuous mode with a defocused beam. In these cases, the electrocautery probe is an essential adjunct to the laser for obtaining surgical hemostasis.

Electrosurgery as a stand-alone method has undergone technical refinements in recent years, and these improvements have eliminated some of the inherent disadvantages of electrosurgical procedures. For example, thermal tissue damage can be substantially reduced by irrigating the surgical site with water. Good clinical results have been achieved by applying a continuous stream of noble gas to the tissue to be coagulated (argon beamer, argon plasma coagulation). This technique permits optimum electrocoagulation of the tissue while preventing carbonization. It has become an accepted alternative to laser surgery, particularly for operations on the nose and paranasal sinuses. So far there has been little clinical experience with argon plasma coagulation in laryngeal surgery, but it is entirely conceivable that the method could be effective in treating vascular lesions located away from the vocal folds.

3.6.3 Vaporization

Aside from the argon plasma coagulation systems described above, there is no alternative to CO_2 laser for tissue vaporization.

3.6.4 Photodynamic Therapy

Laser systems have ideal technical properties for inducing desired photochemical reactions in tissue. PDT would not be possible without lasers. The question is which laser system is the most suitable. This question, just as that of choosing the best photosensitizing agent, is a topic of current research and is beyond the scope of this chapter.

3.7 Anesthesia, Perioperative Care, Adjunctive Medical Therapy

Laser surgery can be done under general endotracheal anesthesia and jet ventilation. Endotracheal intubation is generally preferred in operations where there is likely to be heavy bleeding (tumor resection, arytenoidectomy, laryngeal papillomatosis). Special laser-safe tubes should be used to protect against tube combustion and airway fires.

Because theses tubes are expensive, a number of techniques have been introduced to protect the standard tubes by wrapping them with a protective, nonflammable material. One of the earliest and most effective techniques involved wrapping a 12-mm (0.5 in.) aluminum tape (3M, #425) from the cuff to the proximal end of the tube, in a spiral motion. The entire length at risk of exposure, usually 10–12 cm, is covered for total protection. The wrapping starts at the distal end just proximal to the cuff. A tape cut at 60° allows the first spiral to be applied against the cuff. Each spiral overlaps the previous one by a few millimeters so no bare tube is exposed. At the same time, excessive overlapping is avoided as it makes the tube rigid and unyielding. Copper foil tape (Venture) can also be used. When removing the tube, caution must be taken to avoid injuring the vocal folds with the sharp edge of the aluminum foil.

The foil wrapped-tube is introduced orally because endonasal intubation is too traumatic. To permit swift withdrawal of the tube in case of fire, the proximal end of the tube is not taped to the perioral area contrary to customary anesthetic practice. It is usual to use comparatively small size tubes in microsurgery.

The accidental laser impact on the silver aluminum foil does not cause tube ignition. However, the reflective surface of the foil allows unintentional reflection of laser energy onto nontarget tissue, which may result in secondary "ghost burn." It is necessary for the anesthetist to ensure that the wrapping is adequate. It must be noted that handmade wrapping of the tube is no longer approved by the U.S. Food and Drug Administration (FDA).

Some manufacturers produce factory-wrapped tubes, such as Rüsch and Xomed, of much better quality. Merocel Laser-Guard is a self-adhesive silver foil covered with sponge. It increases the outer diameter of the tube by 2 mm. The sponge must be kept constantly saturated with physiological saline: the Laser-Guard ignites if too dry. Another method for protecting the tube is adhesive copper foil overwrapped with fabric that has to be kept saline-soaked (Laser-Trach).

Cuffs are filled with physiological saline tinted with methylene blue. If the beam perforates the cuff, the saline absorbs the laser, and the dye signals the perforation even if minimal. However, care must be taken to protect the cuff throughout surgery with saturated cotton swabs.

Jet ventilation is preferred during operations for airway stenosis and in many phonosurgical procedures as it provides a better view of the glottis and subglottis. Even extensive endolaryngeal procedures can almost always be done without a prior tracheotomy when surgical lasers are used.

The present authors have achieved good results with routine intravenous administration of 250 mg methylprednisolone before endolaryngeal procedures. Antibiotic prophylaxis (e.g., 3 g ampicillin–sulbactam or 600 mg clindamycin i.v.) is also given for more extensive procedures, especially those involving exposure of laryngeal cartilage. Patients generally require postoperative monitoring in an intensive care unit (ICU) following laser surgery for airway stenosis. For all other procedures, ICU monitoring is generally unnecessary from a surgical standpoint.

3.8 Office-Based Laryngeal Procedures

Office-based procedures will increase in the coming years, including biopsies, injections, and lesion removal. The major reasons office procedures are increasing in popularity are based on patient acceptance. When compared with a procedure that is performed under general anesthesia, an office-based procedure is considered less invasive by patients and physicians.

As the aging in developed countries continues, it is anticipated that the elderly and their need for better voice and swallow function will parallel the disease processes that are due to aging, such as presbyphonia and Parkinson's disease. The search by the patient for better function will drive additional procedures to the office. Office-based procedures that are safe and effective will have an increasing role. For most otolaryngologists, laryngeal biopsy or laryngeal injection is laborious, and the time it takes is not compensated adequately. If the surgeon could use the office setting, this would be a more efficient use of time and resources.

Office delivery of drugs, lasers, and instrumentation will improve. The use of chips in scope technology is superior enough that stroboscopy can be accomplished through a flexible laryngoscope. Such technology was not available until recently. A revisit of the procedures that were mastered many years ago is worth it in light of today's technology. Some of the factors for revival of procedures already well known

and written about since the 19th century are economic, demographic, and technological.

Selecting appropriate patients should be mentioned first. It is better to err on the side of caution than to spend too much time with an anxiety-ridden patient only to have the procedure fail because of patient reluctance. In this regard, proper information on the procedure, its duration, and the patient's feelings after local anesthesia is helpful. The duration of local anesthetic application is around 15 minutes, and it cannot be hurried. The local anesthetic is applied topically by spray into the oropharynx and the hypopharynx. The topical medication that is used may be 10% lidocaine. It is important to spray during inhalation. This is done twice. If the patient coughs, it must be repeated. The patient is asked to hold his or her own tongue and sit forward in a chin-forward position. A cotton ball is used to paint the tonsils, vallecula, and piriform sinuses. When the cotton ball is inserted in the larynx, it occludes the airway partially. The patient is instructed to cough with the cotton ball in the larynx. This ensures better topical application.

A test palpation of the larynx can be done using a probe or the biopsy forceps. Tolerance to passive palpation should be confirmed before procedures that may require biopsy, laser beam delivery, or injection. For vasoconstriction of the nasal cavity, a decongestive spray is used. In some cases, a topical swab in the nose to obtain adequate decongestion is necessary to pass the scope. Being able to lay the patient flat is helpful if the patient feels faint.

3.9 Complications of Endoscopic Laser Surgery

A number of authors have described complications of endoscopic laser surgery in the larynx, trachea, and hypopharynx. These problems mostly involve combustion of ventilation tube materials and anesthetic gas mixtures during surgical laser use in the larynx. The surgeon should consider the possibility of these complications during each laser operation and take appropriate precautions. Combustion of tube materials can be avoided by the use of laser-safe tubes. Ignition of anesthetic gas mixtures during procedures using jet ventilation can be prevented by ventilating the patient with room air (rather than pure oxygen) and by operating in intermittent apnea. On the whole, such incidents can be safely avoided nowadays by selecting suitable materials, operating methods, and analgesic techniques. Reports of airway fires in the current literature must be viewed more as a result of poorly trained operating room personnel than as inherent risks of laser surgery.

Possible laser-associated complications are less important during endolaryngeal surgery than complications caused by the laryngoscope itself. In a study by one of the authors [5], 75% of 339 consecutive microlaryngoscopy patients were found to have small mucosal lesions of the lips, oral cavity, and oropharynx. These lesions caused significant complaints for some time but resolved without sequelae in a few days. Dental injuries occur in approximately 6% of all patients, but they predominantly affect patients who already have significant carious damage to the teeth, preexisting loose teeth, periodontal disease, or a fixed denture. Patients with healthy dentition did not sustain dental injuries in this study. The nature of the denture injuries ranged from simple loosening and enamel fractures to chipped teeth and complete dental displacement. No laser-associated complications were observed. Microlaryngoscopic procedures may be followed by transient functional impairment of the hypoglossal nerve and lingual nerve. By and large, this type of complication cannot be completely avoided during microlaryngoscopic surgery, but the range of complications is definitely more limited than with open laryngeal surgery. In summary, laser surgery of benign lesions of the larynx, pharynx, and trachea can be considered a minimally invasive surgical approach with a low risk of complications.

3.9.1 Tips and Pearls to Avoid Complications

- Preoperative examination of patient's dental situation allows risk assessment with regard to dental injuries during microlaryngoscopic surgery.
- Different positions of the patient's head should be tried in cases of difficult laryngeal exposure.
- Comprehensive surgical equipment, including a variety of laryngoscopes, CO_2 laser, electrocautery, microscope and rigid endoscopes (0°, 30°, 70°) should be available during laryngeal surgery.
- Endolaryngeal exposition of glottic and subglottic structures is best when jet ventilation is used in place of ventilation tubes.
- Special laser-safe tubes should be used to protect against tube combustion and airway fires.
- Intraoperative administration of 250 mg of methylprednisolone avoids laryngeal edema.

References

1. Kleinsasser O (1961) [A laryngomicroscope for the early diagnosis and differential diagnosis of cancers in the larynx, pharynx and mouth.]. Z Laryngol Rhinol Otol;40:276–279
2. Strong MS, Jako GJ (1972) Laser surgery in the larynx. Early clinical experience with continuous CO_2 laser. Ann Otol Rhinol Laryngol;81:791
3. Eckel HE (2003) [Lasers in the larynx, hypopharynx and trachea in benign diseases]. Laryngorhinootologie;82(Suppl 1): S89–S113
4. Remacle M, Lawson G, Watelet JB (1999) Carbon dioxide laser microsurgery of benign vocal fold lesions: indications, techniques, and results in 251 patients. Ann Otol Rhinol Laryngol;108:156
5. Klussmann JP, Knoedgen R, Wittekindt C, Damm M, Eckel HE (2002) Complications of suspension laryngoscopy. Ann Otol Rhinol Laryngol;111:972–976

Endolaryngeal Phonosurgery

4

Gerhard Friedrich

Core Messages

> Phonosurgery is any surgery designed primarily for the improvement or restoration of voice. Phonosurgery is therefore not restricted to one or more surgical techniques but is defined by its intended functional goal.

> A prerequisite for phonosurgery is the adequate diagnosis and documentation of the disordered voice.

> As the pathogenesis of voice disorders is usually multidimensional phonosurgery may form only a part of the holistic treatment of voice disorders, in partnership with various nonsurgical methods.

> Phonosurgery should not focus on the appearance of the vocal folds but, rather should aim for an improvement in voice, adapted to the individual request and needs of the patient.

> Vocal fold surgery is a surgical procedure performed directly on the vocal folds with the aim of improving the vibratory movement and restoration of the normal mucosal wave, or correction of vocal fold position and/or tension.

> The basic principle of vocal fold surgery is to maintain or improve the functional structure of the vocal fold by respecting its layered structure. This is achieved by means of minimal tissue excision, minimal disruption of the superficial layer of the lamina propria and preservation of the epithelium, especially at the vibrating edge.

> This can be accomplished using the microflap technique which has completely replaced the resection of the epithelium previously called "stripping" or "decortication" which now better is termed "subepithelial chordectomy".

Phonosurgery is not a new paradigm. In 1911, Brünings [3] introduced vocal fold augmentation by endolaryngeal injection; and in 1915, Payr [13] developed an external method for vocal fold medialization. Following Billroth's first laryngectomy in 1874, Gussenbauer [10] was the first to use an artificial larynx for voice restoration, and Gluck [9] was the first to use a term roughly translating as "phonosurgery" in his 1930 paper "phonetic surgery of the upper aero-digestive tract and artificial and natural voice restoration." Despite these early forays, however, Hans von Leden's [21, 22] statement remains broadly true, that "during the first 100 years of our specialty, laryngeal surgery was devoted largely to the removal of neoplasms, and any potential improvement in voice was really a by-product of this process." It was also Hans von Leden, together with Gottfried Arnold [21, 22], who defined "phonosurgery" (PS) as it presently applies: any surgery designed primarily for the improvement or restoration of voice. PS is therefore not restricted to one or more surgical techniques but is defined by its intended functional goal. PS comprised a

G. Friedrich
Professor and Chairman, Ear, nose and Throat
University Hospital, Graz, Head of Department of Phoniatrics,
Speech and Swallowing, Medical University of Graz,
Auenbruggerplatz 26-28, A-8036, Graz, Austria
e-mail: phoniatrie.hno@meduni-graz.at

M. Remacle, H. E. Eckel (eds.), *Surgery of Larynx and Trachea,*
DOI: 10.1007/978-3-540-79136-2_4, © Springer-Verlag Berlin Heidelberg 2010

Table 4.1. Classification of (primary) phonosurgery [8a]

Vocal fold surgery (VFS)
Laryngeal framework surgery (LFS)
Neuromuscular surgery (NMS)
Reconstructive surgery (RCS)
– Partial defect of the larynx
– Total loss of the larynx

Table 4.2. Vocal fold surgery – approaches [17]

Endolaryngeal
    Indirect
    Direct
External
    Open neck
    Percutaneous

Table 4.3. Vocal fold surgery – procedures [17]

Incision
Excision
Dissection (microflap)
Augmentation
Injection/implantation
Vaporization
Coagulation
Injection of pharmaceutical agents
Suction
Stenting
Mobilization

Table 4.4. Vocal fold lesions impairing the vibratory movement [17]

Epithelium
Papillomatosis
Chronic hypertrophic laryngitis
    Hyperplasia
    Dysplasia
    Carcinoma in situ
Carcinoma

Lamina propria
Exudative lesions affecting Reinke's space
    Nodule
    Polyp
    Pseudocyst
    Reinke's edema
Cyst
    Epidermoid
    Mucous retention
Sulcus ("open cyst")
Mucosal bridge
Atrophy/scar
    Congenital ("sulcus-vergeture")
    Acquired
    Presbyphonia
Vascular
    Ectasia
    Varicosity
    Hematoma

Arytenoid
Granuloma

Anterior commissure
Glottal web, microweb

great variety of procedures and approaches, which makes it difficult to compare results between and among institutions. The European Laryngological Society (ELS) has therefore established a comprehensive classification system [8a] (Table 4.1).

A prerequisite for phonosurgery is the adequate diagnosis and documentation of the disordered voice [6, 8a]. As the pathogenesis of voice disorders is usually multidimensional, PS may form only a part of the holistic treatment of voice disorders, in partnership with various nonsurgical methods. The phonosurgeon must be skilled in the functional investigation of voice and adjunctive treatment regimens or must work in close cooperation with someone having this knowledge. PS should not focus on the appearance of the vocal folds but, rather, should aim for an improvement in voice, adapted to the individual requests and needs of the patient.

4.1 Vocal Fold Surgery: General Survey

The definition of vocal fold surgery is a surgical procedure performed directly on the vocal folds with the aim of (1) improving the vibratory movement and restoration of the normal mucosal wave, or (2) correction of vocal fold position and/or tension [17].

Most PS on the vocal folds requires magnification afforded by an operating microscope (phonomicrosurgery) or a telescope connected to a video camera, both under general anesthesia. However, PS may also be performed directly or percutaneously under control of a flexible transnasal fiberscope or a transoral telescope, sometimes combined with stroboscopy. The former approach is currently preferred by most phonosurgeons for most procedures (Tables 4.2, 4.6, and 4.7).

Various methods are used for different pathology (Table 4.3). The basic principle of vocal fold surgery is to maintain or improve the functional structure of the vocal fold by respecting its layered structure. This is achieved by means of minimal tissue excision, minimal disruption of the superficial layer of the lamina propria, and preservation of the epithelium, especially at the vibrating edge.

Most glottic lesions affect phonatory function of the larynx. Surgical management aims at removing these lesions and restoring phonation. The procedure should be precise, and the healing process should not result in significant scarring.

Table 4.5. Movement disorders of the vocal folds [17]

Vocal fold immobility
Paralysis/paresis
Cricoarytenoid joint disorders

Neurologic
Tremor/spasmodic dysphonia

Dysfunctional
Hyperfunctional/hypofunctional
Dysphonia plicae ventricularis

For surgery on the vocal fold, the primary aim is to preserve the underlying vocal ligament. The usual morphological anatomy of the vocal fold is described as having a superior and an inferior surface, with intervening free edge. However, the free edge is far from an "edge." The dynamic anatomy of the vocal fold shows three distinct "borders" to the free edge: superior, middle, and inferior. During surgery, if the superior border of the free edge is surgically removed, the mechanical vibration continues from the inferior border to the middle border, and the voice generally recovers within 2–6 weeks. When both the superior and middle borders are removed simultaneously, recovery of the vibration is usually longer, at 4–6 weeks. Removal of all three borders prolongs recovery of the vibration to 8 weeks or more, and the risk of developing a permanent scar is increased. Worse still, the scar may retract within the substance of the fold. To avoid this condition, it is advisable to leave a strip of epithelium intact.

Table 4.6. Vocal fold lesions impairing vibratory movements: phonosurgical procedures aiming at Improvement of vibratory movements/restoration of the normal mucosal wave [17]

Pathology	Procedure	Approach	
Exudative lesions of Reinke's space			
Nodule	Dissection and excision	Endolaryngeal	Direct
Polyp			Indirect
Pseudocyst			
Reinke's edema	Dissection and suction (and excision)	Endolaryngeal	Direct
Cyst			
Epidermoid	Dissection an excision	Endolaryngeal	Direct
Mucous retention			
Sulcus ("open cyst")	Dissection, excision (and augmentation)	Endolaryngeal	Direct
Mucosal bridge	Excision	Endolaryngeal	Direct
	Dissection and gluing		
Atrophy/scar			
Congenital ("sulcus-vergeture")	Dissection, excision (and) augmentation	Endolaryngeal	Direct
Acquired	Implantation		
Presbyphonia	Augmentation	Endolaryngeal	Direct
	Implantation		
Vascular			
Ectasia	Coagulation and/or excision	Endolaryngeal	Direct
Varicosity	Vaporizaton	Endolaryngeal	Direct
Hematoma	Incision and suction	Endolaryngeal	Direct
Arytenoid granuloma	Excision	Endolaryngeal	Direct
	Tension reduction (botulinum toxin injection)		
Glottal web, microweb	Incision (and stenting)	Endolaryngeal	Direct

Table 4.7. Movement disorders of the vocal folds: phonosurgical procedures aiming at correction of the position and/or tension of the vocal folds [17]

Pathology	Procedure	Approach	
Vocal fold immobility			
Paralysis/paresis	Augmentation	Endolaryngeal	Direct
			Indirect
		External	Percutaneous
	Implantation	Endolaryngeal	Direct
		External	Open neck
Cricoarytenoid joint disorders	Augmentation	Endolaryngeal	Direct
			Indirect
		External	Percutaneous
	Implantation	Endolaryngeal	Direct
		External	Open neck
	Mobilization	Endolaryngeal	Direct
			Indirect
		External	Open neck
Neurologic			
Tremor/spasmodic dysphonia	Injection (botulinum toxin)	Transcutaneous	Percutaneous
		Endolaryngeal	Direct
			Indirect
	Thyroarytenoid muscle excision/coagulation	Endolaryngeal	Direct
Dysfunctional			
Hyperfunction	Injection (botulinum toxin)	Endolaryngeal	Direct
			Indirect
Hypofunction	Augmentation	Endolaryngeal	Direct
Dysphonia plicae ventricularis	Excision	Endolaryngeal	Direct
	Injection (botulinum toxin)	Endolaryngeal	Direct
			Indirect

This has led the paradigm of the microflap [4, 20, 1], itself sometimes subdivided into a mini-microflap [20], subepithelial microflap [11], medial microflap [5], and lateral microflap [1]. These techniques have completely replaced the previously employed resection of the epithelium formerly called "stripping" or "decortication" which now better is termed "subepithelial chordectomy" [16]. The microflap technique provides a significant more predictable and better functional outcome.

Two major disease groups are addressed by vocal fold surgery (VFS): *vocal fold lesions* with redundant pathological tissue impairing the vibratory movement (Table 4.4) and *vocal fold movement disorders* with inappropriate position and/or tension of the vocal fold (Table 4.5). As a result of the complex processes involved in the generation of voice, the two groups frequently overlap.

For epithelial lesions, the primary aim of surgery is complete epithelial resection for histological purposes (Table 4.4) and is thus "secondary PS" [8a]. Under the heading "exudative lesion of Reinke's space" [10a, 15], benign vocal fold lesions with the same histological components (fibrosis, vascular ectasia, and edema) are grouped together. In terms of vocal fold movement disorders (Table 4.5), this chapter is restricted to lesions amenable to VFS (Table 4.7).

The various types of VFS in terms of pathology, therapeutic aim, procedure, and approach are listed in Tables 4.6 and 4.7. Surgical instruments (e.g., cold instruments, CO_2 laser, microdébrider) or injectable materials (e.g., fat [2, 12], fascia [19], collagen [7, 14, 18]) are not included, as they are highly operator- and material-dependent.

4.2 Tips and pearls

- A prerequisite for phonosurgery is the adequate diagnosis and documentation of the disordered voice.
- As the pathogenesis of voice disorders is usually multidimensional phonosurgery may form only a

part of the holistic treatment of voice disorders, in partnership with various nonsurgical methods.

- Phonosurgery should not focus on the appearance of the vocal folds but, rather should aim for an improvement in voice, adapted to the individual request and needs of the patient.

- The basic principle of vocal fold surgery is to maintain or improve the functional structure of the vocal fold by respecting its layered structure.

- This is achieved by means of minimal tissue excision, minimal disruption of the superficial layer of the lamina propria and preservation of the epithelium, especially at the vibrating edge.

- The appropriate method to accomplish this is the microflap technique which has completely replaced the resection of the epithelium previously called "stripping" or "decortication" which now better is termed "subepithelial chordectomy".

References

1. Bouchayer M, Cornut G (1992) Microsurgical treatment of benign vocal fold lesions: indications, technique results. Folie Phoniatr (Basel) 44:155–184

2. Brandenburg JH, Kirkham W, Koschkee D (1992) Vocal cord augmentation with autogenous fat. Laryngoscope 102: 495–500

3. Brünings W (1911) Über eine neue Behandlungsmethode der Rekurrenslähmung. Verl Deutsch Laryng 18:93–151

4. Courey MS, Gardner GM, Stone RE, OssoV RH (1995) Endoscopic vocal fold microflap: a three-year experience. Ann Otol Rhinol Laryngol 104:267–273

5. Courey MS, Garrett CG, Ossov RH (1997) Medial microflap for excision of benign vocal fold lesions. Laryngoscope 107: 340–344

6. Dejonckere PH, Bradley P, Clemente P, Cornut G, Crevier L, Buchman G, Friedrich P, Van de Heyning, Remacle M, Woisard V (2001) A basic protocol for functional assessment of voice pathology, especially for investigating the efficacy of (phonosurgical) treatments and evaluating new assessment techniques. Eur Arch Otorhinolaryngol 258:77–82

7. Ford CN, Martin DW, Warner MD (1984) Injectable collagen in laryngeal rehabilitation. Laryngoscope 94:513–518

8. Friedrich G, De Jong FICRS, Mahieu HF, Benninger MS, Isshiki N (2001) Laryngeal framework surgery: a proposal for classification and nomenclature by the Phonosurgery Committee of the European Laryngological Society. Eur Arch Otorhinolaryngol 375:1–8

8a. Friedrich G, Remacle M, Birchall M, Marie JP, Arens C (2007) Defining Phonosurgery: a proposal for classification and nomenclature by the Phonosurgery Committee of the European Laryngological Society (ELS). Eur Arch Otorhinolaryngol 264:1191–1200

9. Gluck Th (1930) Phonetik-Chirurgie der oberen Luft- und Speisewege und künstlicher und natürlicher Stimmersatz (Phonetic – surgery of the upper aero-digestive tract and artificial and natural voice restoration). Monatsschrift für Ohrenheilkunde und Laryngo Rhinologie 64(8): 881–893

10. Gussenbauer C (1874) Über die erste durch Theodor Billroth am Menschen ausgeführte Kehlkopf-Exstirpation und die Anwendung des künstlichen Kehlkopfes (on the first laryngectomy in humans by Theodor Billroth and the usage of an artificial larynx). Arch Klin Chirurgie 343–356

10a. Hantzakos A, Remacle M, Dikkers FG, Degols JC, Delos M, Friedrich G, Giovanni A, Rasmussen N (2009) Exudative lesions of Reinkes space: a terminology proposal. Eur Arch Otorhinolaryngol 266:869–878

11. Hochman II, Zeitels SM (2000) Phonomicrosurgical management of vocal fold polyps: the subepithelial microflap resection technique. J Voice 14:112–118

12. Mikaelian DO, Lowry LD, Sataloff RT (1991) Lipoinjection for unilateral vocal cord paralysis. Laryngoscope 101(5): 465–468

13. Payr E (1915) Plastik am Schildknorpel zur Behebung der Folgen einseitiger Stimmbandlähmung (plastic surgery on the thyroid cartilage for treatment of unilateral vocal fold paralysis). Dtsch Med Wochenschr 43:1265–1270

14. Remacle M, Dujardin JM, Lawson G (1995) Treatment of vocal fold immobility by glutaraldehyde-cross-linked collagen injection: long-term results. Ann Otol Rhinol Laryngol 104(6):437–444

15. Remacle M, Degols JC, Delos M (1996) Exudative lesions of Reinke's space. An anatomopathological correlation. Acta Otorhinolaryngol Belg 50:253–264

16. Remacle M, Eckel HE, Antonelli A, Brasnu D, Chevalier D, Friedrich G, Olofsson J, Rudert HH, Thumfart W, Wustrow TP (2000) Endoscopic cordectomy. A proposal for a classification by the Working Committee, European Laryngological Society. Eur Arch Otorhinolaryngol 257:227–223

17. Remacle M, Friedrich G, Dikkers FG, De Jong F (2003) Phonosurgery of the vocal folds: a classification proposal. Eur Arch Otorhinolaryngol 260:1–6

18. Remacle M, Lawson G, Jamart J, Delos M (2006) Treatment of vocal fold immobility by injectable homologous collagen: short-term results. Eur Arch Otorhinolaryngol 263: 205–209

19. Rihkanen H (1998) Vocal fold augmentation by injection of autologous fascia. Laryngoscope 108:51–54

20. Sataloff RT, Spiegel JR, Heuer RJ, Baroody MM, Emerich KA, Hawkshaw MJ, Rosen DC (1995) Laryngeal mini-microflap: a new technique and reassessment of the microflap saga. J Voice 9:198–204

21. Von Leden H (1971) Fono-cirujia. Acta ORL Iber-Am 22: 292–299

22. Von Leden H (1993) The history of phonosurgery. In: Gould WJ, Sataloff RT, Spiegel JR (eds) Voice surgery. Mosby, St. Louis, pp. 65–95

Microphonosurgery Using Cold Instruments

4a

Gerhard Friedrich

Core Messages

> In microlaryngoscopy the surgeon and the anaesthesiologist share the same area, therefore a good collaboration between them is mandatory.

> Endoscopic surgery relies first on exposure. The largest-caliber laryngoscope that can be comfortably placed should be used.

> A large variety of laryngoscopes are available and there is not a single "best" one that fits all situations. The surgeon must become familiar with several types and identify those in which he or she is most comfortable.

> Elevating the head so it resembles the sniffing ("Boyle-Jackson") position eases the insertion of the laryngoscope and exposure of the endolarynx particularly the anterior commissure.

> The precision of the surgery is enhanced with magnification, therefore the highest magnification adapted to the individual situation should always be used.

> The delicate microsurgery in the endolarynx requires specially designed, sharp, precise and small instruments.

> To enhance the surgeon´s manual dexterity and maintaining instrument stability it is generally recommended to use armrests in phonomicrosurgery.

G. Friedrich
Professor and Chairman, Ear, Nose and Throat,
University Hospital, Graz, Head of Department of Phoniatrics,
Speech and Swallowing, Medical University of Graz,
Auenbruggerplatz 26-28, A-8036 Graz, Austria
e-mail: phoniatrie.hno@meduni-graz.at

Shortly after introduction of the laryngeal mirror by Türck [30] and Czermak [30] into clinical medicine, laryngology developed as a new specialty. Within a short time, mirror laryngoscopy was used not only for diagnosis but for indirect operations in the endolarynx. Especially after the introduction of topical anesthesia with cocaine by Jelinek [28], use of this technique spread and became standard. For this purpose, a great variety of indirect instruments were designed. For indirect laryngoscopic surgery the patient is generally seated. Topical anesthesia is applied, and the endolarynx is visualized with a laryngeal mirror, laryngeal telescope, or flexible fiberoptic laryngoscope. Injections into the vocal folds (e.g., collagen, botulinum toxin) may be performed transorally or externally by passing the needle through the cricothyroid membrane. Advantages of these techniques include relatively easy access, avoidance of the need for an operating room, and immediate evaluation of the functional result, particularly in combination with intraoperative stroboscopy [9, 22, 24]. With indirect surgery it is also not necessary to exert considerable force on the orophayngeal tissues during exposure, which can result in injuries and complications [13, 17, 18, 23, 32, 34]. However, the precision is not as good as that accomplished with microlaryngoscopy under general anesthesia. Although the importance of indirect endolaryngeal surgery declined after the introduction of suspension laryngoscopy, the procedure is still invaluable and should be in the armamentarium of the phonosurgeon [9, 20, 24]. For phonosurgical purposes, recently more sophisticated instruments were designed by Sataloff [27]. Nowadays, with the improvement of flexible endoscopes, indirect surgery on the vocal folds can also be performed using flexible fiberoptics with flexible instruments [29].

The area of direct phonomicrosurgery started during the early 1960s with the introduction of micolaryngoscopy by Kleinsasser [15]. Responsible for this breakthrough were adoption of the Zeiss microscope with a 400 mm focal length, the development of special enlarged and tapered laryngoscopes, and the appearance of long-handled laryngeal instruments for precision surgery on the vocal folds together with Storz (Storz, Tuttlingen, Germany). In 1968, Kleinsasser [16] published his comprehensive textbook on microlaryngoscopy. During the same period, parallel advances were being made by laryngologists in the United States. Geza Jako developed an improved laryngoscope for binocular diagnosis and bimanual surgery [12]. He developed a series of well designed microlaryngeal instruments with Stümmer (Stümmer, Würzburg, Germany).

Usually, general anesthesia is used for microlaryngoscopy. As the surgeon and the anesthesiologist share the same area, a good collaboration between them is mandatory. Typically anesthesia is performed by intubation with a small endotracheal tube that does not interfere with surgery in the anterior two-thirds of the vocal folds. Endotracheal intubation provides the safest ventilation and enables a stable operating field for precision surgery, as required in phonosurgery. For special indications, jet ventilation is a useful and sometimes indispensable technique [11a, 21] (Table 4a.1).

Endoscopic surgery, like other surgical techniques, relies first on exposure. The largest-caliber laryngoscope that can be comfortably placed in the patient is used. A large variety of laryngoscopes are available, and there is not a single "best" one that fits all situations. The surgeon must become familiar with several types and identify those with which he or she is most comfortable. In general, the laryngoscope should be as wide as possible at the proximal end to permit binocular viewing and to allow working space for at least two microlaryngeal instruments simultaneously. The contact area with the upper teeth should be flat so the pressure is distributed to minimize the risk of injury to the teeth. The original Kleinsasser laryngoscopes are rounded along the whole length, whereas more modern types of laryngoscopes are triangular at the distal end. This respects more the anatomical configuration of the glottis and eases exposure of the anterior commissure, which always is the critical area. Many laryngoscopes have an upward flair at the distal tip, which although designed for easier exposure of the anterior commissure can push this region out of the visual field [32] (Fig. 4a.1). Anatomical differences among patients require dexterity on the part of the surgeon to achieve optimal exposure [7].

Table 4a.1. Jet ventilation: advantages,disadvantages, indications, and contraindications

Advantages
- Unimpaired access for the surgeon
- No tracheostomy because of anesthesiology
- No danger of tube fire
- Operating field smoke-free
- No contamination with anesthetic gases
- Anesthesia accurate control

Disadvantages
- Fixed postion of the laryngoscope
- Smoke concentration in the operating room
- Dirtying of the microscope lens or laser mirror
- Vibration and exsiccation of the tissue
- Loss of body heat
- Danger of aspiration

Favorable indications
- Stenoses and narrow anatomical situation
- Lesions at the posterior glottis, subglottis, trachea
- Laser surgery
- Minor/superficial procedures

Less favorable indications
- Lesions at the anterior glottis, i.p. phonosurgery
- Supraglottic lesions, extralaryngeal extension
- Major procedures
- Adipositats permagna

Contraindications
- Insufficient exposure of the larynx
- Danger of major bleeding
- Increased danger of infection (hepatitis C, HIV)

From Friedrich [11], with permission

Once the laryngoscope is inserted, application of the suspension device with complete patient relaxation provides a stable field for inspection, manipulation, and surgical intervention. Historically, Kirstein introduced the suspension laryngoscopy in 1897, and it allowed for the first time bimanual instrumental manipulation of the surgical field [14]. In those days, the suspension gallows technique was too complex and anesthesia techniques were not always optimal. These problems led to the development of the fulcrum technique by Brünings in 1912 [5] and Seiffert in 1922 [25], which has been adopted widely. After the development of proper laryngoscopes in combination with a laryngoscope holder by Kleinsasser, this method became standard [16]. The laryngoscope holder originally was positioned at the chest of the patient, although nowadays most surgeons prefer a chest support (Fig. 4a.2). The main difference between the two techniques is that fulcrum-based techniques use the maxilla as a point to produce a lever force. Suspension gallows exert force on the soft tissues associated with the mandible and are

Fig. 4a.1. Exemplary selection of different types of laryngoscopes. (**a**) Kleinsasser laryngoscopes (Storz). (**b**) Bouchayer laryngoscope (Microfrance). (**c**) Zeitels Glottiscope (Endocraft)

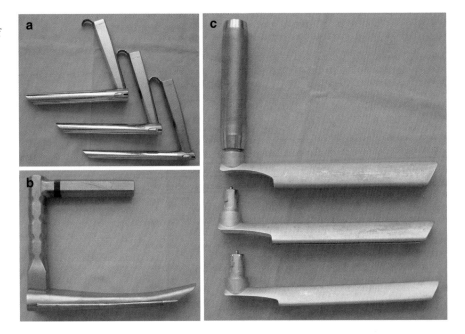

not a lever system [34]. True suspension devices in the tradition of Kirstein exert force on the soft tissues associated with the mandible, whereas common fulcrum-holder stabilizers use the maxilla as a point to produce a lever force [34]. This, of course, has considerable effects on force proportions. The use of gallows suspension subjects the patient to different force vectors when compared to the rotation-based suspension devices: Pressure is taken off the teeth, in contrast to rotation based-fulcrum laryngoscopes, where dental injuries are a well described injury. The fulcrum at the teeth forces the head toward the table, thus extending the head and neck. Former studies have pointed out that elevating the head so it resembles the sniffing ("Boyle-Jackson") position used for indirect laryngoscopy eases insertion of the laryngoscope and exposure of the endolarynx, particularly the anterior commissure [13, 31]. In contrast, Kleinsasser in his textbook advocated for a position of the head flat on the operating table [16]. In accordance with some American authors [13, 31], we could show that flexing the cervical spine allows better access to the endolarynx with less force required [11b]. For positioning the head of the patient, a headrest that allows variable adjustment of the patient's head even with the laryngoscope inserted is useful (Fig. 4a.2) [11b, 13a]. Even with the best technique, however, exposure of the endolaryngeal structures during direct laryngoscopy inevitably demands exerting pressure on the oropharyngeal and laryngeal tissues [11c, 13a]. These forces can lead to tissue

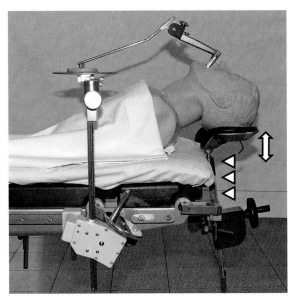

Fig. 4a.2. Setting during microlaryngoscopy. Head is elevated using a headrest (Haslinger-Lemoine; Storz 10900) (*arrowheads*), which allows variable adjustment of the patient's head (*double arrow*). The arm of the laryngoscope holder (Storz 8575GK) rests on the chest support (Storz; 8575K) [13 a]

trauma, with the consequence of tooth fracture, hematoma, swelling, mucosal injury, bleeding, and nerve injuries—all of which must be addressed when establishing informed consent [17, 18, 23].

The preservation of surrounding normal tissue with as little disruption as possible is crucial to the return of normal laryngeal function postoperatively. To achieve this goal, surgical precision is aided by magnification and delicate laryngeal instrumentation. Typically, assessment of vocal fold pathology inspection starts using magnifying laryngeal telescopes (0°, 30°, sometimes 70°). They allow the surgeon to visualize lesions in great detail, to appreciate the limits of lesions in three dimensions, and to have a look into obscure areas such as the laryngeal ventricle. Binocular vision is next obtained with the use of an operating microscope. Typically, a 400 mm focal length lens provides good visualization and allows adequate working space. Some surgeons, however, are more comfortable with a 350 mm focal lens [3, 4]. Because the precision of surgery is enhanced with the magnification, the highest magnification adapted to the individual situation should always be used [7, 24].

Delicate microsurgery requires specially designed, sharp, precise, small instruments. Instruments should be long enough to be manipulated easily in the laryngoscope but not so long that they can bump into the microscope. Bouchayer, in collaboration with Microfrance, must be credited for the development of the first comprehensive set of instruments specially designed for phonomicrosurgery [3, 4] (Fig. 4a.3). Currently, several further developed, invaluable instrument sets, in particular from Sataloff and Benninger (Medtronic Xomed, Microfrance) (Fig. 4a.4) and other companies (Storz), are on the market. Benninger [2] has designed new reverse-action instruments that are operated by the thumb of the surgeon and allow increased precision. A typical set for phonosurgery includes scissors (straight up, up-biting, curved left, curved right), small grasping cupped forceps (straight, up-biting, right, left), larger cupped forceps (straight and up-biting, at least), alligator forceps (straight, right, left), knifes, right-angle, and oblique blunt ball-tipped dissectors, spatula, scalpel, and suction. Cutting instruments should be sharp at all times [7, 24, 26, 33].

Maintaining instrument stability has become an increasingly important requirement of successful surgery. The long (22–30 cm) instruments must be precisely manipulated within the narrow laryngoscope. This lever arm effect greatly magnifies the motion caused by tremor, which is present in varying degree in every individual. A number of maneuvers are used to minimize tremor. Kleinsasser [16] suggested resting the instrument on the lip of the endoscope. Other investigators have advocated extending the index finger on

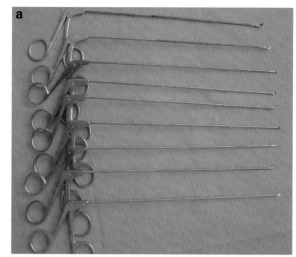

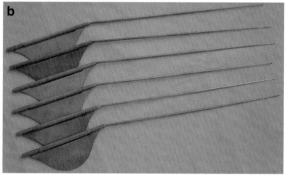

Fig. 4a.3. Bouchayer phonosurgery instruments (Medtronic Xomed, Microfrance)

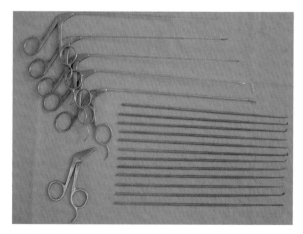

Fig. 4a.4. Sataloff phonosurgery instruments (Medtronic Xomed, Microfrance)

the instrument [1]. It is generally recommended armrests be used for delicate surgery to enhance the surgeon's manual dexterity [33]. An interesting development is a special laryngoscope instrument stabilizer [1]. Another alternative technique for reducing tremor is to use "no-touch" surgical techniques, in particular like the use of the laser controlled by a joystick.

Powered laryngeal surgery is a relatively new concept. The role in laryngeal surgery is not defined completely, but powered laryngeal surgery is clearly useful for treating some conditions such as papillomas and neoplasm [10]. Especially for endolaryngeal keel fixation Lichtenberger [19] has developed an endo-extralaryngeal needle carrier that is an invaluable instrument for a variety of procedures (i.e., treatment of glottic webs).

4a.1 Tips and Pearls

- In endolaryngeal phonomicrosurgery a good collaboration between the surgeon and the anaesthesiologist is mandatory.
- The largest-caliber laryngoscope that can be comfortably placed should be used.
- There is not a single "best" laryngoscope that fits all situations. The surgeon therefore must become familiar with several types.
- Elevating the head eases the insertion of the laryngoscope and exposure of the endolarynx particularly the anterior commissure.
- For maximum precision of surgery the highest magnification adapted to the individual situation should always be used.
- The delicate microsurgery in the endolarynx requires specially designed, sharp, precise and small instruments.
- To enhance the surgeon´s manual dexterity and maintaining instrument stability it is generally recommended to use armrests in phonomicrosurgery

References

1. Armstrong WB, Karamzadeh AM, Crumley RL, Kelley TF, Jackson RP, Wong BJF (2005) A novel laryngoscope instrument stabilizer for operative Microlaryngoscopy. Otolaryngol Head Neck Surg 132(3):472–477
2. Benninger MS (2003) Laryngeal microinstrumentarium: a novel design to reduce movement. Otorhinolaryngol Head Neck Surg 129(3)
3. Bouchayer M, Cornut G (1988) Microsurgery for benign lesions of the vocal folds. Ear Nose Throat J67(6):446–449, 456–464
4. Bouchayer M, Cornut G (1992) Microsurgical treatment of benign vocal fold lesions: indications, techniques, results. Folia Phoniatrica 44(3–4):155–184
5. Brünings W (1912) Direct laryngoscopy, bronchoscopy, and esophagoscopy. Bailliere, Tindall, & Cox, London
6. Cornut G, Bouchayer M (1989) Phonosurgery for singers. J Voice 3(3):269–276
7. Courey MS, Ossof RH by Rubin SJ, Sataloff RT, Korovin GS (2006) Diagnosis and treatment of voice disorders. Plural Publishing, San Diego, CA/Oxford
8. Czermak JN (1858) Über den Kehlkopfspiegel, Wiener med. Wochenschr 8(27):196–198
9. Dikkers FG, Sulter AM (1994) Suspension microlaryngoscopic surgery and indirect microlaryngostroboscopic surgery for benign lesions of the vocal folds. J Laryngol Otol 108(12):1064–1067
10. Flint PW (2000) Powered surgical instruments for laryngeal surgery. Otolaryngol Head Neck Surg 122(2):263–266
11. Friedrich G, Mausser G, Nemeth E (2002) Development of a jet-tracheoscope. Clinical significance of superimposed high-frequency jet-ventilation (SHFJV) in endoscopic respiratory tract surgery (Entwicklung eines Jet-Tracheoskops, Wertigkeit und Einsatzmöglichkeit der superponierten Hochfrequenz-Jet-Ventilation (SHFJV) in der endoskopischen Chirurgie der Atemwege). HNO 50:719–726
11a. Friedrich G, Mausser G, Gugatschka M (2008) Jet Ventilation in laryngotracheal surgery, Die Jet-Ventilation in der operativen Laryngologie (orig. in german),, HNO 56:1197–1206
11b. Friedrich G, Gugatschka M (2009) Influence of head positioning on the forces occurring during microlaryngoscopy, Eur Arch Otorhinolaryngol. 266:999–1003
11c. Friedrich G, Kiesler K, Gugatschka M Curved rigid laryngoscope: missing link between direct suspension laryngoscopy and indirect techniques? Eur Arch Otorhinolaryngol. (accepted for publication)
12. Leden von H (2005) The evolution of phonosurgery. In: Sataloff RT (ed.) Professional voice: the science and art of clinical care, vol. III. Plural Publishing, San Diego, CA/Oxford
13. Hochman I, Zeitels SM, Heaton JT (1999) Analysis of the forces and position required for direct laryngoscopic exposure of the anterior vocal folds. Ann Otol Rhinol Laryngol 108:715–724
13a. Gugatschka M, Gerstenberger C, Friedrich G (2008) Analysis of forces applied during Microlaryngoscopy: a descriptive study. Eur Arch Otorhinolaryngol. 265:1083–1087
14. Kirstein A (1897) Autoscopy of the larynx and trachea (direct examination without mirror). F.A. Davis, Philadelphia, PA, pp. 57–58
15. Kleinsasser O (1964) Mikrochirurgie im Kehlkopf. Arch Ohrenheilk 183:428–433
16. Kleinsasser O (1968) Mikrolaryngoskopie und endolaryngeale Mikrochirurgie. Technik und typische Befunde. 1. Auflage Schattauer Verlag, Stuttgart
17. Klussmann JP, Knoedgen R, Damm M, Wittekindt C, Eckel HE (2002) Complications of suspension laryngoscopy. Ann Otol Rhinol Laryngol 111(11):972–976

18. Knoedgen R et al (2002) Complications of suspension laryngoscopy. Ann Otol Rhinol Laryngol 111:972–976

19. Lichtenberger G (1983) Endo-extralaryngeal needle carrier instrument. Laryngoscope 93:1348–1350

20. Mahieu HF, Dikkers FG (1992) Indirect microlaryngostroboscopic surgery. Arch Otolaryngol Head Neck Surg 118(1):21–24

21. Mausser G, Friedrich G, Schwarz M (2007) Airway management and anaesthesia in neonates, infants and children during endolaryngotracheal surgery. Pediatr Anesth 17: 942–947

22. Milutinovic Z (1990) Advantages of indirect videostroboscopic surgery of the larynx. Folia Phoniatr 42:77–82

23. Rosen CA, Filho PA, Scheffel L, Buckmire R (2005) Oropharyngeal complications of suspension laryngoscopy: a prospective study. Laryngoscope 115:1681–1684

24. Sataloff RT (2005) Voice surgery. In: Sataloff RT (ed.) Professional voice, the science and art of clinical care, vol. III. Plural Publishing, San Diego, CA/Oxford

25. Seiffert A (2003) Apparat zur direkten Untersuchung, 2. Jahresversammlung der Ges. dtsch. Hals-Nasen-Ohrenärzte, 1922 in Feldmann H, Bilder aus der Geschichte der Hals-Nasen-Ohren-Heilkunde. Median-Verlag von Killisch-Horn GmbH, Heidelberg

26. Shapshay SM. Healy GB (1990) New microlaryngeal instruments for phonatory surgery and pediatric application. Ann Otol Rhinol Laryngol 98:821–823

27. Simpson CB, Amin MR (2004) Office-based procedures for the voice. Ear Nose Throat J 83(Suppl. 2):6–9

28. Skopec M, Majer EH (1998) History of oto-rhino-laryngology in Austria. Christian Brandstätter Verlag & Edition, Wien

29. Tsunoda K, Kikkawa YS, Yoshihashi R, Sakai Y (2002) Detachable forceps for flexible fibre-optic surgery: a new technique for Phonosurgery in cases where rigid laryngoscopy is contraindicated. J Laryngol Otol 116(7):559–561

30. Türck L (1858) Der Kehlkopfspiegel und die Methode seines Gebrauchs. Z Ges der Ärzte zu Wien 28(26)

31. Vaughan CW (1993) Vocal fold exposure in phonosurgery. J Voice 7:189–194

32. Zeitels SM (1999) Universal modular glottiscope system: the evolution of a century of design and technique for direct laryngoscopy. Ann Otol Rhinol Laryngol 108(Suppl. 179):2–24

33. Zeitels SM (2001) Atlas of phonomicrosurgery and other endolaryngeal procedures for benign and malignant disease. Singular/Thomson Learning, San Diego, CA

34. Zeitels SM, Burns JA, Dailey SH (2004) Suspension laryngoscopy revisited. Ann Otol Rhinol Laryngol 113:16–22

Laser-Assisted Microphonosurgery

4b

Marc Remacle

Core Messages

> Carbon dioxide (CO_2) laser should be regarded as complementing the existing instrumentation. It is not meant to replace well-established microlaryngoscopic techniques.

> Newcomers to laser technology must first be competent in the microlaryngoscopic technique. Then they can learn the lasers and their tissue effects as continuing professional development.

> Thanks to the development of the high-powered pulsed waves, the micromanipulator Acuspot, and the scanning device, laser-assisted surgery can be approached in a safe way provided that the parameters are strictly respected.

Most glottic lesions affect phonatory function of the larynx. Surgical management aims at removing of these lesions and restoring phonation. The procedure should be precise, and the healing process should not result in significant scarring. Microlaryngoscopic technique with high-quality instruments and their proficient use by skilled surgeons has done much to achieve this goal during the past few decades [4]. The use of lasers in phonomicrosurgery was first described three decades ago [7].

M. Remacle
Department of Otorhinolaryngology and Head & Neck Surgery,
University Hospital of Louvain at Mont-Godinne,
Dr. G. Therasse avenue 1, 5530 Yvoir-Belgium
e-mail: Marc.remacle@uclouvain.be

Introduction of CO_2 laser [17] should be regarded as complementing the existing instrumentation. It is not meant to replace well established microlaryngoscopic techniques. Recognizing this limited but important role of laser, a term "laser-assisted procedure" seems more appropriate than "laser surgery." It is thus obvious that a newcomer to laser technology must first be competent in microlaryngoscopic technique and then learn the lasers and their tissue effects as continuing professional development.

With surgery on the vocal cord, the primary aim is to preserve the underlying vocal ligament. The usual morphological anatomy of the vocal fold is described as having a superior and an inferior surface, with an intervening free edge. However, the free edge is far from an "edge." The dynamic anatomy of the vocal fold shows three distinct "borders" to the free edge: superior, middle and inferior.

If the superior border of the free edge is surgically removed, the mechanical vibration continues from the inferior border to the middle border, and the voice generally recovers within 2–6 weeks. When both the superior and the middle borders are removed simultaneously, recovery of the vibration usually takes longer, 4–6 weeks. Removal of all three borders prolongs recovery of the vibration to 8 weeks or more, and the risk of developing a permanent scar is increased. Worse still, the scar may retract within the substance of the fold. To avoid this condition, it is advisable to leave a strip of epithelium intact.

Thanks to the development of the high-powered pulsed waves (SuperPulse or UltraPulse) and the micromanipulator Acuspot, laser-assisted surgery can be approached in a safe way provided the parameters are strictly respected. This is even more true with the robotic or digital scanning device (see Chapter 3).

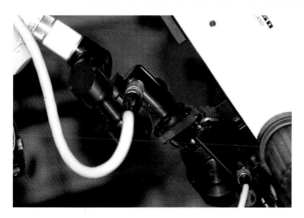

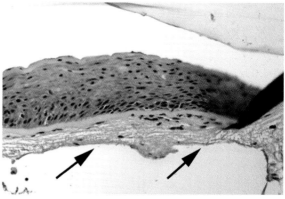

Fig. 4b.1. Scanning device connected to the laser arm and the micromanipulator. The scanning device is guided by the Acublade software

Fig. 4b.2. Histological specimen from a nodule resected with a CO_2 laser scanning system. Coagulation at the margin (arrows) is no more than 20 μm. (H&E, ×20)

Recommended laser settings in phonosurgery without the scanner are SuperPulse or UltraPulse, 0.1-second exposure duration of 2–3 W with a focused beam that has a 250 μm spot size for a working distance of 400 mm. If microvasculature coagulation is required (e.g., chorditis vocalis or Reinke's edema) before incising the epithelium, the laser is set at 0.05-second pulsed exposure of 1 W with a slightly defocused beam.

With the scanning system (Fig. 4b.1), the proposed parameters for phonosurgery are depth of 0.2 mm, 10 W, single pulse, 0.10 s for SuperPulse and two passes, 10 W, single pulse, 0.10 second for UltraPulse. The length of the incision line or the diameter of surface to ablate was 1–2 mm depending on the lesion.

Beam parameters are for guidance only. A number of factors affect the ultimate effect of the beam on the pathological (and normal) tissue. The type of laser used, the lifespan of the device, the make, and the experience of the surgeon all have a bearing on the outcome.

The CO_2 laser controls bleeding from blood vessels up to 0.6 mm by shriveling the tissue. Oozing can be controlled by ice-cold cottonoids held in position for a few seconds or swabs soaked in suitable decongestant. Any bleeding from large vessels is controlled by monopolar diathermy, which is incorporated in the forceps. Dilated and varicose vessels can be obliterated by defocusing the beam slightly. In the defocused spot, the energy concentration is reduced, and tissue is coagulated.

The thickness of thermal-damaged tissue in the case of benign lesions of the vocal fold is usually no

more than 20 μm [12] (Fig. 4b.2). This explains the stroboscopically observed reduction in postoperative healing time, compared with that obtained with cold instruments.

Laser phonomicrosurgery for benign lesions is functional surgery, and careful selection of patients is critical for a successful outcome. Particular care should be taken with voice performers because even the most minor anatomical removal may not restore the quality of voice on which the performers have built their careers. The extent of scarring from the excision can be controlled by meticulous attention to details, particularly regarding the laser effects that are beyond visual control [3]. Furthermore, the eventual healing by scar tissue and its effect on vibratory margin cannot be predicted with any degree of certainty. It is necessary to convey this to the patient unequivocally in a way that he or she understands, so that he or she is in a position to give informed consent.

Microsurgery of the phonatory disorder and voice therapy are inseparable [8]. This dual management strategy varies according to the lesion. In some cases, voice therapy is the initial treatment. When voice therapy fails or symptoms return because of recurrence, surgery is inevitable. In other cases, surgery is the initial treatment, followed by a course of voice therapy. The following examples illustrate the difference.

• When hoarseness is due to nodules that are formed owing to dysfunctional dysphonia, a course of voice therapy resolves the condition in most cases. Similarly, adequate improvement follows voice therapy in cases where hoarseness is due to minor sulcus, scar, or chorditis vocalis. Surgical intervention should be considered only in cases that fail to respond or that recur.

- Hoarseness due to Reinke's edema, cyst, or extensive sulcus requires initial surgical management. After a period of voice rest, a course of voice therapy is undertaken.

The choice of the surgical instrument depends on the experience and expertise of the phonosurgeon [10]. In the hands of some surgeons, skillful surgery with cold instruments can produce acceptable results [15]. For certain lesions, such as nodules, edematous polyps, mucous retention cysts, and epidermoid cysts, CO_2 laser has no particular advantage over the cold instruments. However, the authors prefer laser instrumentation for certain conditions such as hemorrhagic polyps, Reinke's edema, and sulcus or sulcus vergeture [14].

The continuous mode should never be used because of increased irradiance of tissues in this mode. In the pulse mode, the thermal damage is only a few microns deep. The absence of an adverse deep thermal effect after a CO_2 laser-assisted micropoint incision or dissection is demonstrated by Andrea's contact endoscopy [1], showing persistence of microvasculature flux of erythrocytes in Reinke's space.

Microsurgery is preferable under general anesthesia for a number of reasons. Preoperative assessment, based on videostroboscopy, may identify the vibratory disorders, but the precise nature and the extension of the pathology may not be fully apparent. "Instrument palpation" carried out under general anesthesia is useful for accurate, precise assessment. The cords should be routinely everted and the subglottis examined. A 70° telescope passed through the cords shows any lesions in the subglottis and upper trachea. An examination of the upper aerodigestive and lower respiratory passages must be carried out in cases of recurrent respiratory papillomatosis (RRP) to exclude their involvement.

There is a major trend [2, 11, 16] among North American laryngologists to perform office-based procedures whenever possible, including injection of materials for glottic gap, injection of *Botulinium* toxin for spasmodic dysphonia, biopsies, PDL laser-assisted procedures such as vaporization of papilloma, lesions of the free edge such as nodules, or polyps. The financial advantage is obvious, but the risk of poor

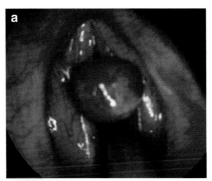

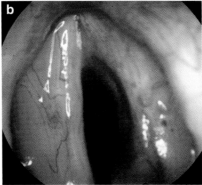

Fig. 4b.3. Angiectatic polyp. (**a**) Before surgery. (**b**) After resection)

functional results in comparison with the procedures performed under general anesthesia and the criteria of selection are not yet evaluated.

Two techniques are employed most extensively: excision and dissection. Excision is indicated for nodules, polyps, small sulcus (referred to as opened cysts by Cornut and Bouchayer), a mucosal bridge, mucous retention cysts, epidermoid cysts, and granulomas. The lesion is grasped with a Bouchayer microforceps (Bouchayer; Micro-France, Paris, France) and stretched toward the midline to define the plane between it and the vocal ligament. The laser is used in pulse mode to cut the stretched fibers in the plane (Fig. 4b.3a, b).

In contrast, dissection is preferred for Reinke's edema, a large sulcus, and a scar. For Reinke's edema, the microvasculature on the superior surface of the vocal cord is coagulated first. The epithelium is then incised close to the lesion, along the length of the superior surface, from the vocal process to within 2–3 mm from the anterior commissure [6, 14]. Once the incision is made, the free margin is drawn toward the midline with the Bouchayer microforceps, and the gelatinous material is aspirated. The microflap is then

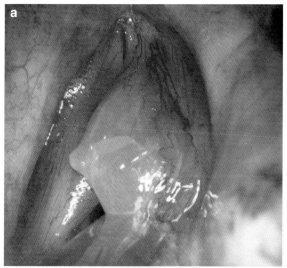

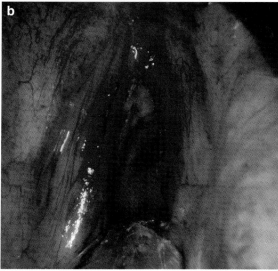

Fig. 4b.4. Reinke's edema. (**a**) Before surgery. (**b**) After dissection and suction of the glue. The excess epithelium has been cut

re-draped. The excess epithelium, if any, is trimmed to achieve the best possible approximation of the incision edges. Provided a 2- to 3-mm strip of intact mucosa close to the anterior commissure is spared, surgery may be carried out simultaneously on the two sides (Fig. 4b.4a, b)

For the sulcus or a scar, the technique developed by Bouchayer [5] is employed. The incision begins on the superolateral edge of the lesion. Then, using the Bouchayer microforceps, the inner edge of the incision is grasped, and careful dissection is performed along the epithelium. During the dissection, it is advisable to grasp the entire dissected epithelium to separate it from

the vocal ligament all the way to the inferior surface of the vocal cord. Small cottonoid pledgets, soaked in a solution of physiological saline and epinephrine cooled to 5°C, are used to control minor superficial bleeding and remove tissue debris. After completing the surgery, a few drops of slow-setting fibrin glue (Tissucol; Immuno, Vienna, Austria) is applied, either for covering the excision field or for re-draping the microflap. The specimen is systematically oriented and sent for histological examination. An accurate histological examination is not impaired by the presence of char and coagulation, which extends only a few microns deep.

Although the use of fibrin glue is somewhat empirical, the authors subscribe to the view of Bouchayer [4] that it is useful for covering the site of the operation. It possibly acts as scaffolding for regeneration of epithelium and discourages any potential to granuloma formation. To date, no short-term or permanent side effects have been observed.

Following phonosurgery, strict 8-day vocal rest is prescribed. Medical treatment consists of steroid aerosols and oral antibiotics for 8–10 days, at the end of which time assessment takes place. Thereafter, the patient may resume phonation under the supervision of a speech therapist. The postoperative stroboscopic examination of small lesions shows a good recovery of vibration amplitude and return of the mucosal wave along the superior surface of the vocal cord. The vibration is usually symmetrical after surgery for a nodule. However, the vibration may remain slightly asymmetrical following an intervention for a polyp, a mucous retention cyst, an epidermoid cyst, or a small sulcus. This asymmetry, however, does not result in diplophonia.

The recovery time is directly related to the extent of the surgical procedure. The more extensive the dissection, the longer the recovery of the vibration: 3–4 weeks for Reinke's edema and 3–4 months for a large sulcus or a sulcus vergeture [13]. In the case of a sulcus vergeture, although the vibration improves it is not normal. The spindle-shaped glottic aperture is smaller but still apparent. Even if the amplitude returns to normal, the vibration frequently remains asymmetrical during phonation. At times, a mucosal wave can be identified.

The minimum follow-up period is 3 months for Reinke's edema, a polyp or a mucous retention cyst; 4 months for a small sulcus; 5 months for a scar or a sulcus vergeture; and 6 months for a nodule.

Following phonomicrosurgery, voice therapy is indispensable [9, 18]. The duration varies according to the severity of the surgery and the individual patient. The sulcus vergeture requires prolonged speech therapy (up to 6 months) because the therapy must suppress the hyperkinetic compensatory mechanisms adopted by the patient before surgery. Furthermore, although the aim of the surgery is to correct the glottic gap and fibrosis, surgery itself induces a certain degree of fibrosis (although always less than the preoperative state). Following surgery for a nodule, a polyp, a mucous retention cyst, or a small sulcus, there is subjective recovery to a normal voice. The outcome is maintained provided any functional dysphonic element is properly corrected by voice therapy. After surgery for Reinke's edema, the pitch of the voice improves, particularly in women, and the voice quality remains satisfactory provided the patient discontinues smoking.

After an intervention for sulcus vergeture, the patient perceives improved phonatory ease, reduced vocal fatigue, and a steady improvement in timbre. Breathiness, hoarseness, and the episodes of vocal instability decrease. The projected voice improves, but it does not return to normal. Complete anatomical and physiological restoration of the vocal cord cannot be achieved. It is therefore necessary to tell the patient the limitations of the phonatory outcome and ensure compliance to extensive voice rehabilitation.

4b.1 Tip and Pearls

- Recommended laser settings in phonosurgery without the scanner are SuperPulse or UltraPulse, 0.1 second exposure duration of 2–3 W, with a focused beam with a 250 μm spot size for a working distance of 400 mm.
- If microvasculature coagulation is required (e.g., chorditis vocalis or Reinke's edema) before incision of the epithelium, laser is set at 0.05-second pulsed exposure of 1 W with a slightly defocused beam.
- With the scanning system, the proposed parameters for phonosurgery are a depth of 0.2 mm, 10 W, single pulse, 0.10 second for SuperPulse; and two passes, 10 W, single pulse, 0.10 second for UltraPulse. The length of the incision line or the diameter of the surface to ablate was 1–2 mm depending on the lesion.

- Continuous mode should never be used because of increased irradiance of tissues in this mode.
- Beam parameters are for guidance only. A number of factors affect the ultimate effect of the beam on the pathological (and normal) tissue. The type of laser used, the lifespan of the device, the make, and the experience of the surgeon have a bearing on the outcome.

References

1. Andrea M, Dias O, Santos A (1995) Contact endoscopy of the vocal cord: normal and pathological patterns. Acta Otolaryngol 115(2):314–316
2. Bastian RW, Delsupehe KG (1996) Indirect larynx and pharynx surgery: a replacement for direct laryngoscopy. Laryngoscope 106(10):1280–1286
3. Benninger MS (2000) Microdissection or microspot CO_2 laser for limited vocal fold benign lesions: a prospective randomized trial. Laryngoscope 110(2 Pt 2):1–17
4. Bouchayer M, Cornut G (1992) Microsurgical treatment of benign vocal fold lesions: indications, technique, results. Folia Phoniatr (Basel) 44(3–4):155–184
5. Bouchayer M, Cornut G, Witzig E, Loire R, Roch JB, Bastian RW (1985) Epidermoid cysts, sulci, and mucosal bridges of the true vocal cord: a report of 157 cases. Laryngoscope 95(9 Pt 1):1087–1094
6. Desloge RB, Zeitels SM (2000) Endolaryngeal microsurgery at the anterior glottal commissure: controversies and observations. Ann Otol Rhinol Laryngol 109(4):385–392
7. Frèche Ch, Piquet JJ, Traissac L, Romanet P, Guerrier B, Brasnu D, et al (1993) Le laser en ORL. Arnette, Paris
8. Giovanni a, Remacle M, Robert D (2000) Phonochirurgie des tumeurs bénignes des cordes vocales. - 16p. Paris, Editions scientifiques et médiacles Elsevier SAS. Encycl Med Chirur, techniques chirurgicales - Tête et cou 46–350
9. Johannsen HS (2001) Phoniatric aspects in microsurgical removal of benign vocal cord changes. Laryngorhinootologie 80(4):226–233
10. Keilmann A, Biermann G, Hormann K (1997) CO_2 laser versus conventional microlaryngoscopy in benign changes of the vocal cords. Laryngorhinootologie 76(8):484–489
11. Milutinovic Z (1990) Advantages of indirect videostroboscopic surgery of the larynx. Folia Phoniatr (Basel) 42(2):77–82
12. Remacle M, Hassan F, Cohen D, Lawson G, Delos M (2005) New computer-guided scanner for improving CO(2) laser-assisted microincision. Eur Arch Otorhinolaryngol 262(2): 113–119
13. Remacle M, Lawson G, Degols JC, Evrard I, Jamart J (2000) Microsurgery of sulcus vergeture with carbon dioxide laser and injectable collagen. Ann Otol Rhinol Laryngol 109(2): 141–148
14. Remacle M, Lawson G, Watelet JB (1999) Carbon dioxide laser microsurgery of benign vocal fold lesions: indications,

techniques, and results in 251 patients. Ann Otol Rhinol Laryngol 108(2):156–164

15. Sataloff RT, Spiegel JR, Heuer RJ, Baroody MM, Emerich KA, Hawkshaw MJ, et al (1995) Laryngeal mini-microflap: a new technique and reassessment of the microflap saga. J Voice 9(2):198–204

16. Simpson CB, Amin MR (2004) Office-based procedures for the voice. Ear Nose Throat J 83(7 Suppl. 2):6–9

17. Strong MS, Jako GJ (1972) Laser surgery in the larynx. Early clinical experience with continuous CO_2 laser. Ann Otol Rhinol Laryngol 81(6):791–798

18. Woo P, Casper J, Colton R, Brewer D (1994) Diagnosis and treatment of persistent dysphonia after laryngeal surgery: a retrospective analysis of 62 patients. Laryngoscope 104(9): 1084–1091

Laryngeal Framework Surgery

5

Gerhard Friedrich

Core Messages

> Laryngeal framework surgery (LFS) is a unique phonosurgical concept that enables us to influence the laryngeal biomechanics by changing the shape/position of the laryngeal cartilages.

> LFS is performed by an external approach, which minimizes the risk of damaging the delicate structures of the vocal folds with the consequences of scarring and stiffening.

> LFS is performed under local anesthesia, and the phonatory function therefore can be monitored during surgery. The surgery can be tailored to the individual patient's situation on the operating table, which often requires a combination of techniques.

> LFS procedures can be favorably combined with one another but also with other phonosurgical methods, and they are usually reversible and correctable.

> LFS is an essential technique in phonosurgery and offers a safe, highly effective, usually long-lasting method for voice improvement and/or adjustment.

5.1 Introduction

Every surgery performed directly on the vocal folds inevitably carries the risk of damaging the delicate structures of the vocal folds, leading to a risk of unfavorable postoperative results due to scarring and stiffening. The idea of influencing the endolaryngeal biomechanics and consequently improving the voice without touching the vocal folds by just changing the shape or position of the laryngeal cartilages is not new. As early as 1915, Payr [88] published a method for external vocal fold medialization using a transthyroidal approach (Fig. 5.1). Although his ingenious idea was recognized and various modifications were developed, mostly using paraglottic implantation of cartilage, external approaches for vocal fold medialization did not gain general acceptance [3, 18, 19, 59, 63, 74, 86, 87, 94, 99, 113]. It was Isshiki during the 1970s who

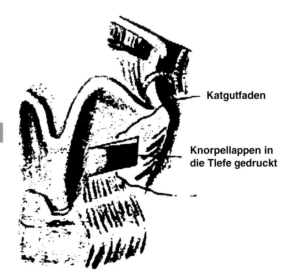

Katgutfaden

Knorpellappen in die Tlefe gedruckt

Fig. 5.1. Original depiction of Payr's medialization. (From Payr [88], with permission)

G. Friedrich
Professor and Chairman, Ear, Nose and Throat University Hospital Graz, Head of Department of Phoniatrics, Speech and Swallowing, Medical University of Graz, Auenbruggerplatz 26-28, A-8036 Graz, Austria
e-mail: gerhard.friedrich@klinikum-graz.at
www.uni-graz.at/phoniatrie/

M. Remacle, H. E. Eckel (eds.), *Surgery of Larynx and Trachea,*
DOI: 10.1007/978-3-540-79136-2_5, © Springer-Verlag Berlin Heidelberg 2010

took up this idea and, based on his fundamental research on vocal fold biomechanics, systematically developed the functional concept of laryngeal framework surgery (LFS), which added a new dimension to the field of phonosurgery (PS). He also defined four types of "thyroplasty" (TPL) [46, 47, 51, 53, 55]. To establish unambiguous terminology for the various procedures in this dynamic field, the European Laryngological Society (ELS) in 2001 published a definition and classification proposal [35] (Tables 5.1 and 5.2).

Table 5.1. Laryngeal framework surgery: definition

- Surgery for improvement or restoration of voice
- Performed on the laryngeal skeleton and/or inserting muscles
- For correction of position and/or tension of the vocal folds

From Friedrich et al. [35] with permission

Table 5.2. Laryngeal framework surgery: classification and nomenclature

Approximation laryngoplasty
Medialization thyroplasty
(Thyroplasty type I (Isshiki [46, 47])

Arytenoid adduction
Rotation (pull) techniques (Isshiki [48])
(LCA pull technique (Iwamura [57]))
Fixation techniques (Morrison [78], Maragos [70])
(Adduction arytenopexy (Zeitels [118]))

Expansion laryngoplasty
Lateralization thyroplasty
Lateral approach
(Thyroplasty type IIa (Isshiki [46, 51])
Medial approach
(Thyroplasty type IIb, expansion of the anterior commissure, midline lateralization thyroplasty (Isshiki [46, 51, 54]))

Vocal fold abduction
Suture technique (Isshiki [51])
Resection technique (Woo [116])

Relaxation laryngoplasty
Shortening thyroplasty
Lateral approach
(Thyroplasty type III [51])
Medial approach
(Anterior commissure retrusion (Tucker [106–108]))

Tensioning laryngoplasty
Cricothyroid approximation
(Thyroplasty type IVa (Isshiki [46]), cricothyroid subluxation (Zeitels [119]))

Elongation thyroplasty
Lateral approach
(Thyroplasty type IVb (Isshiki [49–51])
Medial approach
(Springboard advancement (Le Jeune [65]), anterior commissure advancement, anterior commissure laryngoplasty (Tucker [105, 106, 108]))

From Friedrich et al. [35], with permission

5.2 Indications and Preoperative Workup

Laryngeal framework surgery is a phonosurgical procedure, and therefore its intentions clearly differ from those of traditional laryngeal surgery, which mostly is performed because of vital indications. It is therefore necessary to define basic principles for the indications for LFS [30]. One precondition is a sufficient diagnosis and documentation of the disordered voice. For this purpose, the ELS has defined a basis protocol [17, 30, 36]. PS, in general, is only one part of the complex treatment of voice disorders and must be combined with various nonsurgical methods together in a complex/global rehabilitation program. The phonosurgeon must have knowledge of functionally oriented investigations of voice/vocal organ and additional/alternative treatment regimens, or he or she must work in close cooperation with someone having this knowledge. Indications for PS must be based on a functional point of view, not on morphology, aiming to improve a voice adapted to the individual requests and needs of the patient. As PS is not vitally indicated, counseling and informed consent must be oriented to focus on functional surgery rather than on surgery for laryngeal cancer, for example. Note that it is always the patient who sets the indications [25, 29]. Ishikki described various manual tests regarding the indications and for estimating the results of the operation [51]. By exerting pressure on the laryngeal skeleton, these tests are able to mimic the functional effects that can be obtained after various surgical procedures [12] (Figs. 5.5, 5.18).

5.3 Surgical Techniques

5.3.1 General Factors

Usually LFS procedures are carried out under local anesthesia. This has a major advantage in that it enables intraoperative fine-tuning of the patient's voice. Furthermore, the technique(s) can be modified on the operating table on a trial-and-error basis. Usually, a preoperative medication (e.g., midazolam), single-dose intravenous cortisone (150–250 mg prednisolone), and a broad-spectrum antibiotic are administered approximately 30 minutes preoperatively. We also give proton pump inhibitors perioperatively as a standard regimen. Intraoperatively, the patient is monitored continuously by the anesthesiologist, and narcotics and analgesics are administered on demand.

It is mandatory for the surgeon to have a clear concept and distinct knowledge of the anatomical landmarks and how the endolaryngeal structures project onto the laryngeal skeleton. Based on morphological measurements, we have developed a scale model that includes absolute and relative dimensions that allow direct correlation and application for individual surgery (Fig. 5.2). In contrast to the absolute dimensions, the relative proportions are much more constant and are not sex-specific [26, 27, 31].

At the beginning of the surgery, the various structures of the laryngeal skeleton are located by careful palpation. Local anesthesia usually is performed with lidocaine 1% with epinephrine 200,000. In case of drilling out the cartilage, continuous irrigation with local anesthetic has proved to be beneficial. Use of loupe spectacles or an operating microscope may be helpful. The intraoperative functional result is checked primarily by listening to the voice of the patient while performing tasks such as counting, prolonged vowels /a/, coughing [11, 47]. Additionally, the effect of the surgery can be monitored by an inserted fiberscope [23, 40, 41, 51, 60, 80, 114]. In special cases, the operation can be carried out under general anesthesia. As an endotracheal tube would impair the surgery, we use a laryngeal airway mask with a fiberscope inserted in these cases.

5.4 Approximation Laryngoplasty

The principle of this group of operations is to bring the vocal fold in a more medialized position to enable better glottic closure. As insufficient glottic closure is one of the most common causes of dysphonia, glottal narrowing procedures are the most widely performed types of LFS. Mostly, the glottic insufficiency is caused by a unilateral vocal fold paralysis; but scars, atrophy, and sulcus/vergeture can also be treated successfully and often in combination with other LFS procedures (i.e., tensioning or relaxation laryngoplasty, or LPL) [4, 5, 32, 33]. An increasing indication is aspiration due to insufficient glottic closure [10, 13, 21, 59].

5.4.1 Medialization TPL

According to Isshiki's original description of what he called TPL type I, a rectangular cartilage piece out of the thyroid cartilage is mobilized and medialized using a properly shaped piece of Silastic [45, 47] (Figs. 5.3 and 5.4).

Essential to the success of the operation is an optimal position of the implant, which is determined by proper localization of the cartilage window [32, 33, 51] (Fig. 5.6). The midpoint between the superior and inferior thyroid notches corresponds to the endolaryngeal insertion of Broyle's tendon in the endolarynx. Starting at this point, the free margin of the vocal fold projects parallel to the inferior border of the thyroid [31–34, 51]. The window should be outlined, with the vocal cord line being the upper line of the rectangle [32, 51]. According to Isshiki, the anterior vertical line should be about 5–7 mm from the median line of the thyroid cartilage. Based on our morphological and functional studies, we recommend that anatomical landmarks be used rather than absolute dimensions for positioning the window [31, 34]. The inferoposterior corner of the cartilage window should be placed in the area of the oblique line [31, 32]. We therefore prefer to position the window further dorsal than recommended by Isshiki [51]. Considering these landmarks, an optimal implant position can be achieved with the posterior edge of the titanium vocal fold medializing implant (TVFMI) located lateral to the vocal process, resulting in physiological medialization of the entire vocal fold [32].

Different techniques and modifications regarding the surgical technique and the implant have been described [9, 16, 75–77]. There is also some demand for a ready-made, standardized implant system that shortens the operating time and eases the application (Table 5.3) [16, 75, 76]. At the moment, three implant systems are on the market. One is the Montgomery Thyroplasty Implant System, consisting of different sizes and shapes of shims made of Silastic [75, 76]. The VoCom System also contains a set of different sizes and shapes of implants made out of hydroxyapatite [16] and TVFMI, which comes in two sizes and is made of pure titanium [34]. As this operation is not vitally indicated, the safety of the implant system and avoidance of negative side effects should be of major interest. In this respect, the TVFMI has fulfilled our expectations because of the superb biocompatibility

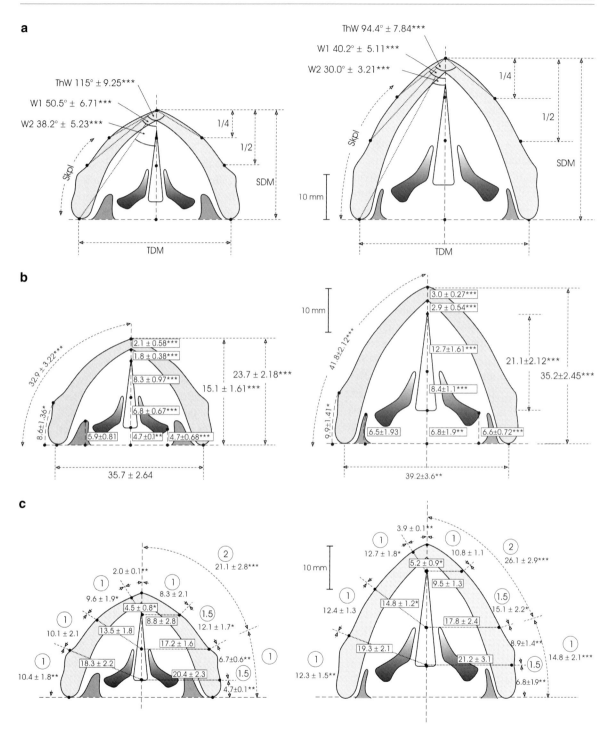

Fig. 5.2. Surgical anatomy of the larynx. Given are each mean with standard deviation and significance level on comparing the corresponding sex-related values. (**a**) Thyroid angles in males and females, reference points for measurement. *SDM*, sagittal diameter; *TDM*, transverse diameter; *Skpl*, thyroid plate. (**b**) Dimensions in the glottic plane. (**c**) Projection of the endolaryngeal structures onto the thyroid surface. *Right*, lateral projection. *Left*, projection perpendicular to the thyroid cartilage. (**d, e**) Thickness of the thyroid cartilage, location of the oblique line, and ventral extension of the piriform sinus at different levels in females (**d**) and males (**e**). (**f**) Location of the superior and inferior thyroid tubercles, course of the oblique line, and projection of the ventral extension of the piriform sinus. *VK*, mucosa of anterior commissure; *PV*, vocal process; *PM*, muscular process. (**g**) Projection of the fixation of the anterior commissure tendon and of the free margin of the vocal fold in a lateral view. (**h**) Topographical relations between the cricoid and thyroid cartilage with respect to the free margin of the vocal fold. (From Friedrich and Lichtenegger [31], with permission)

d   **e**

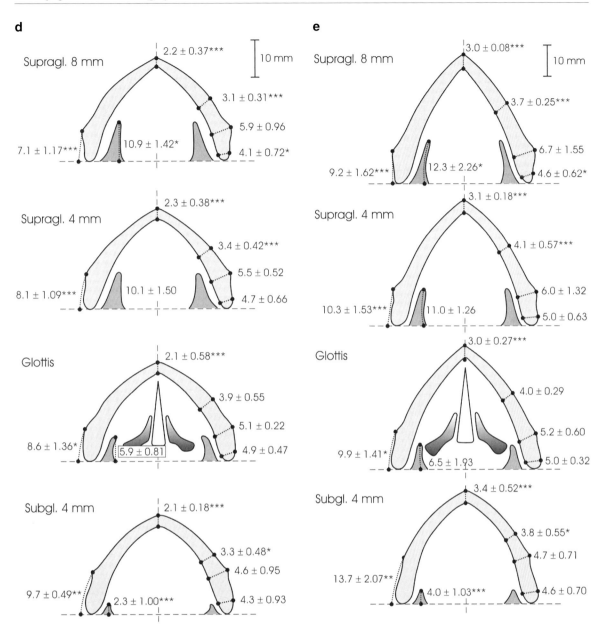

Fig. 5.2. (continued)

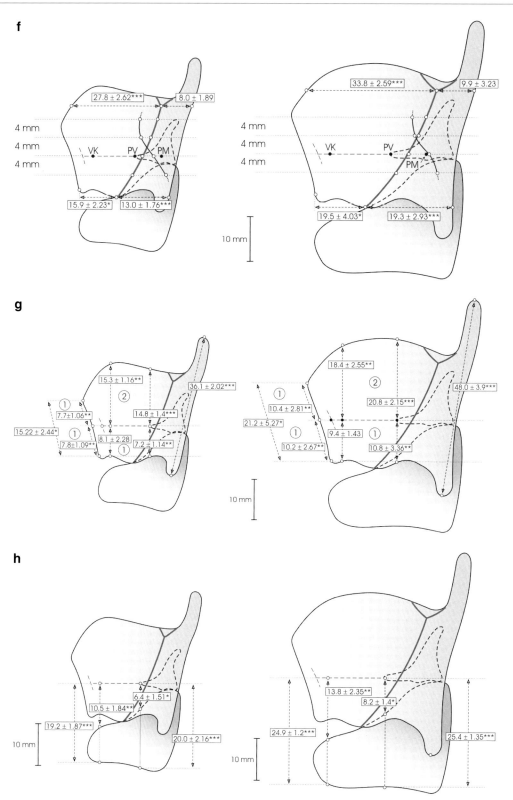

Fig. 5.2. (continued)

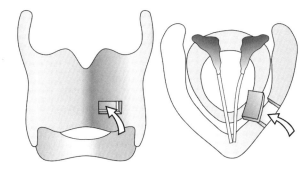

Fig. 5.3. Medialization thyroplasty. (From Friedrich et al. [35], with permission)

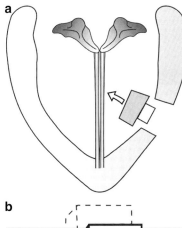

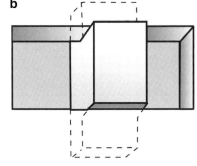

Fig. 5.4. Proto-type thyroplasty type I according to Isshiki (**a**) using a Silastic shim (**b**). (From Isshiki [51], with permission)

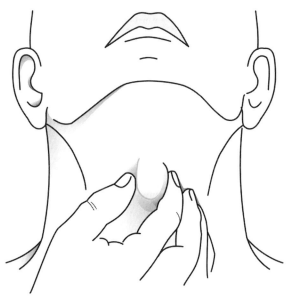

Fig. 5.5. Manual compression test for medialization thyroplasty. (From Isshiki [51], with permission)

the loudness of the voice increased. Often, additional fat injections are necessary to reach an acceptable result.

5.4.2 Arytenoid Adduction

In the case of an abducted or tilted arytenoid cartilage, a large posterior glottic chink, or a level difference of the vocal folds, the arytenoid adduction technique can be a good option. It first was described by Morrison as reverse King operation [78], and its principle is to mimic the pull of the lateral cricoarytenoid (LCA) muscle by a suture through the muscular process of the arytenoid (Fig. 5.12). The disadvantages are mainly due to technical problems: more complicated surgical procedure, longer operating time, difficulty locating the muscular process, danger of hypopharyngeal perforation, pronounced postoperative swelling, and increased airway obstruction, with a higher tracheostomy risk. Moreover, it is an irreversible procedure, and so the indication must be more strict. To obtain access to the arytenoid cartilage, Isshiki [48] described dislocation of the cricothyroid joint. In contrast, Maragos [68, 70, 71] introduced resection of the posterior rim of the thyroid plate, thus avoiding dislocation of the cricothyroid joint and the possible negative consequences on

of the titanium and the secure fixation of the implant, preventing dislocation and extrusion (Fig. 5.7–5.10).

A special problem is vocal fold medialization after cordectomy. The dense, thin scar tissue in the endolarynx makes mobilization difficult, and there is an increased danger of perforation and implant extrusion, which is the reason why using autogenous cartilage can be favorable [100] (Fig. 5.11). Good results have been reported [89] using the TVFMI in patients after endoscopic cordectomy. The results, in general, are not as good as in patients with paralytic dysphonia, but usually the loss of air during phonation can be diminished and

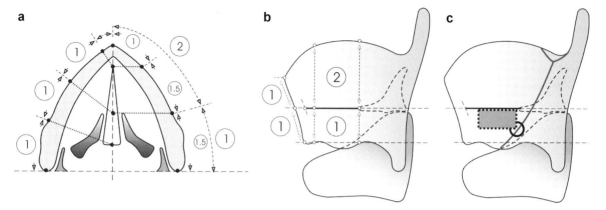

Fig. 5.6. Proportions of larynx and anatomic landmarks for positioning the cartilage window for a titanium vocal fold medializing implant (TVFMI). (**a**) Projection of endolaryngeal structures onto the thyroid cartilage surface. *Right*, lateral projection. *Left*, perpendicular to the thyroid plate. (**b**) Localization of the free margin of the vocal fold in a lateral projection. (**c**) Positioning thecartilage window using projection of the free margin of the vocal fold and an oblique line (*circle*). (From Friedrich [34], with permission)

Table 5.3. Medialization thyroplasty: materials and implant systems

Alloplastic	Autogen
Silicone (Isshiki [46, 47])	Cartilage (Payr [88], Kleinsasser [59], Denecke [64], Meurman [74], Seiffert [99], Sittel [100])
Polyethylene (Berghaus [6, 7])	Fascia (Tsunoda [103])
Ceramic (Sakai [92])	Fat (Dedo)
Gore-Tex (McCulloch [73], Giovanni [38], Sataloff [93], Zeitels [120])	
Hydroxyapatite (Cummings [16])	
Titanium (Friedrich [33, 34])	

Free-formed	Preformed
Silicone (Isshiki [46, 47])	Montgomery [75, 76]
Polyethylene (Berghaus [6, 7])	Cummings [16]
Gore-Tex (McCulloch [73], Giovanni [38], Sataloff [93], Zeitels [120])	Friedrich [33, 34]
Autogen implants	(Desrosiers, [20]) (not on the market)

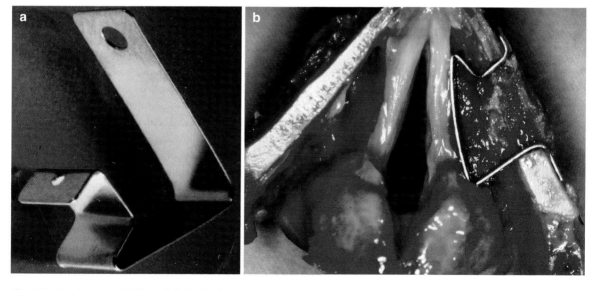

Fig. 5.7. Titanium vocal fold medializing implant (TVFMI). (**a**) Alone. (**b**) Inserted in a specimen. (From Friedrich [34], with permission)

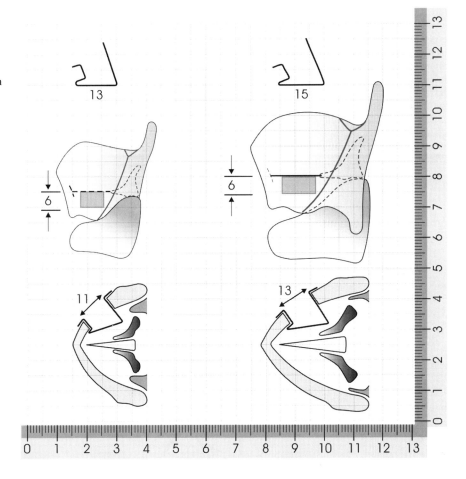

Fig. 5.8. Scale model, in millimeters, of average male and female thyroid cartilage configurations. Location of the cartilage window and correct positioning of 13-mm and 15-mm titanium vocal fold medializing implants (TVFMIs), respectively. (From Friedrich [34], with permission)

the biomechanics of the larynx. Concerning the technique of arytenoid adduction, two types can be distinguished: The arytenoid rotation (pull) techniques [48, 57, 81, 101], uses a suture through the muscular process or attached muscles, whereas the arytenoid fixation technique [70, 71, 78, 118] fixates the whole arytenoid cartilage by sutures onto the cricoid plate. Arytenoid adduction fails to correct a bowed membranous vocal fold, so usually it has to be combined with a medialization TPL using any type of implant [8, 51, 72, 101].

5.5 Expansion LPL

The indication for expansion LPL is a too tight glottic closure when the glottis is functionally overclosed, such as with adductor spasmodic dysphonia. Although some of the procedures are similar to operations used to treat glottic stenoses or bilateral vocal fold paralysis,

it is important to note that the aim of the procedure is to improve the voice, not to improve respiratory status.

5.5.1 Lateralization Thyroplasty

Lateralization of the vocal folds can be achieved by expanding the thyroid cartilage in the transverse diameter whether by a lateral or a medial approach. The lateralization TPL by a lateral approach is surgically performed by first exposing the thyroid cartilage in its anterior part. It is then cut vertically at the line between the anterior one-third and the posterior two-thirds (Fig. 5.13). The incised edges are overlapped, with the lateral side over the median side so the vocal fold is displaced laterally [51].

The medial approach for lateralization TPL (expansion of the anterior commissure, midline lateralization TPL) recently has been reported by Isshiki to be

Fig. 5.9. Inserting the TVFMI. (**a**) Situation after excision of cartilage and incision of inner perichondrium at the dorsal rim. (**b**) Inserting TVFMI ventrally. (**c**) Introducing TVFMI into the endolarynx with slight tension. (**d**) TVFMI correctly inserted and fixated with sutures dorsally. (From Friedrich [34], with permission)

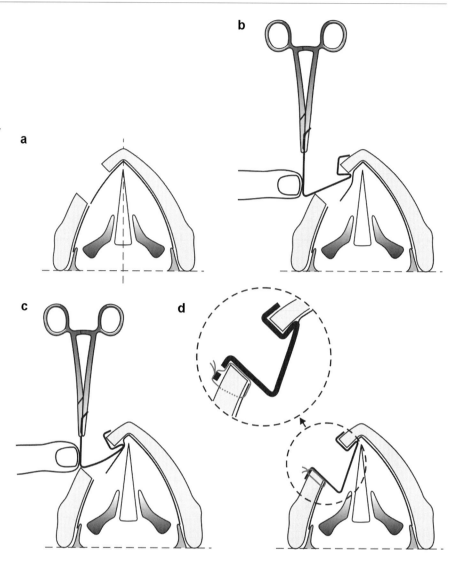

successful in the treatment of spasmodic dysphonia (Fig. 5.14). Surgically, the anterior part of the thyroid cartilage is exposed, and a midline laryngofissure is performed. A Silastic block is inserted between the two edges of the thyroid plate [51, 54]; recently, a special titanium implant for this purpose has been developed [56]. We use titanium miniplates, which can be bent properly quite easily (Fig. 5.15).

5.5.2 Vocal Fold Abduction

Another option for lateralizing the vocal folds is to perform a direct abduction by an approach through the thyroid cartilage [51]. Technically, these operations are similar to medialization TPL; that is, a thyroid cartilage window is created, giving direct access to the vocal fold muscles. The lateralization can be performed by sutures going through the membranous and/or cartilaginous portion of the vocal folds (Fig. 5.16). Another technique is to resect part of the vocalis muscle through this cartilage window whether by cold instruments, electrosurgery, or laser. A modification is just to section the laryngeal recurrent nerve branches to the adductory muscles with or without resecting muscle [51, 116].

5.6 Relaxation LPL

One indication for relaxation LPL is an inappropriately high-pitched voice, especially in men, such as is seen in mutational voice disorders [46, 49, 50, 53, 108]. As these

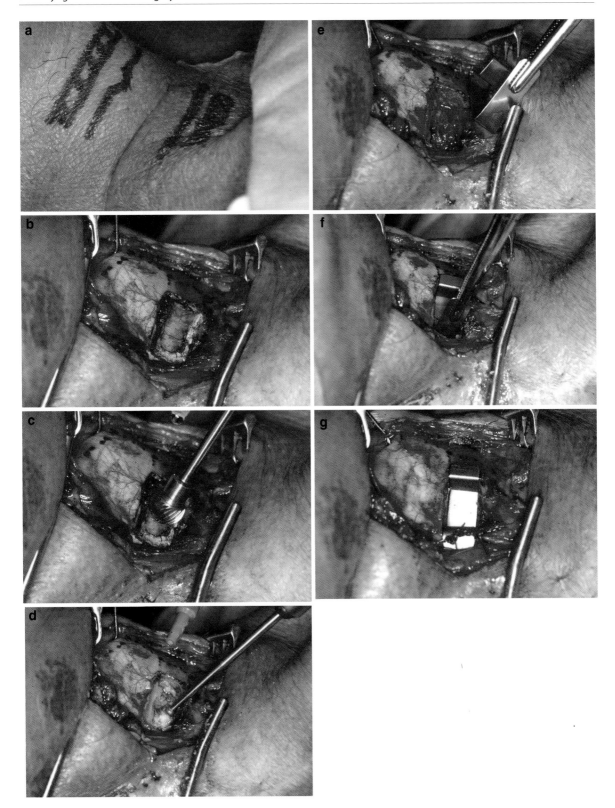

Fig. 5.10. Vocal fold medialization using the TVFMI. (a) Marking the laryngeal structures on the skin. (b) Outlining and positioning the window. (c) Drilling out the outlined window. (d) Using a diamond bur and irrigation with local anesthetics near the inner perichondrium. (e) TVFMI prior insertion. (f) TVFMI inserted. (g) Fixation with sutures. (From Friedrich [34], with permission)

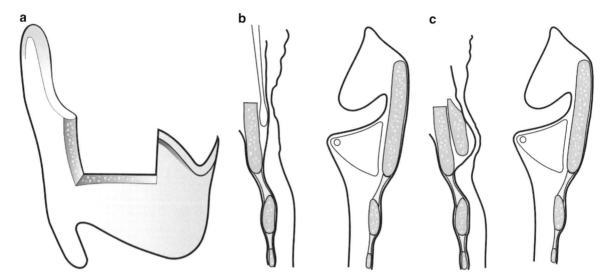

Fig. 5.11. Vocal fold medialization after laser chordectomy. (**a**) Donor site of autologous cartilage graft. (**b**) Preparation of a pocket in the subperichondrial space from the superior direction.

(**c**) Cartilaginous strut placed in the subperichondrial space, forcing the scarred site of the laser resection into a more medial position. (From Sittel et al. [100], with permission)

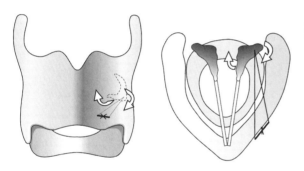

Fig. 5.12. Arytenoid adduction (rotation technique). (From Friedrich et al. [35], with permission)

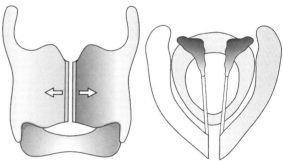

Fig. 5.14. Lateralization thyroplasty (medial approach). (From Friedrich et al. [35], with permission)

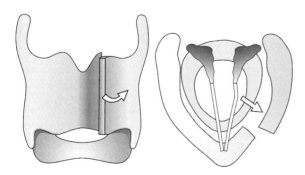

Fig. 5.13. Lateralization thyroplasty (lateral approach). (From Friedrich et al. [35], with permission)

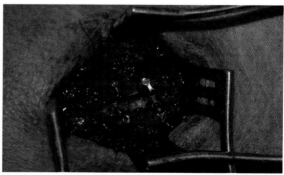

Fig. 5.15. Lateralization thyroplasty (medial approach), usage of miniplates.

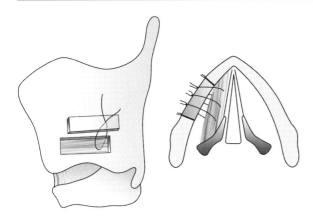

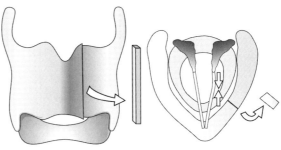

Fig. 5.17. Shortening thyroplasty (lateral approach). (From Friedrich et al. [35], with permission)

Fig. 5.16. Vocal fold abduction. (From Isshiki [51], with permission)

disorders usually react well to voice therapy, this always is the first choice treatment [54]. At least in a certain group of patients with mutational voice disorders that have been diagnosed as "functional" after common clinical examinations, there is evidence that they have an underdeveloped larynx; thus, there is also a structural basis for the dysphonia [28]. Another indication are stiff vocal folds with a narrow chink during phonation often resulting from surgical trauma, irradiation, chronic laryngitis, or sulcus vocalis/vergeture [51]. The functional results usually are not as good as for structurally normal vocal folds, and often the procedures have to be combined (e.g., with medialization TPL). A third indication is abductor spasmodic dysphonia [106]. In these cases, the operation mostly is performed in combination with a lateralization TPL. In general, relaxation LPL mostly is part of combination framework surgery (Isshiki [69, 72, 85]. The common principle of all these operations is it to shorten the distance between the vocal fold attachments at the thyroid plate and the arytenoid cartilage, thereby reducing tension of the vocal folds.

5.6.1 Shortening TPL

The shortening TPL can be performed using a lateral or medial approach (Fig. 5.17). The operative settings for this surgery are essentially the same as those for the other TPL procedures. The thyroid ala is incised at about the junction of the anterior and middle one-third, and a 2- to 5-mm cartilage strip is excised [51]. Medial or lateral overlapping of the cartilage edges without excision results in a combination between relaxation

and approximation or expansion LPL, respectively [51]. Tucker created an anterior cartilage flap and retrused it into the larynx for treatment of adductor spasmodic dysphonia [105, 106, 108].

5.7 Tensioning LPL

The tensioning LPL is the antagonistic procedure to relaxation LPL. The main indication for it is an inappropriately low-pitched voice in women (androphonia). This can be associated with hormonal diseases, side effects of hormonal drugs (i.e., anabolic agents, androgen hormones), or male-to-female transsexualism. [46, 49, 51, 53, 67, 82, 83]. Other indications are abnormal lax or bowed vocal folds (e.g., in presbyphonia) and paralysis of the cricothyroid muscle. In these cases, tensioning LPL usually is combined with medialization TPL [46, 49, 51–54, 111]. The basic principle of the operation is to increase the distance between the vocal fold attachments and thus raise the tension of the vocal fold.

5.7.1 Cricothyroid Approximation

Cricothyroid approximation increases the vocal pitch by simulating the contraction of the cricothyroid muscle with sutures (TPL type IV) [46] (Figs. 5.18 and 5.19). According to Isshiki's original description, four nonabsorbable monophilic sutures are placed to draw the cricoid and thyroid cartilages together. In thyroid cartilage, bolsters should be used to prevent cutting through the sutures. The cricoid and thyroid cartilage is approximated as closely as possible because postoperative reversion toward

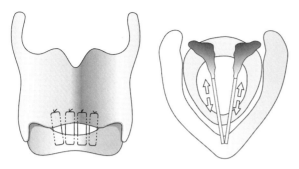

Fig. 5.18. Cricothyroid approximation. (From Friedrich et al. [35], with permission)

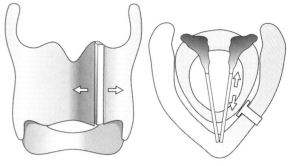

Fig. 5.20. Elongation thyroplasty (lateral approach). (From Friedrich et al. [35], with permission)

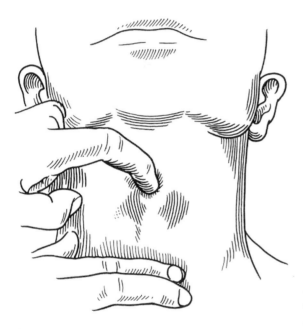

Fig. 5.19. Manual cricothyroid approximation to determine the indication for surgically elevating the vocal pitch. (From Isshiki [51], with permission)

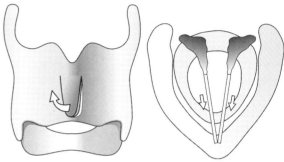

Fig. 5.21. Elongation thyroplasty (medial approach). (From Friedrich et al. [35], with permission)

The lateral approach, sometimes also called TPL type IV, requires an implant for permanent extension of the thyroid ala [49, 51] (Fig. 5.20). A vertical incision is made at the junction of the anterior and middle one-third of the ala, as in surgery to lower the vocal pitch, and a Silastic implant is fixed between the cartilage edges by two mattress sutures. If pitch elevation is insufficient, the same procedure may also be performed on the contralateral side.

The medial approach, first described by Le Jeune as "springboard advancement" [65], tightens flaccid vocal folds (Fig. 5.21). The indication for the surgery is mainly a breathy voice due to bowed vocal folds. After exposure of the anterior portion of the thyroid cartilage, an inferiorly based cartilage flap is formed so as to include the anterior commissure. The upper end of the flap is held in position by a tantalum shim. Tucker [105] in 1985 modified Le Jeune's [65] technique by reversing the pedicle and called it anterior commissure LPL or anterior commissure advancement (Fig. 5.21). He also used the flap to lower the vocal pitch by displacing the flap in the dorsal direction.

a lower pitch to some extent is inevitable. Several modifications have been described, especially using different suture techniques or miniplates [82, 83]. A new modification was recently published by Zeitels as cricothyroid subluxation [119].

5.7.2 Elongation TPL

Elongation TPL is the antagonistic procedure to shortening TPL utilizing the same surgical technique [46, 51].

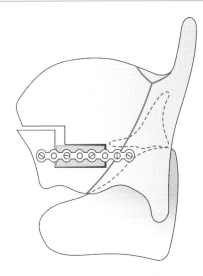

Fig. 5.22. Combination of medialization thyroplasty and elongation thyroplasty (medial approach). (From Friedrich [32], with permission)

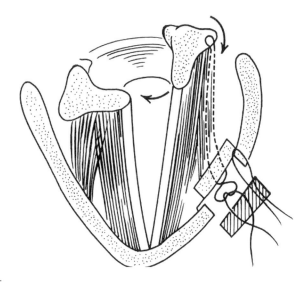

Fig. 5.24. Combination of arytenoid adduction with medialization thyroplasty. (From Isshiki [51], with permission)

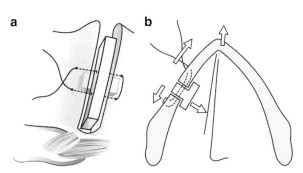

a   **b**

Fig. 5.23. Combination of medialization thyroplasty and elongation thyroplasty (lateral approach). (From Isshiki [51], with permission)

may be indicated on an individual basis according to the local situation and the wish and requests of the patient. In fresh paralysis or sulcus vocalis patients, we prefer to start with a fat injection; in the case of a too high resorption rate, we perform a thyroplasty as the second step. On the other hand, sometimes after thyroplasty progressive muscle atrophy occurs, leading to glottic insufficiency. In these cases, an additional fat injection is highly effective. A combination of approximation and tensioning LPL is particularly well suited for treating superior laryngeal nerve paralysis [79].

5.8 Combination LPL

A major advantage of LFS is that during the procedure under local anesthesia the functional outcome can be assessed and adapted individually (Figs. 5.22–5.24). Often different LFS procedures have to be combined for an optimal result. Maragos showed some typical combinations and favorable indications (Table 5.4). There is also no conflict between LFS and other phonosurgical procedures (e.g., injection augmentation) or neuromuscular surgery [107]. Especially for vocal fold medialization, both techniques should be available and

5.9 Postoperative Care and Complications

Laryngeal framework surgeries are usually considered safe procedures with low complication rates [1, 15, 24, 40, 60, 61, 90, 104, 108, 109, 110]. Possible complications are swelling due to edema and or hematoma with respiratory distress, infections, bleeding, and entering the airway. Long-term complications can be caused by implant dislocation, perforation, and extrusion. Table 5.5 clearly shows that life-threatening respiratory distress occurs exclusively after arytenoid adduction, which makes it clear that this is a more

Table 5.4. Combination laryngoplasties

Combination	Purpose	Indications
Medialization TPL + arytenoid adduction (rotation)	Medialization of the entire vocal cord (anterior and posterior)	Open posterior glottis High vagal paralysis RLN paralysis with lateralized arytenoid Nonrotating arytenoid
Bilateral medialization TPL	Medialization of both membranous vocal cords	Open anterior glottis Bilateral vocal cord weakness (e.g., presbyphonia) Bilateral loss of muscle mass Tremor-induced AbSD
Medialization TPL + tensioning LPL	Stretching of vocal cord with medialization of affected side	Unilateral SLN weakness
Medialization TPL + arytenoid adduction (fixation)	Medial vocal cord fixation	Anterior dislocation of arytenoid cartilage; arytenoid fracture Failed arytenoid adduction (rotation) (cricoarytenoid joint ankylosis)
Bilateral relaxation LPL	Relaxation of both vocal cords	Too high-pitched male voice Stable AdSD in males
Medialization TPL + relaxation LPL	Relaxation and increased mass of one vocal cord	High-pitched, presbyphonic male voice

Modified after Maragos [72], with permission
RLN, recurrent laryngeal nerve; SLN, superior laryngeal nerve; AdSD, abductor spasmodic dysphonia

Table 5.5. Rates of severe complications in medialization TPL and arytenoid adduction according to various authors

Complications	Medialization TPL	Medialization TPL + arytenoid adduction	Author
Severe dyspnea	–	2	Abraham et al. [1], $n = 237$
Extrusion	3	–	
Severe dyspnea	–	7	Weinman and Maragos [115], $n = 630$
Extrusion	1	–	Laccourreye and Hans [64], $n = 27$
Severe dyspnea	–		Cotter et al. [15], $n = 58$
Extrusion	5		
Extrusion	1		Giovanni et al. [38], $n = 13$
Extrusion	102		Rosen [91], $n = 12644$

invasive procedure and the indications should be carefully considered. Usually, the implants used (silicone, hydroxyapatite, Gore-Tex, titanium, ceramic) have excellent biocompatibility and do not cause an inflammatory reaction or granuloma formation [22, 38, 64, 73, 92, 120]. There is one report of an allergic reaction to a silicone implant after medialization TPL [44]. The biggest advantage of LFS compared to other methods (e.g., injection augmentation) is that in case of adverse effects the implant can be removed completely without causing further destruction or voice deterioration [2]. In case of severe dyspnea, intravenous administration of a high dose of cortisone is the first choice of treatment. If it does not lead to relief, a tracheostomy may be necessary. Informed consent has to be established

prior to surgery regarding this possibility. A meta-analysis showed that there is a learning curve and that complication rates are higher with inexperienced surgeons [91].

Most important for a low complication rate is atraumatic preparation, in particular when performing the endolaryngeal mobilization, carefully avoiding entering the airway. If this occurs, the perforation must be repaired using sutures and a local tissue flap. Preoperative application of broad-spectrum antibiotics minimizes the danger of wound infections. Preparation of the endolaryngeal tissue should not exceed 30 minutes; if it takes longer, the increasing endolaryngeal edema makes it difficult to estimate the quality of the postoperative voice [16, 40, 41, 51, 52, 61].

Slight postoperative edema and hematoma are normal and are not considered complications. Nonsteroidal antiinflammatory medications are administered as needed (except aspirin, which is also avoided preoperatively) as well as saline inhalants. Relative voice rest should be applied until the swelling abates. Breathing should be monitored for at least 48 hours. Phonation can temporarily deteriorate during the first postoperative days because of edema. Evaluation of the surgical outcome is possible after 3 weeks at the earliest; voice improvement reaches the 80th–90th percentile of the final result in 2 months, although further improvements are possible for up to 1 year. Postoperative voice therapy may lead to further improvement and should be indicated for the individual patient, starting not earlier than 3 weeks postoperatively [66].

Among nearly 300 LFS procedures we have not experienced any serious perioperative complications, and we never had to perform a tracheostomy. In one operated and irradiated patient, the anterior part of the titanium vocal fold medializing implant (TVFMI) perforated the external skin and had to be covered with a small skin flap. In three cases (two after cordectomy) there was perforation of the implant in the endolarynx and the implants had to be removed. They were replaced by a small muscle flap, and the vocal outcome was satisfactory in all cases. We never experienced dislocation or extrusion of the TVFMI, but there were three cases of dislocation of Silastic shims on the mobilized cartilage islands respectively. This was a major reason that we have developed the TVFMI and stopped using Silastic.

5.10 Results and Prognosis

5.10.1 Approximation LPL

Medialization TPL can result in the degree of glottic insufficiency being reduced significantly, with the consequence that all voice function parameters can be improved significantly (Tables 5.6 and 5.7). Especially for evaluating the voice after medialization TPL, we introduced the Voice Dysfunction Index, which has shown statistically significant improvement after TPL (Table 5.8 and 5.6) [32–34, 64, 95, 96]. The grade of glottic insufficiency and the Voice Dysfunction Index showed a significant correlation ($r = 0.45$, $p < 0.05$) [32, 33]. This is in accordance with Omori [84, 85] and proves that the grade of glottic insufficiency is the determining factor for the severity of dysphonia. By means of aerodynamic measures, it could be demonstrated that the medialization procedure does not cause an increase in laryngeal resistance during breathing [98].

Subjective self-evaluation of the voice is of growing importance in daily clinical practice [17, 23, 40, 43, 52, 58]. Usually a significant improvement in the patient's vocal communication skills in his/her everyday and/or professional life can be observed [24, 33, 40, 52, 97, 112] (Table 5.6).

Generally, the medialization TPL results are better in patients suffering from paralytic dysphonia than in those with glottic insufficiency due to sulcus/vergeture or scars. Nevertheless, both conditions are good indications

Table 5.6.	Results	Preop.	p	Postop.
Functional results of medialization TPL	Glottic gap (0–3 scale)	2.2	< 0.001	0.5
	Mean fundamental frequency (fem)	202.1 Hz	n.s.	210.4 Hz
	Mean voice intensity (fem)	59.7 dB	< 0.01	65.2 dB
	Mean fundamental frequency (male)	109.3 Hz	n.s.	127.8 Hz
	Mean voice intensity (male)	60.4 dB	n.s.	66.0 dB
	Intensity range	27.4 dB	< 0.001	39.2 dB
	Pitch range	14.2 ST	< 0.001	21.6 ST
	Hoarseness (0–3 scale)	2.1	< 0.001	0.6
	Roughness (0–3 scale)	0.5	< 0.001	0.1
	Breathiness (0–3 scale)	2.2	< 0.001	0.6
	Maximum phonation time	7.3 s	< 0.001	13.2 s
	Impairment of vocal comm. skills (0–3 scale)	2.3	< 0.001	0.6
	Voice Dysfunction Index (0–3 scale)	2.2	< 0.001	0.8

Data are from Friedrich [32, 33]

Table 5.7. Grading of glottic insufficiency

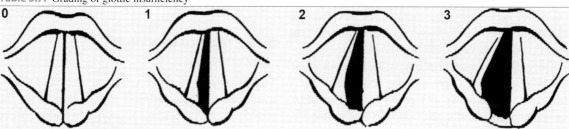

From Friedrich [32, 33], with permission

Table 5.8. Calculation of the Voice Dysfunction Index

Grade of hoarseness	2	Index	2	0	1	2	3
Frequency range	20	ST	1	> 24	24–18	17–12	< 12
Intensity range	31	dB(A)	2	> 45	45–35	34–25	< 25
Maximum phonation time	13	seconds	1	> 15	15–11	10–7	< 7
Impairment of vocal communication skills	1	Index	1	0	1	2	3
Voice Dysfunction Index (Σ/5)			1,4				

From Friedrich [33, 34], with permission
Example is printed in boldface and shaded in gray.
Range of the index: min = 0 (normal voice), max = 3 (extreme deviant voice)

for the procedure, and patients usually appreciate the increased endurance and intensity range of the voice [5, 23, 33, 42, 52, 62, 89, 114].

A clinically relevant question is whether early medialization leads to better results or, conversely, after a certain period does the prognosis deteriorate. Statements in the literature regarding this are inconclusive [37, 41, 117]. We found no significant correlation ($r = 0.07$, n.s.) between the results and the preoperative time [32]. According to our experience medialization TPL can be performed even decades after the onset of paralysis with good results. Interestingly, we found a significant correlation between the age of the operated patient and the functional result ($r = 0.35, p < 0.01$) in that older patients show a better functional outcome. This means that higher age is no contraindication, and good functional results are to be expected even in elderly patients [33].

Unfavorable results may be due to overcorrection or undercorrection. Undercorrection can be caused by intraoperative edema, which after resorption leaves a remaining glottic gap. Quick, atraumatic preparation diminishes the danger of excessive edema, which can be enabled by using a prefabricated implant [16, 34, 76]. Medialization on the operating table should be done until a slightly pressed voice is produced; that is,

after reaching an optimum voice result, a 1- to 2-mm medialization should be added. Undercorrection that occurs after an initially good result can be due to muscular atrophy. In these cases, we found that performing an additional fat injection as a first step, rather than change the implant immediately, was met with success. The major reason for unsatisfactory results is improper placement of the implant. If the implant is located too far anteriorly, the vocal fold edge becomes S-shaped with an anterior bulge causing insufficient glottic closure at the posterior part. If the implant is located too high, the ventricular fold is medialized, also causing insufficient glottic closure.

As in the available literature and our own experience, there are no significant differences in the functional outcome with different techniques and implants, provided the surgeon can achieve good medialization of the vocal fold [33, 34, 77, 95–98].

Another effective method for vocal fold medialization is the arytenoid adduction procedure. Several authors believe that the indications for this operation are a large posterior glottic chink, level differences, and a tilted arytenoid [9, 45, 67, 101, 102, 121]. Although some report superior functional results compared to the medialization TPL, the indications and benefits of each procedure are controversial. Mahieu [67] reported that according to his experience in approximately 30% an arytenoid adduction had to be performed additionally to medialization TPL; in our series this rate was less than 10%. In any case, arytenoid adduction is a more invasive procedure with a higher complication rate, and the indications should be carefully considered (Table 5.5). A meta-analysis indicated no clear benefit of arytenoid adduction and medialization TPL compared with medialization TPL alone [14].

5.11 Expansion LPL

The major indication for this type of operation is treatment of spasmodic dysphonia. In contrast to botulinum toxin injections, LPL offers the option of permanent voice improvement. Isshiki has reported good, and so far permanent, results using a midline lateralization TPL [54].

5.12 Relaxation LPL

One indication for relaxation LPL is lowering an inappropriately high-pitched voice, especially in those with mutational voice disorders. Isshiki lowered the pitch in nine patients from 239 Hz preoperatively to 138 Hz postoperatively [51]. This is in accord with the results from Guo-Dong Li [39], who found that after the operation the voice frequency was significantly decreased ($p < 0.5$). Tucker also reported good results after treating spasmodic dysphonia with a medial approach to shortening TPL [105, 106].

5.13 Tensioning LPL

A major indication for tensioning LPL is voice pitch elevation in male-to-female transsexuals. Usually, vocal pitch elevation is substantial after cricothyroid approximation. On average, the medium speaking voice can be raised by 5 semitones and in 39% of patients by more than 12 semitones [82, 83]. Isshiki reported that the voice pitch could be changed, on average, from 163 Hz preoperatively to 215 Hz postoperatively [51]. In some patients, progressive tension loss is observed, causing lowering of the pitch in the long run. Sataloff [93]

developed an alternative technique that fuses the cricoid and thyroid, which should provide better long-term results. The vocal pitch range of the voice is narrowed after the operation; practically, however, the speech does not sound more monotonous, and patients have not complained about it [51, 82, 83]. For bowed vocal folds (e.g., in presbyphonia or vocal fold atrophy) elongation LPL, whether by a medial or a lateral approach, gives good results, sometimes in combination with bilateral medialization TLP [52, 62, 65, 105].

5.14 Tips and Pearls to Avoid Complications

- Careful preoperative assessment and reliable indications
- Meticulous information and properly informed consent
- Clear definition of goals and realistic prognosis
- Preoperative administration of antibiotics and cortisone
- Exact palpation and location of anatomical landmarks
- Clear concept of underlying anatomy and the intended procedure
- Atraumatic preparation, carefully avoiding entering the airway
- Postoperative monitoring for at least 48 hours
- Postoperative voice therapy based on individual indications

References

1. Abraham MT, Goen M, Kraus DH (2001) Complications of type I thyroplasty and arytenoid adduction. Laryngoscope 111(8):1322–1329
2. Al-Yousuf A, Jain A, Parker AJ (2006) Postthyroplasty implant extrusion. Folia Phoniatrica et Logoppaedica 58: 139–142
3. Beck C, Richstein A (1982) Medianverlagerung einer paretischen Stimmlippe durch partielle Schildknorpelkompression. Laryngol Rhinol Otol 61:251–253
4. Benninger MS, Crumley RL, Ford CN, Gould WJ, Hanson DG, Ossoff RH, Sataloff RT (1994) Evaluation and treatment of the unilateral paralyzed vocal fold. Otolaryngol Head Neck Surg 111(4):497–508
5. Benninger MS, Alessi D, Archer S, Bastian R, Ford Ch KoufmanJ, Sataloff RT, Spiegel JR, Woo P (1996) Vocal fold scarring: current concepts and management. Otolaryngol Head Neck Surg 115(5):474–482

6. Berghaus A (1987) Verfahren zur Unterfütterung von Stimmlippen. HNO 35:227–233

7. Berghaus A (1992) Alloplastische Implantate in der Kopf-Halschirurgie. Eur Arch Otol Rhinol Laryngol Suppl 1: 53–95

8. Bielamowicz S, Berke GS (1995) An improved method of medialization laryngoplasty using a three-sided thyroplasty window. Laryngoscope 105:537–539

9. Bielamowicz S, Berke GS, Gerratt BR (1995) A comparison of type I thyroplasty and arytenoid adduction. J Voice 9(4): 466–472

10. Bigenzahn W, Denk DM (1999) Oropharyngeale dysphagien. Thieme, Stuttgart/New York

11. Blaugrund St M, Carroll LM (1993) Technique and perioperative quantitative analysis of thyroplasty type I. Operat Tech Otolaryngol Head Neck Surg 4(3):186–190

12. Blaugrund St M, Taira T, Isshiki N (1991) Laryngeal manual compression in the evaluation of patients for laryngeal framework surgery. In: Gauffin JU, Hammarberg B (eds) Vocal fold physiology. Singular Publishing, San Diego, CA

13. Carrau RL, Pou A, Eibling DE (1999) Laryngeal framework surgery for the management of aspiration. Otolaryngol Head Neck Surgery 21(2):139–145

14. Chester MW, Stewart MG (2003) Arytenoid adduction combined with medialization thyroplasty: an evidence-based review. Otolaryngol Head Neck Surg 129:305–310

15. Cotter CS, Avidano MA, Crary MA, Cassisi NJ, Gorham MM (1995) Laryngeal complications after type 1 thyroplasty. Otolaryngol Head Neck Surg 113(6):671–672

16. Cummings C, Purcell L, Flint P (1993) Hydroxylapatite laryngeal implants for medialization. Preliminary report. Ann Otol Rhinol Laryngol 102:843–851

17. Dejonckere PH, Bradley P, Clemente P, Cornut G, Crevier-Buchmann L, Friedrich G, Van De Heyning P, Remacle M, Woisard V (2001) A basic protocol for functional assessment of voice pathology, especially for investigating the efficacy of (phonosurgical) treatments and evaluating new assessment techniques. Eur Arch Otorhinolaryngol 258:77–82

18. Denecke HJ (1961) Korrektur des Schluckaktes bei einseitiger Pharynx- und Larynxlähmung. HNO (Berl.) 9:351–353

19. Denecke HJ (1964) Stimmverbesserung bei einseitiger Rekurrenslähmung mit larynxeigenem Material. Z Laryngol Rhinol Otol 43:221–225

20. Desrosiers M, Ahmarani C, Bettez M (1993) Precise vocal cord medialization using an adjustable laryngeal implant: a preliminary study. Otolaryngol Head Neck Surg 109(6): 1014–1019

21. Flint PW, Purcell LL, Cummings CW (1997) Pathophysiology and indications for medialization thyroplasty in patients with dysphagia and aspiration. Otolaryngol Head Neck Surg 116:349–354

22. Flint WP, Corio RL, Cummings CW (1997) Comparison of soft tissue response in rabbits following laryngeal implantation with hydroxylapatite, silicone rubber, and teflon. Ann Otol Rhinol Laryngol 106:399–407

23. Ford Ch N, Bless DM, Prehn RB (1992) Thyroplasty as primary and adjunctive treatment of glottic insufficiency. J Voice 6(3):277–285

24. Ford ChN, Inagi K, Khidr A, Bless DM, Gilchrist KW (1996) Sulcus vocalis: a rational analytical approach to diagnosis and management. Ann Otol Rhinol Laryngol 105:189–200

25. Freidl W, Friedrich G, Egger J, Fitzek T (1993) Psychosocial aspects of functional dysphonia. Scand J Log Phon 18:115–119

26. Friedrich G, Kainz J (1988) Morphometrie des Kehlkopfes an Horizontalschnitten. Basisdaten für die quantitative Auswertung von modernen bildgebenden Verfahren. Laryngol Rhinol Otol 67:269

27. Friedrich G, Kainz J, Freidl W (1989) The laryngeal skeleton: anomalies and their clinical relevance. Arch Otorhinolaryngol 246:433

28. Friedrich G (1991) Schröckenfuchs M., Kehlkopfmorphologie bei postmutationellen Stimmstörungen. Sprache Stimme Gehör 3(15):79–124

29. Friedrich G (1993) Modelltheoretische Aspekte der Ätiopathogenese funktioneller Dysphonien. Sprache Stimme Gehör 17:114–118

30. Friedrich G (1995) Grundprinzipien für die Indikationsstellung zur Phonochirurgie Laryngol Rhinol Otol 74:663–665

31. Friedrich G, Lichtenegger R (1997) Surgical anatomy of the larynx. J Voice 11(3):345–355

32. Friedrich G (1998) Externe Stimmlippenmedialisation - operative Erfahrungen und Modifikationen [External vocal fold medialization: surgical experience and modification] Laryngol Rhinol Otol 77:7–17

33. Friedrich G (1998) Externe Stimmlippenmedialisation: Funktionelle Ergebnisse [external vocal fold medialization: functional results]. Laryngol Rhinol Otol 77:18–26

34. Friedrich G (1999) Titanium vocal fold medializing implant – introducing a novel implant system for external vocal fold medialization. Ann Otol Rhinol Laryngol 108:79–86

35. Friedrich G, De Jong FICRS, Mahieu HF, Benninger MS, Isshiki N (2001) Laryngeal framework surgery: a proposal for classification and nomenclature by the Phonosurgery Committee of the European Laryngological Society. Eur Arch Otorhinolaryngol 375:1–8

36. Friedrich G, Dejonckere PH (2005) Das Stimmdiagnostik-Protokoll der European Laryngological Society (ELS) – erste Erfahrungen im Rahmen einer Multizenterstudie – the voice evaluation protocol of the European Laryngological Society (ELS) - first results of a multicenter study. Laryngol Rhinol Otol 84:738–743

37. Gacek M, Gacek RR (1996) Cricoarytenoid joint after chronic vocal cord paralysis. Laryngoscope 106:1528–1530

38. Giovanni A, Vallicioni J, Gras R, Zanaret M (1999) Clinical experience with Gore-Tex for vocal fold medialization. Laryngoscope 198:284–288

39. Guo-Dong L, Liancai M, Shilin Y (1999) Acoustic evaluation of Isshiki type III thyroplasty for treatment of mutational voice disorders. J Laryngol Otol 113:31–34

40. Harries ML, Morrison M (1995) Short-term results of laryngeal framework surgery - thyroplasty type 1: a pilot study. J Otolaryngol 24(5):281–287

41. Harries ML (1997) Laryngeal framework surgery (thyroplasty). J Laryngol Otol 111:103–105

42. Hirano M, Tanaka S, Yoshida T, Hibi S (1990) Sulcus vocalis: functional aspects. Ann Otol Rhinol Laryngol 99:679–683

43. Hogikyan N, Sethuraman G. Validation of an instrument to measure voice-related quality of life. J Voice 13(4):557–569

44. Hunsaker DH, Martin PJ (1995) Allergic reaction to solid silicone implant in medial thyroplasty. Otolaryngol Head Neck Surg 113:782–784

45. Inagi K, Connor NP, Suzuki T, Ford CN, Bless DM, Nakajima M (2002) Glottal configuration, acoustic and aerodynamic changes induced by variation in suture direction in arytenoid adduction procedures. Ann Otol Rhinol Laryngol 111:861–870

46. Isshiki N, Morita H, Okamura H, Hiramoto M (1974) Thyroplasty as a new phonosurgical technique. Acta Otolaryngol 78:451–457

47. Isshiki N, Okamura H, Ishikawa T (1975) Thyroplasty type I (lateral compression) for dysphonia due to vocal cord paralysis or atrophy. Acta Otolaryngol 80:465–473

48. Isshiki N, Tanabe M, Sawada M (1978) Arytenoid adduction for unilateral vocal cord paralysis. Arch Otolaryngol 104: 555–558

49. Isshiki N, Taira T, Tanabe M (1983) Surgical alteration of the vocal pitch. J Otolaryngol 12:5

50. Isshiki N, Ohkawa M, Goto M (1985) Stiffness of the vocal cord in dysphonia – its assessment and treatment. Acta Otolaryngol (Stockh) 419:167–174

51. Isshiki N (1989) Phonosurgery – theory and practice. Springer, Tokyo

52. Isshiki N, Kojima H, Shoji K, Hirano S (1996) Vocal fold atrophy and its surgical treatment. Ann Otol Rhinol Laryngol 105:182–188

53. Isshiki N, Taira T, Tanabe M (1998) Surgical treatment for vocal pitch disorders. In: Fujimura O (ed.) Vocal physiology: voice production, mechanisms and functions. Raven, New York

54. Isshiki N (2000) Progress in laryngeal framework surgery. Acta Otolaryngol 120:120–127

55. Isshiki N, Yamamoto Y, Tsuji DH, Iiziuka Y (2000) Midline lateralization thyroplasty for adductor spasmodic dysphonia. Ann Otol Rhinol Laryngol 109:187–193

56. Isshiki N, Yamamoto I, Fukagai S (2004) Type 2 thyroplasty for spasmodic dysphonia: fixation using a titanium bridge. Acta Otolaryngol 124:309–312

57. Iwamura S (1996) A newer surgical treatment of one vocal fold paralysis – lateral cricoarytenoid muscle pull technique - methods and results. Abstract: the Second International Symposium on Laryngeal and Tracheal Reconstruction, Monte Carlo, 182: 26

58. Jacobson B, Johnson A, Grywalski C, et al (1997) The Voice Handicyp Index (VHI). Am J Speech Lang Pathol 6:66–70

59. Kleinsasser O, Schroeder H-G, Glanz H (1982) Medianverlagerung gelähmter Stimmlippen mittels Knorpelspanimplantation und Türflügelthyreoplastik. HNO 30: 275–279

60. Koufman JA (1986) Laryngoplasty for vocal cord medialization: an alternative to teflon. Laryngoscope 96(7):726–731

61. Koufman JA (1988) Laryngoplastic phonosurgery. In: Johnson JT (ed.) Instructional courses, American Academy of Otolaryngology Head and Neck Surgery, vol. 1. Mosby, St. Louis, pp. 339–350

62. Koufman JA (1989) Surgical correction of dysphonia due to bowing of the vocal cords. Ann Otol Rhinol Laryngol 98: 41–45

63. Kramer FM, Som ML (1972) Correction of the traumatically abducted vocal cord. Arch Otolaryngol 95:6

64. Laccourreye O, Hans S (2003) Endolaryngeal extrusion of expanded polytetrafluoroethylene implant after medialization thyroplasty. Ann Otol Rhinol Laryngol 112(11):962–964

65. Le Jeune FE, Guice CE, Samuels MP (1983) Early experiences with vocal ligament tightening. Ann Otol Rhinol Laryngol 92:475–477

66. Leder St B, Sasaki CT (1994) Long-term changes in vocal quality following Isshiki thyroplasty type I. Laryngoscope 104:275–277

67. Mahieu HF (2000) Laryngeal framework surgery. In: Ferlito A (ed.) Diseases of the larynx. Arnold, London, pp. 437–473

68. Maragos NE (1994) A modification of the Isshiki arytenoid adduction. The Third International Symposium on Phonosurgery-Proceedings. Kyoto, Japan, International Association, Phonosurg, pp. 62–6

69. Maragos NE(1997) Combination medialization thyroplasty: theory and practice. XVI World Congress of Otolaryngol Head Neck Surgery, Sydney, Australia

70. Maragos NE (1999) Arytenoid fixation surgery for the treatment of arytenoid fractures and dislocations. Laryngoscope 109(5):834–837

71. Maragos NE (1999) The posterior thyroplasty window: anatomical considerations. Laryngoscope 109:1228–1231

72. Maragos NE (2000) Combination thyroplasty. Advances in Otolaryngol Head Neck Surgery, Proceedings, Santorin, Greece

73. McCulloch TM, Hoffman HAT (1998) Medialization laryngoplasty with expanded polytetrafluoroethylene. Surgical technique and preliminary results. Ann Otol Rhinol Laryngol 107:427–432

74. Meurman Y (1952) Operative mediofixation of the vocal cord in complete unilateral paralysis. Arch Otolaryngol 55: 544–553

75. Montgomery WW, Blaugrund St M, Varvares MA (1993) Thyroplasty: a new approach. Ann Otol Rhinol Laryngol 102:571–579

76. Montgomery WW, Montgomery SK (1997) Mongomery thyroplasty implant system. Ann Otol Rhinol Laryngol 170:106

77. Montgomery WW, Bunting G, Mclean-Muse A, Hillman R, Doyle P, Varvares M, Eng J (2000) Montgomery® thyroplasty implant for vocal fold immobility: phonatory outcomes. Ann Otol Rhinol Laryngol 109:393–400

78. Morrison LF (1948) The "Reverse King Operation": a surgical procedure for restoration of phonation in cases of aphonia due to unilateral vocal cord paralysis. Ann Otol Rhinol Laryol 57:945–956

79. Nasseri SS, Maragos NE (1999) Combination thyroplasty and the "Twisted Larynx": combined type IV and type I thyroplasty for superior laryngeal nerve weakness. J Voice 14(1):104–111

80. Netterville JL (1990) Evaluation and treatment of complications of thyroid and parathyroid surgery. Otolaryngol Clin North Am 23(3):529–552

81. Netterville JL, Stone RE, Luken ES (1993) Silastic medialization and arytenoid adduction: the Vanderbilt experience. Ann Otol Rhinol Laryngol 102:413–424

82. Neumann K, Welzel C, Berghaus A (2003) Resorbable material for osteosynthesis or titanium for the cricothyroidopexy?. Laryngorhinootologie 82(6):428–435

83. Neumann K, Welzel C (2004) The importance of the voice in male-to-female transsexualism. J Voice 18(1):153–167

84. Omori K, Kacker A, Slavit DH, Blaugrund St M (1996) Quantitative videostroboscopic measurement of glottal gap

and vocal function: an analysis of thyroplasty type I. Ann Otol Rhinol Laryngol 105:280–285

85. Omori K, Slavit DH, Kacker A, Blaugrund St M (1996) Quantitative criteria for predicting thyroplasty type I outcome. Laryngoscope 106:689–693

86. Opheim O (1955) Unilateral paralysis of the vocal cord. Operative treatment. Acta Otolaryngol 45:226–230

87. Parker W (1955) Repair of a persistently patent glottis: report of a case. Ann Otol Rhinol Laryngol 64:924–930

88. Payr E (1915) Plastik am Schildknorpel zur Behebung der Folgen einseitiger Stimmbandlähmung. Dtsch Med Wochenschr 43:1265–1270

89. Remacle M, Lawson G, Hedayat A, Trussart C, Jamart J (2001) Medialization framework surgery for voice improvement after endoscopic cordectomy. Eur Arch Otorhinolaryngol 258:267–271

90. Rosen CA, Murry T, Woodson GE (1996) Migration of the anterior segment following anterior commissure advancement: a case report. J Voice 10(4):405–409

91. Rosen CA (1998) Complications of phonosurgery: results of a national survey. Laryngoscope 108(11):1697–1703

92. Sakai N, Nishizawa N, Matsushima J (1996) Thyroplasty type I with ceramic shim. Jpn Artif Organs 20(8):951–954

93. Sataloff R (2005) Voice surgery in professional voice. In: Sataloff R (ed.) The science and art of clinical care, 3rd ed., vol. III. Plural Publishing, San Diego, CA/Oxford, pp. 1137–2005

94. Sawashima M, Totsuka G, Kobayashi T, Hirose H (1968) Surgery for hoarseness due to unilateral vocal cord paralysis. Arch Otolaryngol 87:289–294

95. Schneider B, Bigenzahn W, End A, Denk DM, Klepetko W (2003) External vocal fold medialization in patients with recurrent nerve paralysis following cardiothoracic surgery. Eur J Cardiothorac Surg 23:477–483

96. Schneider B, Denk DM, Bigenzahn W (2003) Acoustic assessment of the voice quality and after medialization thyroplasty using the titanium vocal fold medialization implant (TVFMI). Otolaryngol Head Neck Surg 128:815–822

97. Schneider B, Denk DM, Bigenzahn W (2003) Functional results after external vocal fold medialization thyroplasty with the titanium vocal fold medializing Implant. Laryngoscope 113:628–634

98. Schneider B, Kneussl M, Denk DM, Bigenzahn W (2003) Aerodynamic measurements in medialization thyrpolasty. Acta Otolaryngol 123(7):883–888

99. Seiffert A (1942) Operative Wiederherstellung des Glottisschlusses bei einseitiger Recurrenslähmung und Stimmbanddefekten. Arch Ohr Nas Kehlkheilk 152:366–368

100. Sittel Ch, Zorowka P, Friedrich G, Eckel HE (2002) Surgical voice rehabilitation after laser surgery for glottic carcinoma. Ann Otol Rhinol Laryngol 111:493–499

101. Slavit DH, Maragos NE (1994) Arytenoid adduction and type I thyroplasty in the treatment of aphonia. J Voice 8(1):84–91

102. Thompson DM, Maragos NE, Edward BW (1995) The study of vocal fold vibratory patterns in patients with unilateral vocal fold paralysis before and after type I thyroplasty with or without arytenoid adduction. Laryngoscope 105: 481–486

103. Tsunoda K, Niimi S (2000) Autologous transplantation of fascia into the vocal fold. Largyngoscope 110(4):680–682

104. Tucker H (1983) Complications after surgical management of the paralysed larynx. Laryngoscope 93:295–298

105. Tucker HM (1985) Anterior commissure laryngoplasty for adjustment of vocal fold tension. Ann Otol Rhinol Laryngol 94:547–549

106. Tucker HM (1989) Laryngeal framework surgery in the management of spasmodic dysphonia. Ann Otol Rhinol Laryngol 98:52–54

107. Tucker HM (1990) Combined laryngeal framework medialization and reinnervation for unilateral vocal fold paralysis. Ann Otol Rhinol Laryngol 99:778–781

108. Tucker HM (1993) Anterior commissure repositioning for adjustment of tension in the vocal cords. Operat Tech Otolaryngol Head Neck Surg 4(3):178–182

109. Tucker HM (1993) Complications of laryngeal framework surgery for phonatory disorders. Operat Tech Otolaryngol Head Neck Surg 4(3):232–235

110. Tucker HM, Wannamaker J, Trott M (1993) Complications of laryngeal framework surgery (phonosurgery). Laryngoscope 103:525–528

111. Tucker HM (1998) Laryngeal framework surgery in the management of the aged larynx. Ann Otol Rhinol Laryngol 97:534–536

112. Uloza V, Pribuisiene R, Saferis V (2005) Multidimensional assessment of functional outcomes of medialization Thyroplasty. Eur Arch Otolaryngol 262:616–621

113. Waltner JG (1958) Surgical rehabilitation of voice following laryngofissure. Arch Otolaryngol 67:99–101

114. Wanamaker JR, Netterville JL, Ossof RH (1993) Phonosurgery: silastic medialization for unilateral vocal fold paralysis. Operat Tech Otolaryngol Head Neck Surg 4(3):207–217

115. Weinmann EC, Maragos NE (2000) Airway compromise in thyroplasty surgery. Laryngoscope 110(7):1082–1085

116. Woo P, Genack S (1995) Thyroarytenoid myectomy: a new surgical alternative for intractable spasmodic dysphonia. Trans Am Broncho-Esophagol Ass 95:187–192

117. Woodson GE, Murry T (1994) Glottic configuration after arytenoid adduction. Laryngoscope 104:965–969

118. Zeitels MS, Hochmann I, Hillman RE (1998) Adduction arytenopexy: a new procedure for paralytic dysphonia with implications for implant medialization. Ann Otol Rhinol Laryngol 107:173, 1–24

119. Zeitels MS, Desloge RB, Hillman RE, Bunting GA (1999) Cricothyroid subluxation: a new innovation for enhancing the voice with laryngoplastic phonosurgery. Ann Otol Rhinol Laryngol 108:1126–1131

120. Zeitels St, Mauri M, Dailey S (2003) Medialization laryngoplasty with Gore-Tex for voice restoration secondary to glottal incompetence: indications and observations. Ann Otol Rhinol Laryngol 112:180–184

121. Zeitels SM, Mauri M, Dailey SH (2004) Adduction arytenopexy for vocal fold paralysis: indications and technique. J Laryngol Otol 118:508–516

Laryngeal Surgery in Children

6

Frederik G. Dikkers, Niels Rasmussen, and Patrick Froehlich

Core Messages

> Laryngeal surgery in children is different from laryngeal surgery in adults and optimally requires a specialized team or staff dedicated to the treatment of children. The anesthesiological approach is related to the age of the patient and is of decisive importance.

> Maturation of the vocal folds is a delicate process, and superficial and intermediate layers are well defined with a mature vocal ligament by age 16.

> *Congenital or acquired cysts* are mostly supraglottic retention cysts.

> Neonates who have been intubated for a long time can have difficulties with detubation due to *intubation granulomas.*

> Congenital laryngeal webs and laryngeal atresia cause stridor. However, *smaller webs* cause hoarseness and breathiness.

> *Subglottic hemangiomas* progressively obstruct the airway within the first few months of life.

> In rare cases, stridor is due to *congenital laryngeal paralysis*, which may be unilateral or bilateral. It can worsen during infancy but may be well tolerated even when bilateral.

> *Juvenile onset of recurrent laryngeal papillomas* is rare but may be suspected in conjunction with progressive dysphonia. Papillomatosis is exceptional before the age of 1 year.

> *Sulcus glottidis* in children seems to be a congenital lesion that deteriorates with increasing age.

> Vocal abuse is frequent in children. The important question is whether the voice problem is the child's problem.

> Gastroesophageal reflux (GER) may cause roughness. The precise pathogenetic role of laryngopharyngeal reflux has not yet been established.

> The preoperative assessment in patients presenting with stridor is important.

> Progressive stridor in infants, degree of suprasternal retraction, and failure to thrive are elements that lead to the decision for performing endoscopy under general anesthesia. Some give antacids at least for as long as stridor is not controlled and/or appropriate surgical treatment has not been performed.

6.1 Introduction

This chapter deals with the indications for surgery and surgical treatment of benign pathology of the larynx excluding congenital laryngeal lesions with stenosis and laryngomalacia, which is dealt with in chapter XXX. Laryngeal surgery in children is different from laryngeal surgery in adults. It optimally requires a specialized team of staff dedicated to the treatment of children.

F. G. Dikkers (✉)
Department of Otorhinolaryngology, University Medical Center Groningen, University of Groningen,
P.O. box 30001, 9700 RB Groningen, The Netherlands
e-mail: f.g.dikkers@kno.umcg.nl

M. Remacle, H. E. Eckel (eds.), *Surgery of Larynx and Trachea,*
DOI: 10.1007/978-3-540-79136-2_6, © Springer-Verlag Berlin Heidelberg 2010

Diagnostic procedures, expected pathology, and treatment depend on the age of the patient. The possibilities for communicating with the child and the use of more sophisticated examination procedures increase with age. In relation to the surgical procedures, the anesthesiological approach is related to the age of the patient and is of decisive importance; it is dealt with in further detail later. When delineating the indications for surgery, the small size of the larynx in small children must, of course, be taken into account. The total vocal fold length is 6–8 mm in the infant; it increases to 12–17 mm in the adult woman and to 17–23 mm in the adult man [8].

Maturation of the vocal folds is a delicate process. Superficial and intermediate layers are well defined with a mature vocal ligament by age 16 [5]. This has consequences for the pathology or the importance of the pathology depending on the age of the patient. Voice mutation is most active between ages 12 and 14 and is usually complete in both sexes by age 15 [9].

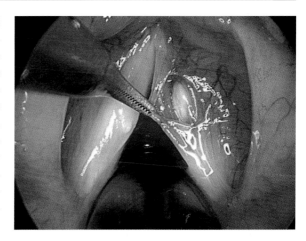

Fig. 6.1. Subepithelial cyst in a 12-year-old boy. Epithelium is held with a small alligator forceps angled to the right

6.2 Indications

Children considered for elective laryngeal surgery are patients with hoarseness and/or increasing stridor. These symptoms may be caused by a number of lesions and must be distinguished from nonorganic conditions due to improper use of the voice.

Congenital or acquired cysts can cause hoarseness. Pediatric cysts, especially in the young infant, are mostly supraglottic retention cysts. In the older infant (from the age of approximately 6 years), epithelial cysts and retention cysts on the vocal folds do exist (Fig. 6.1). Subglottic cysts in premature children can cause distress after several months, especially when intubation was necessary during the neonatal period.

Neonates who have been intubated for a long time can have difficulties with detubation owing to *intubation granulomas* (Fig. 6.2). These granulomas must be addressed when the laryngeal pathology is what is hampering detubation.

Congenital laryngeal webs and laryngeal atresia cause stridor (see Chapter XXX), and *smaller webs* (Fig. 6.3) cause hoarseness and breathiness. They may easily be overlooked during flexible laryngoscopy. This makes it a not uncommon finding during elective direct laryngoscopy under general anesthesia.

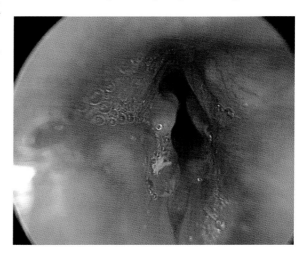

Fig. 6.2. Intubation granulomas in a 3-month-old boy immediately after detubation

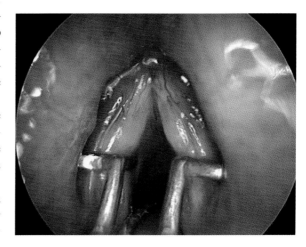

Fig. 6.3. Microweb in an anterior commissure in a 6-year-old boy. The vocal folds are spread using the anterior commissure retractor

Subglottic hemangiomas progressively obstruct the airway within the first few months of life. They may be suspected in children presumed to have laryngitis within the first 3 months of life when episodes are repeated or persist. They can be associated with cutaneous hemangiomas. Beard-shaped hemangiomas, however, are almost constantly associated with laryngeal hemangiomas. Extension downward to the trachea or upward to the glottis and supraglottic region can limit surgical control.

In rare cases stridor is due to *congenital laryngeal paralysis*, which may be unilateral or bilateral. It can worsen during infancy but may be well tolerated even when bilateral. Stridor is associated with dysphonia. The diagnosis is difficult by fiberlaryngoscopy in the outpatient clinic owing to difficulties associated with cooperation with the patient. It may be difficult under general anesthesia as well, as it has to be performed without relaxation to be able to examine laryngeal motility.

Juvenile onset of recurrent laryngeal papillomas (Fig. 6.4) is also rare but may be suspected in progressive dysphonia. Papillomatosis is exceptional before the age of 1 year. In such early cases it appears to be correlated with the presence of condylomas in the genital region of the mother at the time of delivery. In these cases, increasing stridor is frequently the cause for examination and treatment. In children older than 2 years, stridor increasingly becomes a secondary sign as the progressive dysphonia itself usually brings the child to the laryngologist.

Sulcus glottidis (Fig. 6.5) seems to be a congenital lesion that deteriorates with increasing age. The sulcus, which runs parallel to the edge of the vocal fold, may be short or run the entire length of the vocal fold. It can be localized just below the edge of the vocal fold but may also appear on the horizontal part or the inferior part. It may occur together with *cysts* and *epithelial bridges* and may be unilateral or bilateral. It may cause hoarseness, breathiness, difficulty when singing due to high-pitch problems, and vocal fatigue. Frequently, the sulcus is not detected during videolaryngostroboscopy, as the sulcus may appear only as a faint line on the epithelial surface or may not be visible (when it occurs on the inferior aspect of the vocal cord). The indications for surgery are heavily debated as is whether it should be done during childhood or the growth development of the larynx should be finished before surgery [3].

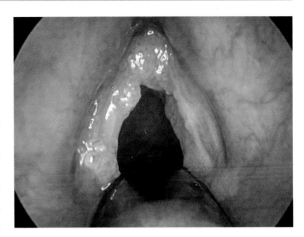

Fig. 6.4. Juvenile onset laryngeal papillomatosis in a 7 year old boy with many years of hoarseness that aggravated during the preceding 6 months, seen with the rigid telescope

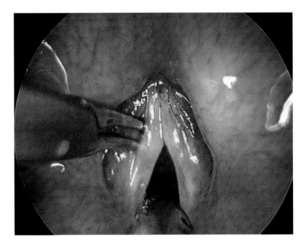

Fig. 6.5. Bilateral sulcus glottitis in a 6-year-old boy, with small alligator forceps to the right in the left sulcus

Vocal abuse is frequent in children. This may be due to a number of reasons, such as social background, family habits, participation in certain sports, and imitation of popular but noisy cartoon characters from television. If the child is unable to use the voice in a balanced quantity, the price may be hoarseness. In a number of cases, the condition leads to formation of *vocal fold nodules* (i.e., bilateral lesions on the border of the anterior and middle third of the vocal folds) (Fig. 6.6). Some children have a larynx that seems predisposed to the development of vocal fold nodules (Fig. 6.7). The coincidence of both an anterior commissure web and vocal fold nodules has been described in adults [2, 7].

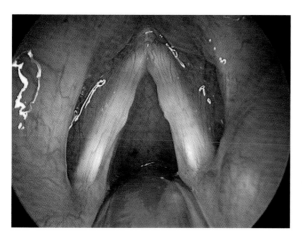

Fig. 6.6. Vocal fold nodules in an 11-year-old boy

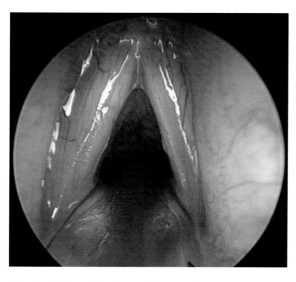

Fig. 6.7. Microweb in the anterior commissure and vocal fold nodules in a 5-year-old girl

Gastroesophageal reflux (GER) may cause roughness. A degree of physiological GER exists in infants. The prevalence of laryngopharyngeal reflux in hoarse children was calculated using the mode of presentation of the hoarseness, associated symptoms, endoscopic findings, laboratory testing, and therapeutic interventions and their outcomes [1]. The conclusion was that laryngopharyngeal reflux appeared to be a common cause of hoarseness in children. However, as with laryngeal disease in adults, the precise pathogenetic role of laryngopharyngeal reflux has not yet been established.

6.3　Preoperative Assessment

6.3.1　Patients Presenting with Stridor

Progressive stridor in infants, the degree of suprasternal retraction, and failure to thrive are elements that lead to the decision to perform endoscopy under general anesthesia. Depending on the local custom, a diagnostic approach may be made in the outpatient clinic by visualizing the larynx using a fiberlaryngoscope with a diameter of ≤ 2 mm.

Treatment of associated reflux varies among institutions. Some give antacids at least as long as stridor is not controlled and/or appropriate surgical treatment has not been performed. Ultrasonography, including assessment of the vascular flow, is useful for diagnosing tracheal compression due to vascular anomalies such as a double aortic arch or an innominate artery. Vascular anomalies such as a "vascular ring" can also be suggested by barium swallow radiography.

The use of endoscopy under general anesthesia depends on the efficiency of antacids and evolution of the stridor, on outpatient fiberlaryngoscopy, the age at which stridor developed, and its severity. Endoscopy can be useful to determine the diagnosis and for treatment.

6.3.2　Patients Presenting with Voice Problems

Preoperative assessment depends on the age of the child. The following age groups are relevant: sucklings and toddlers, infants 2–5 years old, infants 5–7 years old, children 8 years old to puberty (Table 6.1).

Sucklings and toddlers rarely need elective voice surgery, so the preoperative assessment has not been standardized. The second age group is the infant—old enough to give answers personally but too young to read and write. This age group is approximately 2–5 years old. The third age group consists of children learning to read and write but still young and easily frightened, approximately 5–7 or 8 years old. Preoperative assessment is limited in this group. The fourth and final age group consists of the older child, who can reason (approximately 8 years and older). The larynx should be considered as a pediatric larynx up to the time of voice mutation. Of course, the age groups may be adjusted.

Table 6.1. Preoperative assessment in children with voice problems, depending on the age group

Parameter	Sucklings and toddlers	Infants (2–5 years)	Young children (6–8 years)	Children (9–15 years)
History	+	+	+	+
Voice-related interests (e.g., choir, shouting during sporting activities)	–	–	+	+
GRBAS	–	–	+	+
Posture of patient, breathing pattern, resonance, articulation	–	+	+	+
Voice analysis on an extended vowel	–	±	+	+
Voice range profile	–	±	+	+
Phonation times	–	–	+	+
Investigation of functional tasks	–	–	+	+
Rigid laryngostroboscopy	–	–	+	+
Ability to read and write	–	–	+	+

GRBAS is a psychoacoustic evaluation, where G refers to grade, R to roughness, B to breathiness, A to asthenicity, S to strain

History taking should include a description of the voice problem, voice use, previous voice training, and differences between the speaking and singing voices. The important question is whether the voice problem is the child's problem (one cannot understand the child), the teacher's problem (difficulties at school), or the parent's problem (feeling ashamed of the child's voice). When and why did the problems start? Have intubations been performed—how many and when? What irritating factors are present (passive smoking, allergy)?

All external factors negatively influencing the voice can be captured under Voice Related Interests (Table 6.1). These interests can be clear and obvious (i.e., the child is a lead singer in the school's musical) or hidden (i.e., the child is the third child in a family with a handicapped sibling who receives major parental attention). Of course, sporting activities (Is the child captain of the soccer team?) should be included in the history taking.

GRBAS is depiction of the psychoacoustic evaluation [4]. G refers to grade, R to roughness, B to breathiness, A to asthenicity, S to strain. All qualities can be scored 0 (normal) to 3 (extremely abnormal). GRBAS is scored by the speech and language therapist (SLT). For this assessment, the international GRBAS score is used while the patient is reading a standard text loudly as well as during spontaneous speech. The posture of the patient, the breathing pattern, resonance, and articulation are described by the SLT.

An electronic voice analysis is done by examining the signal produced when singing an open //a// ("extended vowel") and calculating a number of measures such as perturbation factors: jitter and shimmer.

Ideally, the assessment continues by creating a Voice Range Profile (Phonetogram) in which dynamic and melodic ranges are reproduced graphically. Measuring the Phonation Time (s) is performed on /aa/, /zz/, and /ss/. Finally, various functional Voice Tasks are investigated to determine if any change in voice quality can be heard. This is performed to predict the potential learning ability of the patient concerning speech therapy.

Rigid laryngostroboscopy can be performed in most children ≥ 10 years of age. Depending on the level of confidence of the child in the physician, laryngostroboscopy can be tried in children as young as 6 years, sometimes even younger. Using modern recording devices, a fair description of the larynx can be provided in an image of <1 second. Of course, an optimal laryngostroboscopic examination requires a much longer recording time. New devices associating stroboscopy and fiberscopy are now available.

The ability of the child to read and write is assessed indirectly. At some clinics, all elective interventions are postponed until the child is able to write so the child is able to communicate during the immediate postoperative period without using the voice.

6.4 Anesthesiology Considerations

The preferred anesthesiology technique depends on the local anesthesiology teams. All techniques have advantages and disadvantages for the surgeon. Typically, elective surgery on the larynx in the pediatric patient takes place under general anesthesia. Patients are exposed to routine monitoring (body temperature, pulse oximetry, capnography, electrocardiography, respiratory rate). Venous access is applied.

Hemodynamic and respiratory data as well as ventilator settings are recorded. Induction and maintenance of anesthesia are accomplished through the airway and intravenously. During the induction of anesthesia the laryngologist is in the operating theater to secure the airway in case of emergency. Depending on local routines and the specific setting determined by the clinical problem, dynamic evaluation of the airway is performed at that phase. This can be accomplished with a fiberscope or under direct vision, allowing a diagnosis to be made, (i.e., supraglottic obstruction and laryngeal mobility). Laryngeal mobility may also be evaluated at the end of endoscopy as the child wakes up.

The airway is sprayed with lidocaine 4% (with a maximum of 4 mg/kg) by the laryngologist when a profound level of anesthesia has been attained. A first assessment of the intubation possibilities can thus be obtained. If a standard orotracheal intubation is performed, the tube is moved to the left corner of the mouth. Anesthesiology tubes and cables are kept on the left side of the patient, as the typical setting has the surgical team on the right and the anesthesiology team on the left (Fig. 6.8).

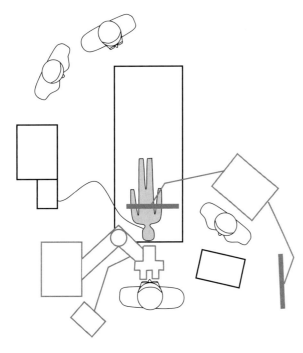

Fig. 6.8. Typical setting during elective laryngeal surgery in children

6.4.1 Spontaneous Ventilation Technique

Surgery on patients with an airway problem should be performed with a so-called dynamic airway. The patient is asleep but breathes spontaneously. Anesthesiology requirements are presented in Chapter XXX. Spontaneous ventilation allows a full endoscopic view of the airway for both stridor and voice problems. It has the advantage of allowing endoscopic surgery of the larynx on all areas and using several tools in the field. It requires an anesthesiology team that is specifically trained and remains familiar with the technique. Maintaining spontaneous ventilation can be difficult in neonates of low weight and in premature infants. Intermittent apnea can occur when obstruction makes ventilation difficult. A first step of ventilation through a bronchoscope or an endotracheal tube can help make spontaneous ventilation feasible.

6.4.2 Endoscopy with Endotracheal Intubation and Relaxation

The conventional orotracheal tube may be preferred when the patient suffers from heart-lung disease, making a closed ventilation circuit desirable; when access to the larynx is difficult; or when complications causing prolonged ventilation are anticipated. If necessary, the orotracheal tube can be elongated. For this purpose, the proximal end of a small tube can be inserted in the distal end of a tube two sizes larger (e.g., a 3.5 tube in a 4.5 tube). Detubation should be performed before cough reflexes return. A technique called "deep detubation" may be applied. Here, the patient remains paralyzed and ventilated, and the tube is removed by the surgeon under direct vision. In this way, manipulation of the vocal fold with the cuff of the endotracheal tube can be controlled by the surgeon. After removing the tube, mask ventilation is resumed until the patient awakes without phonating or coughing.

6.4.3 High-Frequency Jet Ventilation

The technique of high-frequency jet ventilation (HFJV) may be used in all cases other than those already discussed. It has the advantage of giving the surgeon more working space inside the larynx, especially in relation to

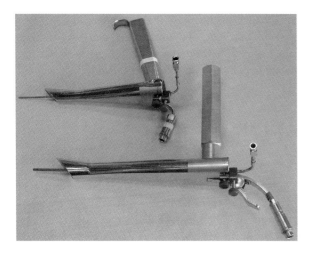

Fig. 6.9. Example of jet ventilation laryngoscopes with a steel tube that is passed through the glottis. The two laryngoscopes (one for children and one for adults) are sufficient to cover all age groups

the posterior commissure. It can be performed using a thin catheter introduced through the nose and passed through the larynx by the anesthetist; or it may be performed using a thin steel tube mounted inside the laryngoscope (Fig. 6.9) and inserted by the laryngologist. The steel tube may be passed through the glottis or be positioned with the end placed inside the laryngoscope. Using a steel tube has two advantages. First, it makes it easier to keep the tube away from the pathology to be operated on. Second, it is nonflammable when using laser. The HFJV technique does not prevent blood, mucus, or other debris from entering the trachea from the larynx, but the air stream blowing from the trachea through the larynx limits this problem in most cases. In patients with severe GER, HFJV may not be suitable owing to the risk of aspiration of gastric juices to the unprotected lower airways. However, as there is no cuff, HFJV eliminates the possibility of accidental puncture of the cuff during laser surgery and manipulation of the vocal cords with the deflated cuff during detubation.

6.4.4 Intermittent Apnea Technique

The intermittent apnea technique may be used in cases of foreign bodies or pathology that can be easily removed under direct vision. In cases of impossible detubation due to suspicion of intubation granulomas, inspection may reveal that these granulomas are the only probable cause for the detubation difficulties.

6.5 Instrumentation

Surgical instruments used for elective laryngeal surgery in children are similar, but smaller, than the instruments used in adults. However, frequently adult laryngoscopes can be used in young patients from the age of 4–5 years, which makes instrumentation easier. For stridor surgery, laryngoscopes that are open on one side make it easier to introduce the instruments into the field. Several models are available with a ventilation canal. It allows administering the anesthetic gas at the tip of the laryngoscope, close to the larynx. Various sizes are available, from those that are appropriate for neonates to others that can be used in teenagers. One should be equipped with a wide range of laryngoscopes, appropriate for each age group. Many fine laryngoscopes have been developed, and many surgeons prefer their own laryngoscopes, so no names of instruments are mentioned here. A sufficient number of telescopes should be readily available for documentation.

The laryngoscope is suspended using a chest support, which should be mounted on a table just above the chest of the patient (Fig. 6.10) so it does not hamper chest excursions during ventilation.

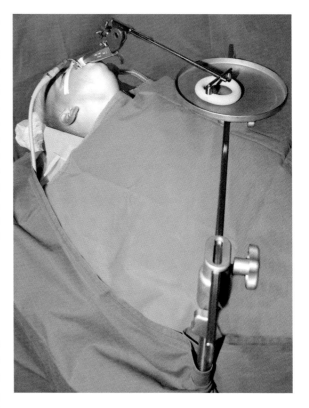

Fig. 6.10. Chest support is mounted on a table just above the patient's chest

Surgery takes place with a surgical microscope or with a telescope and a video monitor. The magnification can be calculated as

$$M_t = (F_{tub}/F_{obj}) \times M_{factor} \times M_{eyepiece}$$

where M_t = the magnification total; F_{tub} = the focal length of the tube; F_{obj} = the focal length of the objective; M_{factor} = the factor of magnification of the zoom; $M_{eyepiece}$ = the magnification factor of the eyepiece.

Standard values are F_{tub} = 170 mm, F_{obj} = 400 mm, M_{factor} = 2.4, and $M_{eyepiece}$ = 12.5. Using this calculation, a total magnification of 12.75 can be obtained. However, progress in the development of telescopes and the quality of cameras—digital cameras and high-definition cameras—are progressively changing habits in laryngeal surgery for stridor. They might replace or complement the microscope and give a higher quality image on the video screen in combination with greater mobility around the surgical field.

6.5.1 Cold Instrumentation

For the surgery proper, it is necessary to have a basic set of surgical tools.

- Adequate suction (tubes 1, 2, and 3 mm diameter, with side holes distally to prevent aspiration of tissue)
- Small alligator forceps, angled to the left and to the right
- Open heart-shaped forceps, angled to the left and to the right
- Scissors, straight and angled to the left and to the right
- Elevators, 1 mm wide, angled 15 ("degrees") to the left and to the right
- Elevators, 1 mm wide, angled 90 ("degrees") to the left and to the right
- Disposable endolaryngeal knives
- Anterior commissure retractor

6.5.2 Lasers

Several lasers are available, CO_2 lasers being the most frequently used in pediatric laryngeal surgery. Soft fibers are now available for CO_2 lasers. Its limitations are due to diffusion and the size of the spot. YAG and KTP lasers have fewer applications in children and have induced subglottic and supraglottic stenosis. New lasers, such as the thulium laser, with soft fibers are under evaluation.

6.5.3 Microdebriders

Microdebriders with specific laryngeal blades are available and have been proposed for excision of tumors (papillomas, hemangiomas, cysts). They allow excision and suction with the same instrument and have been shown to be highly effective. The technique requires careful use so it does not damage normal structures (i.e., the basic structures of the vocal folds). Therefore, high-definition visualization of the operative field is necessary.

6.5.4 Drugs and Additional Endoscopic techniques

Drugs have been proposed to be applied endoscopically in association with other steps of surgery or as sole use during endoscopy. Topical mitomycin has been used at the end of surgical procedure to limit the risk of scarring and subsequent stenosis. Cidofovir is a nucleoside analogue that is injected within the papillomas during endoscopy combined with excision of papillomas. Narrow-band imaging can be applied. This relies on the principle of depth of penetration of light, with the narrow-band blue light having a short wavelength (415 nm) penetrating into the mucosa and highlighting the superficial vasculature [6].

6.6 Surgical Intervention

Various surgical approaches are available for stridor. When several methods are available for treating stridor with comparable results, a preference is made to avoid tracheostomy and postoperative intubation if possible. Endoscopic methods have been developed in recent years to reach this goal. New tools have been found useful and are part of the explanation for a revival of endoscopic laryngeal surgery.

6.6.1 General Aspects

The patient is lying in a supine position. Essentially, the intervention is carried out as in adults. The patient is under general anesthesia. The head is put in a raised and extended position, also called the sniffing position. The patient's head is in line with the end of the operation table. The back of the head is placed in a surgical cushion, and the neck is supported with a roll. The teeth are protected with a teeth protector, and the laryngoscope is introduced. The laryngoscope is then fixed with a chest support on a table (Fig. 6.10). The camera or the microscope is focused on the larynx, with maximum magnification as indicated earlier. Mucus is sucked away, and appropriate pictures can be taken.

The intervention continues with palpation of the vocal folds, using blunt instruments as well as the anterior commissure retractor (Fig. 6.3). Instruments should be kept in the contralateral hand: scissors curved to the right should be kept in the left hand, and vice versa. Suction should be performed with tubes of 1 or 2 mm diameter. The side holes distally prevent aspiration of tissue.

6.6.2 Subglottic Hemangioma

Several options have been developed to control a *subglottic hemangioma* avoiding a tracheotomy. Endoscopic reduction of hemangiomas was first proposed using CO_2 laser. It proved useful for small lateral hemangiomas but could induce subglottic stenosis in larger ones. Open surgical excision was then developed until other lasers (i.e., KTP and thulium lasers) became available. Microdebriders have also been used to excise hemangiomas under spontaneous ventilation without postoperative intubation or short-term intubation. Whatever technique is proposed, it should limit the risk of adding stenosis. Mitomycin can be applied at the end of the procedure to try to limit this risk.

6.6.3 Bilateral Paralysis

Bilateral paralysis can be critical for the airway. Open laryngoplasty with posterior cricoid graft has given excellent results, which have also been obtained through an endoscopic approach consisting of unilateral or bilateral posterior cordectomy. The debate remains on when to choose a surgical option as spontaneous recovery can be observed during the first years of life. Some teams prefer to wait for this with a tracheotomy in place. Comparison of the morbidity associated with a tracheotomy and that of the various procedures is part of the debate.

6.6.4 Recurrent Papillomatosis

Recurrent papillomatosis of the larynx is managed in different ways from one center to another. Excision can be performed with cold instruments, CO_2 laser, or microdebriders. As the recurrence rate is usually high, one should preserve the vocal cords as much as possible. Cidofovir has been used with interesting short and midterm results without damaging the normal tissues and, in the best cases, allowing the larynx to return to normal. No curative treatment is available so far.

6.6.5 Small Anterior Webs

Small anterior webs can be divided endoscopically. Recurrence of the web may be limited by application of mitomycin at the end of the procedure.

6.6.6 Vocal Fold Nodules and Polyps

Epithelial pathology is cut off using a heart-shaped forceps to the ipsilateral side and a knife or scissors to the opposite side, taking care not to damage the anterior commissure. The intervention can then be terminated.

6.6.7 Cysts, Epithelial Bridges, and Sulcus Glottidis

Subepithelial pathology is removed by performing chordotomy with a disposable knife. Injection of saline or saline with a vasoconstringent such as epinephrine in Reinke's space may be useful. A cyst can be bluntly dissected and displayed nicely (Fig. 6.1). The safest way to treat a sulcus appears to be by simple removal of the deep, adherent part of the sulcus. After chordotomy, the epithelial flap may be glued back using fibrin glue or left to heal spontaneously depending on the extent of loose epithelium.

6.6.8 Intubation Granulomas

Intubation granulomas (Fig. 6.2) may be left to disappear spontaneously, but if their size hampers a free airway—especially during an attempt to extubate—these granulomas should be removed with the intermittent apnea technique. Using the intermittent apnea technique, it is possible to administer mitomycin C. Small pads soaked in mitomycin C (5 mg/ml) are held on the wound for 2 minutes. The patient is then ventilated again, and after reoxygenation the wound is cleaned with pads soaked in 0.9% saline. After this apneic period the patient is awakened.

6.7 Postoperative Care

After surgery for obstructive airway, antacids are generally used to cover at least the healing period. If postoperative intubation was avoided but there is residual stridor, epinephrine and steroids can be given.

After a phonosurgical intervention the patient is generally put on voice rest. The definition of voice rest is under discussion, as is the application. For the first author of this chapter, voice rest means total silence: no speaking, whispering, laughing, or crying. The patient and parents are counseled on total postoperative silence twice: when the indication for intervention is made and the day before the intervention. The child is aware of this, and takes paper or a laptop with him during admission in the hospital. Postoperatively, the child is informed about the surgical findings and is shown pictures made during the intervention; the importance of voice rest is stressed again.

The duration of voice rest depends on the surgical technique applied. In the case of an epithelial intervention there is a small wound, which heals fast. Voice rest is applied for the day of the intervention and the first 2 days afterward. In the case of a subepithelial intervention there is a larger wound, which heals more slowly. In these cases, voice rest is applied for the day of the intervention and the following 5 days.

Two weeks after the intervention the patient is interviewed and seen at the Voice Clinic, where videolaryngostroboscopy takes place. The patient is encouraged to use the voice normally again but is discouraged from using the voice for singing or during sporting activities for an additional 2 or 3 weeks. Typically, no voice therapy is prescribed.

In contrast, the second author believes that there is no age limit for performing elective surgery, and the child and parents are only instructed to speak as little as possible, preferably pointing or gesturing to ask for something, during the same periods mentioned above according to the degree of the pathology. This is because it is presumed that children are basically unable to refrain completely from speaking unless they are strictly brought up. Thus, the patient might feel guilty if the operation is not successful and believe that it was due to him or her speaking. (There is no literature proving the effect of complete voice rest postoperatively.) As with adults, they are also instructed not to shout or whisper during the above-mentioned immediate postoperative period. Singing and/or returning to school should be postponed until complete healing has taken place, which varies from 10 days for small lesions up to 3 weeks for large lesions. Voice therapy may be applied when the healing is complete in cases where vocal abuse is presumed to be of pathogenic importance, such as with the formation of vocal nodules or in patients with continuing hoarseness despite a normal appearance of the vocal cords.

The patient is asked to return 3–4 months postoperatively for the final visit. At that time extensive postoperative voice rating is conducted by the speech and language therapist, comparable to the tests performed preoperatively (Table 6.1).

6.8 Tips and Pearls

• Surgical instruments used for elective laryngeal surgery in children are similar, but smaller, than the instruments used in adults. One should be equipped with a wide range of laryngoscopes, fitted for each age group.

- For the surgery, it is necessary to have a basic set of surgical tools, which have been described in detail in chapter 6.5.1.
- Several lasers are available, with CO_2 lasers being the most frequently used in pediatric laryngeal surgery.
- Microdebriders have shown to be highly effective. The technique requires careful use so normal structures are not damaged.
- After surgery for an obstructed airway, antacids are generally used to cover at least the healing period. If postoperative intubation was avoided but there is residual stridor, epinephrine and steroids can be given.
- After phonosurgical intervention the patient is generally put on voice rest.

References

1. Block BB, Brodsky L (2007) Hoarseness in children: the role of laryngopharyngeal reflux. Int J Ped Otorhinolaryngol 71: 1361–1369
2. Ford CN, Bless DN, Campos G, Leddy M (1994) Anterior commissure microwebs associated with vocal nodules: detection, prevalence, and significance. Laryngoscope 104(11 Pt 1): 1369–1375
3. Giovanni A, Chanteret C, Lagier A (2007) Sulcus vocalis: a review. Eur Arch Otorhinolaryngol 264:337–344
4. Hirano M (1981) Clinical examination of the voice. Springer, New York, pp. 83–84
5. Hirano M, Kurita S, Nakashima T (1981) The structure of the vocal folds. In: Stevens KN, Hirano M (eds) Vocal fold physiology. University of Tokyo Press, Tokyo, pp. 33–44
6. Piazza C, Dessouky O, Peretti G, Cocco D, De Benedetto L, Nicolai P (2008) Narrow-band imaging: a new tool for evaluation of head and neck squamous cell carcinomas. Review of the literature. Acta Otorhinolaryngol Ital 28: 49–54
7. Ruiz DM, Pontes P, Behlau M, Richieri-Costa A (2006) Laryngeal microweb and vocal nodules. Clinical study in a Brazilian population. Folia Phoniatr Logop 58:392–399
8. Sataloff RT, Linville SE (2005) The effects of age on the voice. In: Sataloff RT, ed. Professional voice, the science and art of clinical care, 3rd ed. Plural Publishing, San Diego, pp. 497–511
9. Thurman L, Klitzke CA (1994) Voice education and health care for young voices. In: Benninger MS, Jacobson BH, Johson AF (eds) Vocal arts medicine: the care and prevention of professional voice disorders. Thieme Medical Publishers, New York, pp. 266–288

Surgery for Benign Tumors of the Adult Larynx

7

David G. Grant, Martin A. Birchall, and Patrick J. Bradley

Core Messages

> Benign neoplasms of the larynx are uncommon, with the exception of papillomas, which comprise up to 95% of this group.

> Symptoms associated with these benign tumors reflect site and size; in general, dysphonia, dyspnea, and dysphagia are the most common patient complaints and a cause should be thoroughly sought.

> The diagnosis of a benign laryngeal neoplasm, although suspected by the duration of the history and the physical examination, must be confirmed by biopsy or at least investigation when a vascular neoplasm is suspected (e.g., hemangioma or paraganglioma).

> Certain tumors have a predilection for anatomical sites in the larynx. The supraglottis is the most common site (80%), followed by the glottis and subglottis. This information may hinder the accuracy of the diagnosis if one relies on the clinical examination alone.

> Once diagnosed, most benign neoplasms can be treated by surgical excision. The surgical approach and excision depend on the tumor size and location; but in general, preservation of laryngeal function is the primary aim of treatment in the form of complete excision with tumor-free margins.

> Certain neoplasms—papillomas, oncocytic tumors, pleomorphic adenoma, lymphangiomas, neurofibromas, fibromatosis, paragangliomas, rhabdomyomas—have a tendency to recur, be it months or even years, following incomplete excision.

> Differentiation of benign from malignant tumors is vital. Paragangliomas, neurofibromas, and chondromas, among others, have malignant variants, with certain granular cell tumors, hemangiopericytomas, and others having histological features that mimic those of malignant disease. Reliance on expert histopathologists is crucial for accurate, appropriate treatment.

> With improvements in imaging, histopathology, and surgical techniques—endoscopy, microscopic magnification, application of lasers—there has been marked improvement in the accuracy of diagnosis and the ability to perform precision excision surgery for benign tumors. This means more preservation and restoration of laryngeal function than was previously possible.

7.1 Introduction

7.1.1 Background

The delicate balance between surgery and preservation of organ function can have no greater illustration than within the larynx. Treatment of any laryngeal disorder requires a detailed knowledge of both diagnostic

D. G. Grant (✉)
Specialist Registrar, Bristol Royal Infirmary,
Upper Maudin Street, Bristol BS2 8HW, UK
e-mail: mail@davisgrant.com

and therapeutic surgical interventions and their impact on vocal and laryngeal function. Whereas the objectives of surgery for malignant tumors permit a more pyrrhic approach, surgery for benign laryngeal tumors demands particular consideration and application. Furthermore, a thorough appreciation of the pathological processes at work and their prognostic significance aid surgeons in making the best possible treatment choices for their patients.

7.1.2 General Principles

The presence of a mass lesion in the larynx can provoke numerous acute, chronic, progressive, or even life-threatening symptoms. When assessing the patient with a potential laryngeal tumor, a thorough history should be taken with particular emphasis on the age of the patient, the temporal course of the symptom complex, the presence of infection, any previous surgery or trauma, and the presence or absence of respiratory, vocal, or swallowing symptoms—all of which give clues as to the nature and extent of any tumor. Although the experienced laryngologist may be able to make an accurate clinical diagnosis using a flexible nasendoscope in the outpatient clinic, evidence suggests that the accuracy of diagnosis based on visual examination alone is subject to some variation [10].

The initial decision to operate depends on detailed visual inspection of the lesion, histological diagnosis, and a need to establish that the tumor is not malignant. Also, a contemporary meticulous endoscopic examination of the entire upper aerodigestive tract is required to assess the size, position, consistency, and extent of any tumor, in addition to excluding any concurrent aerodigestive tract pathology. Furthermore, information relating to endoscopic and surgical access and the potential for resection should be carefully considered when planning future definitive surgical management. Indications for surgery beyond this first therapeutic step include failure of conservative measures, symptomatic relief, maintenance of organ function, and concern about any potential for malignant transformation. Ultimately, the method by which resection is done is dependent on both tumor and patient factors, the experience of the operating surgeon, and the facilities available to them.

7.1.3 Classification

The definition of noncancerous or benign tumors of the larynx requires some elaboration. In 1938, New and Erich [51] published the Mayo Clinic experience of 722 patients presenting with benign laryngeal pathology. The authors proposed that as true proliferative neoplasms were often clinically indistinguishable from nonproliferative inflammatory or hyperplastic growths the term *benign tumor* should be used to encompass all abnormal growths of tissue in the larynx that lacked malignant or metastatic properties. In 1951, a similar analysis of 1197 patients with benign laryngeal growths by Holinger and Johnstone [30] assented to the New and Erich recommendation. Since then, some authors have revised the concept, classifying vocal fold nodules, laryngeal polyps, cysts, and nonspecific granulomas to be mucosal reactive inflammatory disorders and therefore nonneoplastic in nature [5].

Notwithstanding these various viewpoints, the principles of management remain analogous. A nomenclature based on the authoritative surgical head and neck pathological tomes [5, 44] is shown in Table 7.1. True benign neoplastic tumors of the larynx are rare (Table 7.2). New and Erich [51] reported around 210 such tumors in a series of 722 patients presenting over a 30-year period. Among them, 194 of the 210 (92%) were squamous papillomas. Holinger and Johnstone [31] reported a similar series collected over 15 years. They reported 125 true benign tumors, of which 115 (92%) were papillomas. In a series from Pittsburgh, Barnes [5] reported 404 true benign neoplasms over a period of 38 years. Among these patients, 326 (81%) had papillomas; the remaining 78 (19%) were classified as nonpapilloma lesions. A combined European series from the university departments in Marburg and Giessen, Germany, reported [23] 181 true benign neoplasms in a series of 2223 benign tumors or tumor-like lesions. Of these tumors, only 32 were not papilloma-related. Contemporary series concur with these early findings and show that the papilloma accounts for up to 95% of all nonmalignant laryngeal tumors [50] (Table 7.2). Thus, otolaryngologists may expect to see only a handful of cases during their careers.

The present chapter concentrates on surgery for those lesions considered "true" benign proliferative neoplastic tumors. We reserve the management of

Table 7.1. Pathological classification of benign laryngeal tumors

Epithelial
Squamous epithelium
    Recurrent respiratory papillomatosis
    Keratinized papilloma
Glandular
    Pleomorphic adenoma
    Oncocytic tumor
Nonepithelial
Vascular
    Hemangioma
    Lymphangioma
Cartilage and bone
    Chondroma
    Giant cell tumor
Muscle
    Leiomyoma
    Rhabdomyoma
    Angiomyoma
    Epithelioid leiomyoma
Adipose
    Lipoma
Neural
    Neurilemoma
    Neurofibroma
    Paraganglioma
    Granular cell
Pseudotumors
    Fibroma
    Inflammatory fibroblastic
    Amyloid
    Laryngeal cysts

reactive mucosal and inflammatory lesions for another discussion.

7.2 Papillomas

7.2.1 General Considerations

Squamous papillomas are the most common benign tumors of the larynx. Barnes (2001) [5] classified papillomas into two histological types: keratinized and nonkeratinized. Keratinized papillomas (papillary keratosis) occur mainly in adults and are mostly solitary lesions that arise from the true vocal cord. Most keratinized papillomas are not related to viral infection but are associated with smoking; they can be associated with malignant transformation. Keratinized papillomas

variably recur following simple excision [5]. Recurrent respiratory papillomatosis (RRP), or nonkeratinized papilloma, is the most frequently occurring benign laryngeal neoplasm. The estimated incidence is around 4 per 100,000 population in children and 1–2 per 100,000 population in adults [13, 56]. A disease of viral etiology, RRP is both a neoplastic and an infectious phenomenon caused by the human papilloma viruses (HPV). More than 90 subtypes of HPV are recognized, with HPV-6 and HPV-11 most commonly found in laryngeal papilloma [76]. RRP occurs in response to mucosal infection with HPV and can develop on any mucosal surface of the upper aerodigestive tract. RRP has a tendency to form at anatomical sites of junctions between squamous and ciliated epithelium: papillomas occur most often at the nasal valve, the nasopharyngeal surface of the soft palate, the laryngeal surface of the epiglottis, the upper and lower margins of the ventricle, the undersurface of the vocal folds, the carina, and at bronchial spurs. The most frequently affected site at diagnosis in both the pediatric and adult populations is the larynx (Fig. 7.1).

The incidence of RRP is bimodal, giving rise to two distinct forms: juvenile onset and adult onset [14]. The juvenile onset variant RRP (JO-RRP) is more aggressive than the adult form. Most investigators consider RRP to be of adult onset if the patient is older than 16–20 years of age at diagnosis. Adult-onset RRP is diagnosed most frequently between the ages of 20 and 40 years and shows a slight male preponderance [13].

In RRP, HPV-11 subtypes have been shown to have a more aggressive clinical course, with higher rates of recurrence, poorer response to adjuvant therapy, greater respiratory spread, and increased need for tracheostomy [21]. Some authors have recommended that all patients with RRP should undergo HPV typing early in the course of the disease. Identification of those patients with high-risk subtypes would theoretically allow modification of treatment regimens, such as by early intervention with adjuvant therapy. The incidence of carcinoma developing in patients with RRP is reported at 1–7% [5, 57]. Laryngeal cancer complicating RRP has an increased association with HPV-11, HPV-16, and HPV-18 infection, previous exposure to radiation, and the JO-RRP variant [5, 22, 57]. As patients with RRP may also be heavy smokers and drinkers, larger studies are required to clarify any causal or synergistic relation that may exist between HPV (and/or its subtypes), RRP, and carcinogenesis. (Fig. 7.2)

Table 7.2. Select series of benign laryngeal tumors

	New	Holinger	Barnes	Narozny	Glanz
Series duration (years)	30	15	38	45	12[b]
Total no. of true proliferative neoplastic tumors	210	125	404	291	171
Squamous papillomas[a]					
Total	194 (92%)	115 (92%)	326 (81%)	277 (95%)	149 (82%)
Nonsquamous papillomas					
Adenoma	1	0	0	1	1
Chondroma/osteochondroma	7	2	3	2	5
Fibroma	6	0	0	0	0
Fibromatosis	0	0	1	0	0
Fibrous histiocytoma	0	0	2	1	3
Granular cell	0	0	12	2	2
Hemangioma	Unknown[c]	4	9	6	8
Lipoma	1	0	3	0	5
Lymphangioma	0	1	2	0	1
Myxoma	Unknown[c]	0	0	0	0
Neurilemoma	0	0	2	1	1
Neurofibroma	1	1	3	1	0
Nodular fasciitis	0	0	1	0	0
Oncocytic	0	0	35	0	0
Other	0	2	0	0	3
Paraganglioma	0	0	2	0	3
Adenoma	0	0	1	0	0
Rhabdomyoma	0	0	2	0	0
Total	16 (8%)[c]	10 (8%)	78 (19%)	14 (5%)	32 (18%)

[a]Includes adult and juvenile variants
[b]Two 6-year series combined
[c]Authors unsure of precise nature of many angiomas and myxomas with most estimated to be of inflammatory etiology and only "a few" true neoplasms

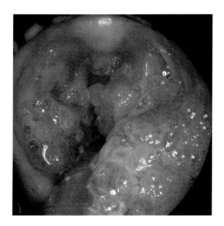

Fig. 7.1. Recurrent respiratory papillomatosis (RRP). Endoscopic view

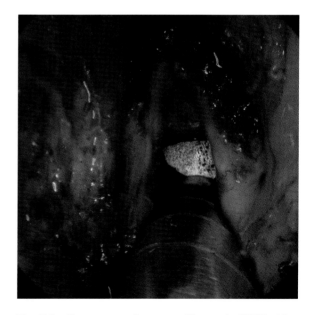

Fig. 7.2. Recurrent respiratory papillomatosis (RRP). After CO_2 laser AcuBlade ablation

7.2.2 Indications

The main indications for surgery in patients with RRP are the need for histological diagnosis, maintenance of an adequate airway, and preservation of laryngeal and vocal function. As RRP represents an as yet undefined alteration of mucosal immunosurveillance rather than a simple mechanical change, surgery for the disease is rarely curative even after en bloc resection of the papillomatous epithelium. Latent HPV DNA has been shown to be present in biopsy specimens from uninvolved sites and from patients in apparent remission. As the epithelium regenerates after surgery, reinfection occurs from virus present in this "normal"-appearing mucosa [58]. The philosophy of surgery for RRP must be altered accordingly. In this situation, the tenet of "less is more" applies. Removal of disease most commonly occurs under general anesthesia. Some patients with mild disease require only a few treatments. Patients with more aggressive variants can require monthly or bimonthly surgery to promote disease regression. This is one reason why office-based procedures are gaining popularity (see below).

7.2.3 Specific Assessment

The most common presenting symptom of RRP in adults is some degree of hoarseness or dysphonia and sometimes shortness of breath. These voice changes may be subtle and can persist for many years. Occasionally, adult-onset RRP behaves like the more aggressive juvenile variant. Here, the patient may develop progressive dyspnea, stridor, and even acute life-threatening airway compromise. Preoperatively, it is useful to evaluate the location and morphology of the papilloma using a flexible nasendoscope. Macroscopically, papillomas are pink or white, sessile or exophytic, pedunculated or broad-based. Occasionally, the papilloma develops across a wide field, appearing like a carpet or velvety sheet of disease, requiring high levels of magnification to localizes it accurately. As the disease can affect different anatomical sites in the larynx, it is important for the surgeon to be comfortable with several surgical methods and instruments. Consideration of these characteristics can guide the surgeon to select the most effective resection technique.

7.2.4 Surgical Techniques

For treating RRP, the menu of surgical options include microsurgical cold steel, carbon dioxide (CO_2) laser, microdébridement, and office-based angiolytic laser treatment. As new techniques have been developed, some investigators have preferred one method over another [20]. The approaches for surgical removal of RRP remain controversial. It should be remembered that no surgical method has been shown to eradicate RRP; therefore, it remains a chronic disease where surgical techniques and instrumentation should be selected to enable the surgeon to achieve the goals of surgery as described above.

7.2.5 CO_2 Laser

The principals of CO_2 laser ablation are relatively simple. At a wavelength of 10,600 nm, light is converted to thermal energy, which is absorbed by water in the target tissues. This causes tissue destruction by vaporization at the molecular level. Two modes—pulsed and continuous—are currently in common use. The pulsed mode produces the fastest vaporization, the least collateral thermal injury, and the least char. Pulsed mode at low power (up to 5 W) allows control over the incision, prevents adjacent thermal damage to the anterior commissure, and avoids a hole of unintended depth (while pausing). Bleeding can be a problem with the pulsed mode, whereas the continuous mode results in more coagulation but with more risk of collateral thermal injury. Manipulation of the laser spot size and "mode" allows the operator to switch between vaporization of large areas of bulky disease or more precise targeted removal of smaller areas.

The CO_2 laser operative techniques are described in detail elsewhere. However, in brief, this is our approach. The operating team consists of a lead scrub nurse, a laser nurse, and a circulating nurse. The laser nurse is free to manage the laser, allowing the other members of the team to concentrate on their duties. All personnel wear protective goggles and approved laser filtration masks with spare goggles and appropriate warning signs placed outside the operating room. The room is set up with the suspension microlaryngoscope system of choice; a selection of laryngoscopes, ventilating bronchoscopes; and Hopkins Rod telescopes; and a set of suction and microlaryngeal instruments. An operating microscope is fitted with a 400-mm lens and a CO_2 laser micromanipulator. A video-endoscope "stack" equipped with a monitor, light source, and digital recording equipment is also used. The anesthesia technique during laser surgery reflects personal preference, experience, and institutional protocols. Nonintubation methods are popular and include spontaneous breathing, apneic, and jet ventilation techniques. The advantages of these methods include no flammable material in the airway so the risk of fire is minimized and there is excellent visibility of the surgical field. Intubation techniques utilize "laser safe," or "armored," endotracheal tubes, and care must be taken to use them in accordance with the manufacturers' recommendations.

Precise operation of the laser depends on the location and morphology of the lesion or lesions. Generally, a defocused spot in continuous mode is utilized for bulky lesions, and a narrow focus spot size in pulsed mode is reserved for areas where minimal damage to laryngeal structures is desired. Andrus (2005) [2] described a "laser brush" technique for sessile papillomatous growth. With this method, the laser is set to the lowest power setting (2–3 W) that allows adequate vaporization of tissue. The time exposure is set at 1 second and the spot size diameter at 0.3 mm. The laser is then applied to the broad surface of the papillomas in brush strokes in an anterior-to-posterior direction. This causes superficial vaporization and carbonization of the surface of the lesion. The char is removed with a saline-soaked neurosurgical pad ("the brush") and microsuction. The depth of removal can easily be assessed at high magnification and the laser used in repeated brush strokes until the uninvolved submucosal layer is identified (Fig. 7.3).

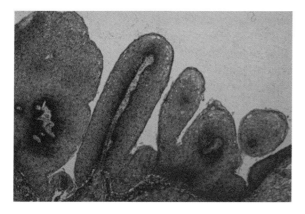

Fig. 7.3. Recurrent respiratory papillomatosis. Microscopic view (H.E)

7.2.6 Angiolytic Laser Treatment

The philosophy of angiolytic laser treatment for RRP appears a sound one. In theory, laser energy between 500 and 600 nm wavelengths is selectively absorbed by intravascular oxyhemoglobin, resulting in coagulation of target tissue vasculature. In contrast, CO_2 laser energy at 10,600 nm is absorbed mainly by water, the primary constituent of most human tissue. Control over CO_2 laser selectivity is therefore limited, and collateral damage to normal tissue is predictable. In 1998, investigators demonstrated application of the 585-nm pulsed dye laser (PDL) to RRP in the human larynx. Early results showed that, compared to the CO_2 laser, PDL was capable of comparable levels of disease regression and reduced risk of normal tissue damage [20]. A further advantage of PDL is that it can be deployed in the office setting under local anesthesia [12, 20].

Treatment with PDL may be associated with some complications, including perivascular extravasation, which appears as a characteristic "purpura" in the surrounding tissues at surgery. Bleeding occurs when blood in the vessel lumen is heated too rapidly, leading to vessel wall rupture before coagulation has occurred. This can be avoided by balancing the relatively short pulse width of the PDL (0.5 ms), the energy settings for that pulse, and delivery of the amount of energy required for coagulation to a moving target (varying fiber-to-tissue distance.) The loss of operative visualization, the patient coughing, and/or the inevitably absorption of laser energy by blood in the surrounding area rather than the target tissues can limit use of the PDL [20].

Issues surrounding the size of the PDL fiber (0.6 mm) and coupling it to the working channel of existing fibreoptic equipment has led to interest in the potassium-titanyl-phosphate (KTP) laser as an alternative angiolytic application. The KTP laser wavelength of 532 nm is strongly absorbed by oxyhemoglobin, and its small fiber diameter of 0.3–0.4 mm allows easier use with existing flexible laryngoscopes. Furthermore, in theory adjusting the pulse width to 15 ms allows slower, more uniform coagulation with less extravasation and collateral photothermal injury [81]. One weakness of both PDL and KTP angiolytic laser therapy is that they are not as effective for bulky disease as conventional surgery.

It may be that utilizing cold steel, microdébridement, or CO_2 laser as an initial treatment strategy with angiolytic laser therapy reserved for maintenance or follow-up surgery will evolve. Some predict that outpatient-based angiolytic laser therapy will supplant CO_2 laser ablation as the primary mode of follow-up surgical management for RRP [2, 81].

7.2.7 Microdébrider

Adaptation of the powered microdébrider system for laryngeal use in RRP was first reported by Myer in 1999 [47]. Equipped with suction, angled oscillating blades, and irrigation, the microdébrider system can be deployed in the larynx under suspension laryngoscopy or in conjunction with a handheld Hopkins rod. Refinements and proliferation of instrument designs have led to the growth in the popularity of this system, and supporters claim several safety advantages over the CO_2 laser. They include the absence of a laser plume, no risk of ocular or other laser injury to the patient or personnel, and no risk of airway fire. Furthermore, use of the microdébrider system is less intensive in terms of equipment charges and operating room staff. Some investigators report a significant reduction in operating times and increased cost-effectiveness compared to similar CO_2 laser procedures. A survey of members of the American Society of Pediatric Otolaryngology showed that use of the microdébrider has overtaken the CO_2 laser as the method of choice for surgical removal of papillomas in the pediatric population [65]. However, those who advocate preservation of as much of the remaining (voice-producing) superficial lamina propria as possible suggest that the technique is insufficiently controlled, especially for patients desiring a career of professional voice use.

7.3 Adjuvant Therapy

7.3.1 General Considerations

Some progress is being made toward developing effective medical treatment for RRP, and these authors hope that the the surgical treatments discussed above will one day be outdated. Current antiviral adjuvant treatments in limited use for RRP include cidofovir, interferon-α, and indole-3-carbinol. Novel agents undergoing Phase III trials include fusion proteins (heat-shock-protein E7,) and cyclooxygenase-2 inhibitors (celecoxib.) Furthermore,

prophylactic immunization against HPV infection, as licensed for cervical HPV infection in young women, is now possible, although large populations would need to be treated to prevent one case. There are currently no formal guidelines, and no substantial randomized controlled trials of adjuvant therapy for RRP. The decision to offer adjuvant therapy therefore must be individualized and based on the frequency of surgical interventions, the morbidity of frequent surgeries, and the recurrence pattern of the papillomas balanced against the possible risks and side effects of these agents (e.g., the possible mutagenic effects of cidofovir). Examination of the available retrospective literature suggests that patients requiring four or more surgical interventions per year for 2 years, suffering from distal, multisite spread of the disease, and/or rapid regrowth with airway compromise might be candidates for adjuvant treatment [14, 65]. Furthermore, as the clinical evidence defining the precise role for these adjuvant therapies is limited, informed consent and consideration of enrollment in clinical trials are important.

7.3.2 Cidofovir

The use of the intralesional antiviral agent cidofovir {1-[(S)-3-hydroxy-2-(phosphonomethoxy)propyl] cytosine dihydrate} (HPMPC) in RRP was first described in 1995 [72]. Since then numerous studies have reported favorable results in terms of disease regression and remission following direct intralesional injection in adults [15, 54]. Interpretation of these and other data is complicated by the wide variation in the total dose given (2–57 mg), the frequency (2–8 weeks) and duration of treatments (months to years), and the concurrent use of surgical and other adjuvant treatments [67]. In addition, the heterogeneity in case series between adult and juvenile populations further confounds the interpretation of outcomes.

The precise dose, frequency of administration, and duration of treatment for cidofovir in adults with RRP is unclear. Systemic toxicity for intralesional cidofovir seems low [68]. Some studies have reported the use of cidofovir in the adult population using concentrations of 2.5–6.5 mg/ml with volumes of up to 6–8 ml per therapeutic session, administered every 2–4 weeks for up to 19 months. Others have utilized higher concentrations (37.5 mg/ml) delivered in smaller treatment volumes (up to 57 mg per therapeutic session) via a percutaneous route [11]. The use of cidofovir therefore remains controversial. We recommend using intralesional cidofovir in moderate to severe disease where there is a need for frequent surgery and deteriorating vocal and airway function. Furthermore, informed consent should be obtained after detailing the potential side effects including nephrotoxicity and carcinogenesis risks. Concerns over long-term efficacy and potential side effects of malignant transformation mandate adequately powered randomized, controlled trials.

7.3.3 Interferon-α

The interferons are a group of natural proteins produced by the body in response to infection. Interferons may be classified as alpha, beta, or gamma and are named after their ability to interfere with viral replication. These substances have been synthesized for clinical use using recombinant DNA techniques. In therapeutic doses, interferon can produce considerable side effects, including flu-like symptoms such as fatigue, headache, and general aches as well as, less regularly, hypothyroidism, arthritis, thrombocytopenia, and psychiatric disturbances. In 1981, Haglund [26] described the use of human leukocyte interferon in a small cohort of patients with RRP. Since then, various studies have demonstrated the usefulness of interferon-α in severe RRP requiring frequent surgical interventions [22, 28, 38]. The long-term effectiveness of interferon-α is still controversial [2, 22, 38]. Combined with its side effect profile and the development of newer adjuvant strategies, the use of interferon-α in RRP seems to be declining [65], and we suggest that it be reserved as a third-line treatment for patients with airway obstruction.

7.3.4 Specific Recommendations According to the Technique

It is important to remember that RRP is not typically cured by surgical removal of disease, and the infectious nature of RRP eventually manifests as a recurrence. An aggressive surgical strategy therefore does not lead to reduced recurrence or a chance of cure. It should also be understood that RRP is limited to the surface epithelium. The principles of surgery, irrespective of the technique chosen, should be tailored to precise, careful

removal of the disease taking into consideration the preservation of underlying structures and vocal function. This is particularly important in relation to the glottis and subglottis, where overly aggressive ablation can result in severe scarring and dysfunction. Preservation of even small areas of mucosa with intact superficial lamina propria may make a huge difference to voice outcomes Extreme care should be taken in the areas of the anterior and posterior commissure. Papillomas should not be removed from both sides of the anterior or posterior commissure simultaneously as it can lead to web formation. An anterior commissure spatula or retractor should be used to protect one side of the anterior commissure while laser ablation or laser excision is performed on the other side.

7.3.5 Recommendations for Follow-Up (Postoperative Care)

We encourage patients with stable disease requiring fewer than three or four procedures per year to self-refer as often as they feel it is necessary. For new patients, frequent office visits are employed to develop trust and a good working relationship. However, the development of more reliable, fast, low-morbidity office-based treatments may alter this stratagem.

7.4 Hemangioma

Laryngeal hemangiomas are rare but important as they may present with significant airway obstructive symptoms. Ferguson [18] classified hemangiomas into two groups: pediatric (10%) and adult (90%) types. The pediatric type is typically subglottic (Fig. 7.4). The pathogenesis of hemangiomas remains controversial as to whether they represent a true neoplasm or a congenital abnormality. Their behavior is sometimes aggressive, in which case it should be considered a malignant neoplastic lesion. When such lesions present in the adult, they usually arise on or above the vocal cords, and patients present with vague, often extended histories of hoarseness and occasional dysphagia. These tumors are seen more frequently in men (60–70%), and most are cavernous-type hemangiomas (the others being capillary type). The tumors are mostly rounded, projecting or pedunculated, purplish growths

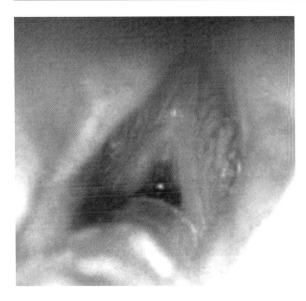

Fig. 7.4. Pediatric subglottic hemangioma (horseshoe shape)

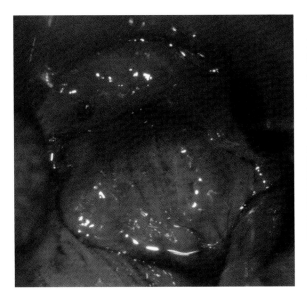

Fig. 7.5. Hemangioma of the left arytenoid of an adult patient

arising on or above the vocal cords. Occasionally, they are larger sessile tumors that extend submucosally into the laryngopharynx (Fig. 7.5) [36]. As a rule, the only symptom is hoarseness, and they rarely progress to the point of causing respiratory narrowing or obstruction. Although most angiomas are benign growths, some are multicentric and the term "hemangiomatosis" is applied; these lesions may be part of a variety of clinical syndromes such as Rendu-Weber-Osler and the Sturge-Weber dyscrasia.

7.4.1 Management

Surgery is the treatment of choice, but the potential for severe hemorrhage during biopsy or excision is well documented [18]. Since the introduction of laser therapy for vascular lesions, the management of laryngeal hemangiomas has proven useful. The use of photocoagulation with Nd:YAG laser has offered the clinician an effective alternative therapy that is minimally invasive and has few complications [80]. Success also has been reported with the use of CO_2 laser excision. Occasionally, use of the laser requires staging and time spacing of the surgical procedure to allow complete resolution of the postoperative laryngeal tissue inflammation and edema. Some patients require a temporary tracheostomy during the course of these laser procedures [41].

7.5 Hemangiopericytoma

Hemangiopericytomas are rare but are highlighted because they can present diagnostic and histological dilemmas (Fig. 7.6) [7]. These lesions present as a supraglottic cyst-like mass that usually has a vascular-type appearance. The mass is firm, solid, pedunculated

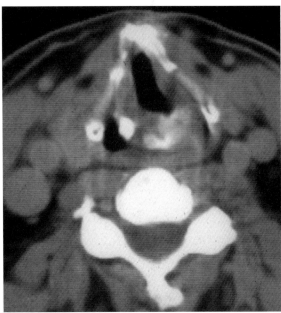

Fig. 7.6. Hemangiopericytoma developed from the subglottic area. Computed tomography (CT) of the right side of the cricoid cartilage

or nodular, usually well circumscribed, in a submucosal location, and is up to 4 cm in greatest diameter. The surface is covered by intact epithelium with dilated vessels. Histologically, the tumor has few mitoses. Occasional increased cellularity, pleomorphism, and mitotic activity are associated with recurrences or metastases in other anatomical locations [49]. The differential diagnosis includes hemangioma, angiosarcoma, glomus tumor, fibrous histiocytoma, leiomyoma, synovial sarcoma, malignant melanoma, leiomyosarcoma, spindle squamous cell carcinoma, and mesenchymal chondrosarcoma [49].

7.5.1 Management

Surgical treatment is recommended and may necessitate total laryngectomy (Fig. 7.7), although lesser surgical procedures have been described. Sadly, long-term follow-up of such cases is lacking to support a laryngeal conservation surgical approach in the light of difficulties with the histopathological diagnosis.

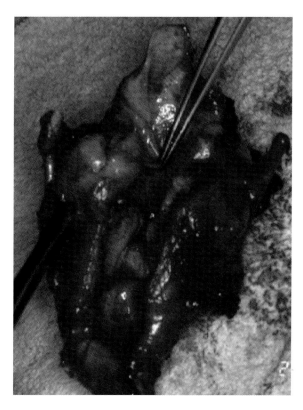

Fig. 7.7. Hemangiopericytoma. Surgical specimen after total laryngectomy

7.6 Leiomyoma

An extremely rare neoplasm, leiomyoma usually occurs in the supraglottic larynx, with the ventricle and false cord most often involved, although leiomyomas of the subglottis and trachea have been described. These tumors arise from smooth muscle and are peculiar in that there is little smooth muscle in the larynx, compared to other parts of the head and neck. The tumors are usually sessile, bulging, or polypoidal red-brown masses that are up to 5 cm in maximum diameter. These masses are usually covered by an intact smooth surface epithelium, with a conspicuous vascular arborizing pattern, although ulceration is noted in larger lesions.

Microscopically, leimyomas are distinctly encapsulated masses located in the submucosa and are composed of spindle cells arranged in fascicles, whorls, and intersecting bundles. Three types of leiomyoma are recognized: the "common" leiomyoma, the vascular leiomyoma (angiomyoma), and the epithelioid (leiomyoblastoma). All three have been identified in the larynx.

The differential diagnosis includes benign peripheral nerve sheath tumors, neurilemomas and neurofibromas, nodular fasciitis, fibromas, and leiomyosarcoma. However, any of the spindle cell tumors (inflammatory myofibroblastic tumor, contact ulcer, fibrosarcoma, spindle cell squamous cell carcinoma, synovial sarcoma) should also be considered.

7.6.1 Management

Surgical excision with clear margins after confirmation of the diagnosis is curative. Because of the vascularity of the angiomas, there is a high risk of significant bleeding, with the possibility of recurrence as a result [1].

7.7 Rhabdomyoma

Rhabdomyomas in the larynx arise from striated muscle and are divided into two subtypes based on their histological features, not on the patient's age at presentation: adult type and fetal cellular type [3]. The current definition of rhabdomyoma is a benign neoplasm of striated muscle tissue, consisting usually of polygonal, frequently vacuolated (glycogen-containing) cells

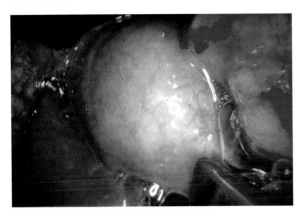

Fig. 7.8. Rhabdomyoma in the aryepiglottic fold

with a fine granular, deeply acidophilic cytoplasm resembling myofibrils cut in cross section [33].

Involvement of the larynx is uncommon [39]. Adult rhabdomyomas occur more frequently in men than women (4:1), with reported ages ranging from 16 to 76 years (mean 52 years). The adult type presents as a single lobulated, polypoidal or pedunculated, nonencapsulated, tan-yellow to deep gray-red-brown mass. Occasionally, these lesions are multifocal, with lesions in more than two locations in the head and neck, including the larynx [40]. They may measure up to 7.5 cm in greatest dimension, but most are 1–3 cm. The lesions have been most frequently located to the supraglottis or vocal cord (Fig. 7.8) [37]. The fetal cellular type of rhabdomyoma has a similar presentation and is usually found in preadolescent patients, although it may affect the head and neck region in elderly men [9]. There is also a fetal myxoid type that is found in the head and neck area of children, especially in the postauricular region, although it has also been reported in the adult larynx [33].

The benign differential diagnosis for the adult type of tumor includes granular cell tumor, oncocytoma, paraganglioma, hibernoma, and alveolar soft-part sarcoma. They are characterized by the presence of a sarcolemma sheath, rod-like cytoplasmic bodies, and cross striations.

7.7.1 Management

Complete surgical excision is curative. Although local recurrences have been reported in more than 33% of cases treated in the head and neck region, which usually result from incomplete resection, it appears not to be associated with rhabdomyomas located in the larynx [31]. Recurrences may present months to years after the initial resection. To date, there has been no documented case of malignant degeneration of the adult-form rhabdomyoma.

7.8 Lipoma

Benign lipomas are commonly encountered in a wide variety of locations throughout the body. It is estimated that 13% of lipomas occur in the head and neck. Laryngeal lipomas are rare, with fewer than 100 cases reported. When present, they are most frequently located in the aryepiglottic fold (Jungehulsing et al. 2005). They are mostly found in adults and primarily affect men, with fewer than 90 cases reported in the literature [75].

In general, these lesions present like cystic lesions: encapsulated, smooth, and usually pedunculated (Fig. 7.9 and 7.10). Symptoms are few and uncharacteristic, making accurate diagnosis difficult. Clinically, they can be confused with other benign lesions, such as retention cysts or laryngoceles [34]. There has been no

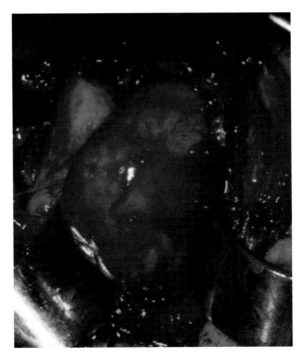

Fig. 7.9. Lipoma. Surgical view during the open neck approach after the laryngeal opening

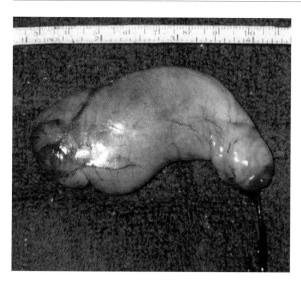

Fig. 7.10. Lipoma. Surgical specimen

report of malignant transformation of a solitary lipoma, although malignant change in multiple lipomas of the larynx and the pharynx has been described [27, 35].

7.8.1 Management

Transoral resection of the lipoma is relatively simple and effective with the use of CO_2 laser. The aim of treatment is always a conservative surgical excision, with preservation of laryngeal function the surgeon's major intent [27]. Although described, recurrence is rare.

7.9 Neurofibromas and Neurilemoma or Benign Schwannomas

Benign neurological lesions are uncommon laryngeal tumors. There are two classes of benign neurogenic tumors of the larynx: schwannomas and neurofibromas, with schwannomas being more frequent. Since the first reported case of laryngeal schwannoma in 1925, more than 130 laryngeal tumors of neural origin had been reported up to 1993 [6], but it is difficult to distinguish the exact number of neurilemomas and neurofibromas.

Most schwannomas present in the parapharyngeal space, with the head and neck accounting for 25–45% identified clinically. The larynx remains a rare site. These tumors in the larynx may present at any age, with a slight female preponderance. Almost all benign neurogenic tumors of the larynx arise in the supraglottis, although the true vocal cord may be involved, with fewer than 10 cases reported [70].

They are more likely to affect sensory nerves than motor nerves and differ from neurofibromas in that the latter are not encapsulated, do not cause symptoms, and may be associated with neurofibromatosis type II (von Recklinghausen's disease) [52]. Neurilemomas affect both sexes equally, and they occur most often during the fifth to sixth decades of life. Neurilemomas typically affect nerve sheaths but not usually the nerve fibers. Neurofibromas may be single or multiple; multiple lesions characterize neurofibromatosis type I [70].

It is important to distinguish between neurofibromas and schwannomas. The recurrence rate is greater for neurofibromas, and malignant transformation from neurofibroma to malignant neurosarcoma occurs in approximately 10% of cases. In contrast, malignant degeneration of schwannomas is extremely rare. Computed tomography (CT) and magnetic resonance imaging (MRI) can help with the diagnosis, revealing not only the extent but the degree of the lipomatous element as well. Compared with CT, MRI offers superior soft tissue definition and better visualization of the laryngeal musculature [69].

The characteristic finding is a round submucosal bulge arising from the false cord and/or aryepiglottic fold, obstructing the view of the ipsilateral true vocal cord. Symptoms depend on the site of origin. Most neurogenic tumors of the larynx originate in either the aryepiglottic fold or the false cord [63]. In these locations, the nerve of origin is likely to be the recurrent laryngeal nerve or the internal branch of the superior laryngeal nerve. As the tumor expands, it distorts the lateral larynx and eventually closes the airway and causes dysphonia. There are no characteristic features suggestive of neurilemoma on simple inspection, although CT and MRI can delineate between benign and malignant conditions in large tumors. The pathological diagnosis is dependent on three criteria: the presence of a capsule, identification of Antoni A and B areas, and a positive reaction of the tumor for S-100 protein.

7.9.1 Management

Ideally, a neurilemoma is totally excised, but anatomical constraints sometimes make this difficult. The preferred method is microlaryngeal endoscopic excision with either conventional microlaryngeal endoscopic instrumentation or the use of CO_2 laser. The open approach may be necessary for large lesions. The treatment should be individualized with alternatives for an open approach via a transhyoid, laryngofissure or a lateral pharyngotomy approach.

7.10 Salivary Gland Tumors

Benign pleomorphic salivary adenoma (PSA) of the larynx has been reported more than 40 times [16], and another series of 11 cases was reviewed in the Japanese literature [64]. Males predominate slightly, with an age range from 15–82 years, with most cases presenting during the fifth to seventh decades. The type and severity of symptoms depends on the size and location of the tumor mass, with dysphonia and dyspnea symptoms being most common; some cases have been diagnosed en passant. The supraglottis is by far the commonest site, followed by the subglottis and the glottis (Fig. 7.11). Within the supraglottis the epiglottis is the most common site, located on the laryngeal surface most commonly. Only one case has involved the whole of one side of the larynx from the valleculae to the ventricle. The tumor presented as a mass with mucosal deformity without ulceration. The tumor may be pedunculated.

The differential diagnosis includes angioma, fibroma, cylindroma, lymphoma, schwannoma, aberrant thyroid, vestigial cyst, and internal laryngocele. Two cases have

been reported in which the carcinoma arose in a pleomorphic adenoma within the larynx [45, 61].

7.10.1 Management

Surgical removal is curative and depends on the location and size of the tumor. Most of these lesions have been approached using a conservation surgical approach with curative intent. They have included endoscopic surgery including laser (Figs. 7.12 and 7.13) an external approach via a laryngofissure, or later pharyngotomy. However, if the tissue analyzed might be misinterpreted or an error made, a more extensive surgical approach may result; several such occasions have been reported. Importantly, the use of radiotherapy alone in a few cases did not shrink the tumor.

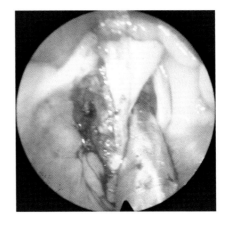

Fig. 7.12. Pleomorphic adenoma (salivary gland tumor) after endoscopic resection that had developed from the left supraglottis

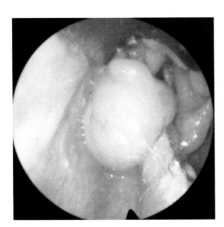

Fig. 7.11. Pleomorphic adenoma (salivary gland tumor) developed from the left supraglottis

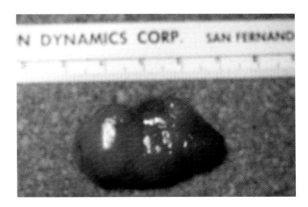

Fig. 7.13. Pleomorphic adenoma (salivary gland tumor) that had developed from the left supraglottis. Surgical specimen

7.11 Oncocytoma

Solitary oncocytomas are extremely rare, with few reported in the literature. Oncocytic hyperplasia, by contrast, is frequently diagnosed in elderly patients and is most commonly reported in the supraglottis [19]. Oncocytic lesions range from solid proliferation to a thin-walled cyst lined by multiple layers of cuboidal epithelium. Oncocytic lesions of the larynx manifest as a morphological spectrum of changes, including surface metaplasia of the respiratory or squamous epithelium, solitary oncocystic "adenomas" (neoplasms), multifocal "hyperplastic" masses, and cysts lined by oncocytes. Each of these entities is within the benign spectrum of oncocytic lesions without any treatment implications. However, oncocytic change/metaplasia can be diagnosed if it is present diffusely or multifocally throughout the larynx. If there is a solid proliferation of oncocytes, the designation "adenoma" can be used. Many cysts of the larynx are lined by oncocytes, and a clear distinction between saccular or ductal cyst and oncocystic papillary cystadenoma is not always possible.

7.11.1 Management

Endoscopic excision is curative [50]; it may be endoscopic, or a laryngofissure approach may be necessary. Recurrences have been reported and are most commonly associated with incomplete excision, although some may be associated with the development of a new lesion from a focus of oncocytic metaplasia previously undetected [19]. Surgery remains the treatment of choice for recurrent disease.

7.12 Necrotizing Sialometaplasia

Two cases of necrotizing sialometaplasia of the larynx have been reported. One case presented in the subglottis and the other in the false cord. It is suggested that this process is associated with other pathologies or processes. Hence, a secondary process occurring in the larynx at the same time or some other cause in the proximity should be sought, such as cancer. It is thought that the likely pathogenesis is vascular compromise of the affected area [73].

7.13 Paraganglioma

Neuroendocrine neoplasms of the larynx can be divided into two main groups: those of epithelial origin (carcinoid and neuroendocine carcinoma) and those of neural type (paraganglioma) [48]. Paragangliomas are uncommon, slow-growing, generally benign tumors. They arise from the paraganglion cells derived from the neural crest as part of a diffuse neuroendocrine system. To date, 76 cases have been identified as fulfilling the specific criteria laid down to make an accurate diagnosis.

In the larynx, there are two-paired paraganglia: the superior and inferior. The superior paraganglia are 0.1–0.3 mm in diameter and are situated in the false cord fold along the course of the superior laryngeal artery and nerve. The inferior paraganglia are 0.3–0.4 mm in diameter and are found near the lateral margin of the cricoid cartilage in the cricotracheal membrane along the course of the recurrent laryngeal nerve.

Typically, these tumors arise from the superior paraganglia (82%) and have a right-side, female predilection (3:1). Only 11 cases of subglottic paraganglia have been reported, again with a female preponderance. An uncommon case with a transventricular location and a fixed vocal cord presented a diagnostic challenge [25]. The age range is 5–90-plus years, although most laryngeal paragangliomas present during the fourth to sixth decades.

Examination reveals a red or blue lobulated, submucosal, smooth mass in the false cord. Rarely, it is associated with a neck mass, unless it is large enough to herniate through the thyrohyoid membrane. The lesion bleeds excessively if biopsied. It can be diagnosed with radiological imaging and angiography [62].

Histologically, paragangliomas are characterized by chief and sustentacular cells. Electron microscopy shows neural secretory granules. Chief cells stain positive for chromagranin and synaptophysin. The presence of mitotic activity does not correlate with the clinical behavior.

7.13.1 Management

The goal of treatment is eradication with preservation of maximal laryngeal function. Cryosurgery has been attempted, but laryngofissure or irradiation has been required following this procedure. No long term follow-up of such cases has been documented. Endoscopic removal has been employed by several authors but has been associated with frequent recurrences. The successful use of CO_2 laser has been reported for a 4 × 4 × 3 cm mass in the supraglottis, with a postintubation period of 2 days, a protracted hospital stay, and a 5-year tumor-free follow-up [66]. Open surgery has in the past achieved excellent tumor control with preservation of laryngeal function, even when the tumor was located in the subglottis. Irradiation has not been reported as successful to date.

7.14 Granular Cell Tumors

Granular cell tumors are uncommon benign lesions that can appear anywhere in the body, although they have a predilection for the upper aerodigestive tract. In fact, 50% of all cases present in the head and neck region. The incidence of granular cell tumors in the larynx is 3–10% of cases in adults, and it is rare in children.

In the head and neck, the anterior tongue and the larynx are the first and second most common sites of these tumors [33, 71]. In the larynx, granular cell tumors are located on the posterior third of the vocal cord (Fig. 7.14). Symptoms depend on the location and size of the tumor, with the most common symptom being dysphonia; frequently, however, they are diagnosed in asymptomatic persons. The histopathological origin and etiology of this tumor are unknown.

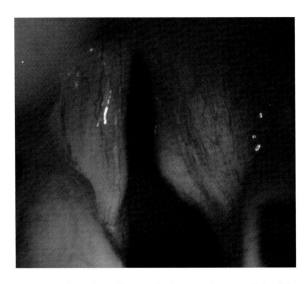

Fig. 7.14. Granular cell tumor in the posterior part of the right vocal fold

Macroscopically, these tumors are described as grayish-yellow, smooth but firm, well circumscribed, and polypoidal or sessile. As many as 50–65% of laryngeal granular cell tumors have pseudoepitheliomatous hyperplasia, which can lead to misinterpretation owing to the similarity of these lesions to squamous cell carcinoma. Granular cell tumors are not malignant, and malignant transformation has so far never been reported; laryngeal malignant granular cell tumors have been recorded, however. They metastasize early, and the prognosis is not good. A 34-year-old man, with a histologically benign granular cell tumor has been reported that recurred with rapid growth. The original tumor was characterized by atypia and pagetoid extensions into the epithelium. It is suggested that such cases be closely followed up. They should be distinguished from benign cases and should be suspected of behaving as a malignancy that has the potential to metastasize [8].

7.14.1 Management

Treatment is local excision by endoscopic, transoral, or laryngofissure methods appropriate to the site of the lesion. The recurrence rate after resection with free margins has been reported to be 8%, but this increases to 21–50% with positive margins. Frozen section analysis has been used to aid endoscopic excision with CO_2 laser and should be considered when there is pathological support for such a technique.

7.15 Giant Cell Tumors

The giant cell tumor is a true neoplasm and is presumed to be part of a series of tumors more frequently reported in long bones—the fibrohistiocytic series. In the larynx, giant cell tumors arise in the osteocartilaginous supporting structures of the larynx proper; they do not seem to be discrete soft tissue masses. One review suggested that 18 true cases have been reported [29]. The lesion involves men in their third to sixth decades; female patients have not been reported to date. Presenting problems include the presence of a slow-growing mass and dysphonia.

On examination, a mass is usually palpable, most commonly originating in the thyroid cartilage. Endoscopically, the lesions have proven to be deeply seated with an intact overlying mucosa. CT scanning reveals a mass with a density intermediate between muscle and fat that may or may not show some central cystic change. The multinucleated giant cell type is more likely to show malignant features than the smaller mononuclear cell type. In all laryngeal giant cell tumors reported, however, tumors with both cell types have been cytologically benign.

7.15.1 Management

Early reports suggested that radiotherapy could be used to control these tumors. Modern therapy, however, suggests that either laryngectomy or hemilaryngectomy can achieve local control and obtain sufficient tissue to confirm the pathological diagnosis.

7.16 Chondroma

Laryngeal chondromas are uncommon and are seen most often during the sixth to seventh decades of life. The most frequent site is the cricoid, followed by the thyroid cartilage and, uncommonly, the epiglottis (Fig. 7.15) [4]. The exact number reported is unknown because it is difficult or impossible to distinguish a benign chondroma from a low-grade chondrosarcoma; it is suggested that the two patterns overlap, and a single tumor can exhibit both patterns. This may have occurred because of the small size of the biopsy specimen and may not be representative of the whole or entire tumor. It is therefore recommended that if a cartilage tumor is suspected the whole of the tumor be excised and subjected to histopathology. The treatment and prognosis of chondroma and low-grade chondrosarcoma is similar [32]. Should an excised chondroma recur, one should seriously doubt the accuracy of the initial diagnosis—it probably had been a low-grade chondrosarcoma all along.

7.16.1 Management

Surgery has always been the treatment of choice for laryngeal cartilage tumors. Most authors claim conservative surgery is the appropriate treatment for both low-grade tumors and chondromas. Even for cricoid

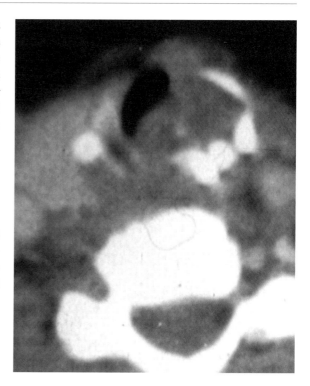

Fig. 7.15. Chondroma (low grade chondrosarcoma) that had developed from the cricoid cartilage. CT scan

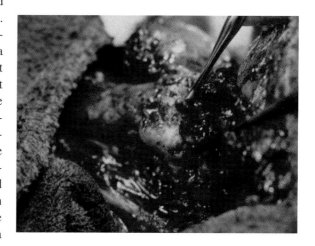

Fig. 7.16. Chondroma (low-grade chondrosarcoma) that had developed from the cricoid cartilage. Surgical view, open neck approach

lesions, conservative treatment through a laryngofissure is possible when the tumor involves less than half the cartilage. Radiotherapy for laryngeal cartilage tumors is controversial; the experience is limited to 12 cases, with only 2 cases of documented long-term follow-up (Fig. 7.16) [4]. Recent reports have described

CO_2 laser therapy as a procedure to deal with recurrences or even the primary lesion [60, 77].

7.17 Nonneoplastic Laryngeal Tumors

7.17.1 Hamartomas

According to the World Health Organization (WHO) classification, a hamartoma is a "developmental anomaly characterised by the formation of a tumor-like mass composed of mature tissue elements that are normally present in the location where it is found but occurring in abnormal proportions or arrangements" [78]. Hamartomas of the head and neck are uncommon but have been described in the sinonasal tract, nasopharynx, oral cavity, oropharynx, larynx hypopharynx, cervical esophagus, ear, parotid gland, trachea, parathyroid gland, and eye. They may be unifocal or multifocal. The term "pleiotropic hamartoma" is used to indicate the presence of multiple hamartomas at different sites in a given patient. Hamartomas of the larynx are rare [59]. Presently, it appears that there are only 11 cases of well documented hamartoma of the larynx. Males are more involved than females, with age peaks during early childhood and middle age (39–56 years). Of the 11 cases accepted as hamartomas of the larynx, 6 of the patients were 16 years of age or older. The main symptoms of laryngeal involvement are similar to those of other benign mass lesions: dysphonia, dyspnea, and dysphagia.

Microscopically, the tissues show a disorganized architectural pattern with mesenchymal derivatives alone or with superadded epithelial elements. Hamartomas of the larynx are mainly composed of cartilage and fibromuscular tissue. Fatty tissue and nerve elements are often seen. No features of malignancy are present. The dominant tissue defines the lesion (e.g., cartilage hamartoma or myxochondromatous hamartoma). Such lesions must be differentiated from choristoma, teratoma, and rhabdomyoma, among others.

7.17.1.1 Management

Treatment consists of local excision, with recurrences usually associated with incomplete removal.

7.18 Pseudotumors or Pseudoneoplastic Lesions

From a practical point of view, pseudoneoplastic lesions of the larynx may be divided broadly into two groups: (1) growths that present clinically as mass lesions but by histological examination are readily diagnosed and are appropriately classified as benign nonneoplastic lesions; and (2) benign lesions that may show histopathological features suggestive of neoplasia. The latter group may be further divided into lesions that are *clinically* suspicious and those that present a *microscopic* dilemma [74]. Some are discussed below.

7.19 Inflammatory Fibroblastic Tumors

Inflammatory myofibroblastic tumors (IMTs) can be polypoid, pedunculated, spherical, lobular, or nodular, with a smooth external appearance. They may be confined to the immediate submucosal region and not truly invading any tissue. They are firm in consistency, fleshy and gritty on cut surface, gray-yellow or tan-white, and may measure up to 3 cm in greatest dimension. To date, only 10 IMTs have been reported in the larynx [24].

The most common site is the vocal cord [17]. These lesions are usually located on the true vocal cord, although the subglottis and upper trachea can be involved. The lesions may have a myxomatous appearance, but they do not exhibit necrosis or hemorrhage. Special histopathological stains confirm the diagnosis. The differential diagnosis centers around spindle cell squamous cell carcinoma, but inflammatory fibrosarcoma, nerve sheath tumors, nodular fasciitis, and nonspecific inflammation must be also excluded [41].

7.19.1 Management

Surgical excision is the treatment of choice [24] but may have to be repeated frequently before the correct diagnosis is confirmed [43].

7.20 Fibroma

Fibromas generally present as polyps or nodules, sessile or pedunculated, and soft or firm; their size depends on the duration and intensity of exposure to the irritating factors. Most lesions are covered by intact epithelium, often exhibiting keratosis, and can measure up to 4 cm. Many fibromas involve Reinke's space (superficial lamina propria) and arise from the anterior two-thirds of the vocal cord. Fibromas probably represent a reactive change and are not true neoplasms. With removal of the putative underlying insult, healing may occur after surgical excision. All lesions removed from the larynx require histopathological examination, with a diagnosis being essential for patient management and prognosis.

7.21 Amyloidosis

Isolated amyloidosis (without plasmactoma) frequently occurs along the false vocal cord, although any portion of the larynx can be affected. The term amyloidosis is used to indicate an extracellular accumulation of homogeneous protein-derived fibrillary and eosinophilic material, with well defined histochemical characteristics. When amyloidosis involves the supraglottic or glottic region, the lesion demonstrates an elevated, smooth or bosselated, polypoidal, mucosa-covered, firm mass. Subglottic amyloidosis presents as a more generalized, diffuse swelling. Multifocal deposits occur quite frequently. Surface ulceration has been reported in more extensive and larger lesions. The mass is firm, with a waxy, translucent cut surface ranging in color from tan-yellow to red-gray [75]. It is reported that up to 15% of patients who demonstrate laryngeal amyloidosis may have amyloid deposits at other head and neck sites.

It is important that when diagnosed with amyloidosis the patient is screened for the possibility that he or she may have tumor-forming amyloid, primary systemic amyloidosis (diagnosed by serum or urine immunoelectrophoresis or by rectal biopsy), secondary amyloidosis (associated with some other predisposing disease), or plasmacytoma, whether it be solitary or part of multiple myeloma. The most common amyloid lesion seen in the larynx is amyloid deposition alone, a localized amyloid deposit, or an amyloid tumor (without associated lymphoproliferative disorder) [55].

7.21.1 Management

Most authors agree that surgery should be the treatment of choice of laryngeal amyloidosis. Surgical procedures include external partial laryngectomy or microlaryngeal excision. An alternative technique is the use of CO_2 laser excision [41].

7.22 Laryngeal Cysts

The gross appearance of cysts in the larynx is often determined by the point of origin in the larynx and the type of cyst (saccular, retention/inclusive, ductal, vascular, traumatic). The cyst can be considered external or internal to the larynx based on the degree of compression of the larynx by the cyst and the extent of the disease in the larynx. Cysts generally do not communicate with the interior of the larynx. A laryngocele (air-filled herniation or dilation of the saccule) can be internal or external to the larynx, communicating with the lumen (Fig. 7.17–7.20). Saccular cysts (anterior or lateral) are submucosal and do not communicate with the lumen but, instead, are filled with mucus or acute inflammatory elements.

Cysts occur in all regions of the larynx, with retention cysts most often located in the epiglottis, saccular cysts in the false cord, and traumatic cysts in the

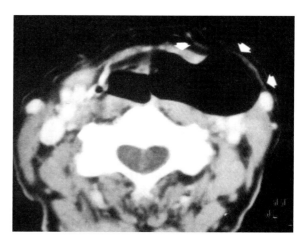

Fig. 7.17. External laryngocele. CT scan

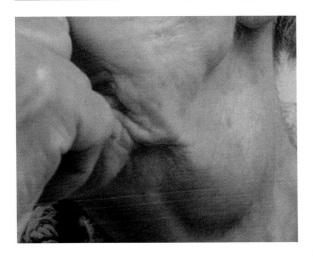

Fig. 7.18. External laryngocele

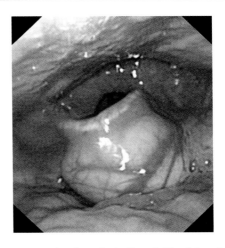

Fig. 7.21. Retentional cyst in the lingual side of the epiglottis

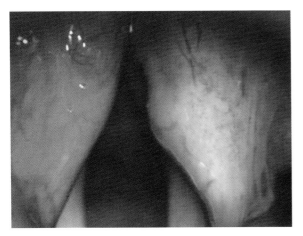

Fig. 7.19. Internal laryngocele that had developed in the right ventricular fold

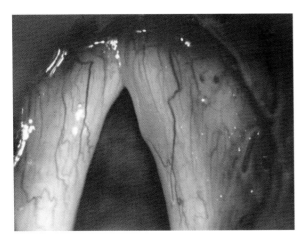

Fig. 7.20. Internal laryngocele that had developed in the right ventricular fold. After endoscopic resection

arytenoid region. The size of the cyst depends on the location; small cysts are usually found on the vocal cords, whereas large cysts are found attached to the epiglottis, pushing the larynx to one side, or projecting into the hypopharynx (Fig. 7.21).

Cyst walls, consisting of fibrous connective tissue, vary in thickness. The lining helps differentiate the cysts into a variety of subtypes. Most cysts are lined by squamous or respiratory epithelium (retention and saccular), and a few cysts are lined by fibrous connective tissue. Those with an admixture of mesodermal and endodermal layers qualify as congenital or embryonal cysts. It has been proposed that all laryngeal cysts can be classified into congenital, retention, and inclusion cysts [3].

7.22.1 Management

All cysts should be considered for a histopathological diagnosis. A biopsy should confirm the clinical suspicion before reassurance is given.

Acknowledgment All illustrations are by courtesy of Marc Remacle.

References

1. Anderson TD, Weinstein GS (2000) Recurrent angiomyoma (vascular leiomyoma) of the larynx after laser excision. Otolaryngol Head Neck Surg 123(5):646–647

2. Andrus JG, Shapshay SM (2006) Contemporary management of laryngeal papilloma in adults and children. Otolaryngol Clin North Am 39(1):135–158

3. Arens C, Glanz H, Kleinsasser O, et al (1997) Clinical and morphological aspects of laryngeal cysts. Eur Arch Oto-Rhino-Laryngol 254(9–10):430–436

4. Baatenburg de Jong RJ, van Lent S, Hogendoorn PCW (2004) Chondroma and chondrosarcoma of the Larynx. Curr Opin ORL-HNS 12:98–105

5. Barnes L (2001) Diseases of the larynx, hypopharynx, and oesophagus. In: Textbook surgical pathology of the head and neck, Chapter 5, 2nd ed. revised and expanded, in Chapter 1. New York/Basel, Marcel Dekker, pp. 151–154

6. Barnes L, Ferlito A (1993) Soft tissue neoplasms. In: Ferlito A (ed.) Neoplasms of the larynx. 1st ed.Churchill Livingstone, Hong Kong, pp. 630–638

7. Bradley PJ, Narula AA, Harvey L, et al (1989) Haemangiopericytoma of the larynx. J Laryngol Otol 103(2):234–238

8. Brandwein M, LeBenger J, Strauchen J, et al (1990) Atypical granular cell tumor of the larynx: an unusually aggressive tumor clinically and microscopically. Head Neck 12:154–159

9. Brys AK, Sakai O, DeRosa J, et al (2005) Rhabdomyoma of the larynx: case report and clinical and pathologic review. Ear, Nose Throat J 84(7):437–440

10. Chau HN,Desai K, Georgalas C, et al (2005) Variability in nomenclature of benign laryngeal pathology based on video laryngoscopy with and without stroboscopy. Clin Otolaryngol 30(5):424–427

11. Chhetri DK, Blumin JH, Shapiro NL, et al (2002) Office-based treatment of laryngeal papillomatosis with percutaneous injection of cidofovir. Otolaryngol Head Neck Surg 126(6):642–648

12. Clyne SB, Halum SL, Kaufman JA, et al (2005) Pulsed dye laser treatment of laryngeal granulomas. Ann Otol Rhinol Laryngol 114(3):198–201

13. Derkay CS (1995). Task force on recurrent respiratory papillomas. A preliminary report. Arch Otolaryngol 121(12):1386–1391

14. Derkay CS (2001) Recurrent respiratory papillomatosis. Laryngoscope 111(1):57–69

15. Dikkers FG (2006) Treatment of recurrent respiratory papillomatosis with microsurgery in combination with intralesional cidofovir--a prospective study. Euro Arch Oto-Rhino-Laryngol 263(5):440–443

16. Dubey SP,Banerjee S, Ghosh LM, et al (1997) Benign pleomorphic adenoma of the larynx: report of a case and review and analysis of 20 additional cases in the literature. Ear Nose Throat J 76(8):548–557

17. Ereno C, Grande J, Santaolalla F, et al (2001) Inflammatory myofibroblastic tumor of the larynx. J Laryngol Otol 115:856–858

18. Ferguson GB (1944) Hemangioma of the adult and infant larynx: a review of the literature and a report of 2 cases. Arch Otolaryngol Head Neck Surg 40:189–195

19. Ferlito AA, Recher G (1981). Oncocytic lesions of the larynx. Arch Otorhinolaryngol 232(2):107–115

20. Franco RA Jr, Zeitels SM, Farinelli WA, et al (2002) 585-nm pulsed dye laser treatment of glottal papillomatosis. Ann Otol Rhinol Laryngol 111(6):486–492

21. Gerein V, Rastorguev EE, Gerein J, et al (2005). Incidence, age at onset, and potential reasons of malignant transformation in recurrent respiratory papillomatosis patients: 20 years experience. Otolaryngol Head Neck Surg 132(3):392–394

22. Gerein V, Rastorguev E, Gerein J, et al (2005). Use of interferon-alpha in recurrent respiratory papillomatosis: 20-year follow-up. Anna Otol Rhinol Laryngol 114(6):463–471

23. Glanz H, Schulz A, Kleinsasser O, et al (1997) Benign lesions of the larynx: basic clinical and histopathological data. In: Kelinsasser O, Glanz H, and Olofsson J (eds) Advances of laryngology in Europe. Elsevier, Amsterdam, pp. 3–14

24. Guilemany JM, Alos L, Alobid I, et al (2005) Inflammatory myofibroblastic tumor in the larynx: clinicopathological features and histeogenesis. Acta Otolaryngol 125(2):215–219

25. Gupta S, Pathak KA, Sanghvi V (2003) Transventriular paraganglioma of the larynx. Eur Arch Otorhinolaryngol 260(7):358–360

26. Haglund S, Lundquist PG, et al (1981) Interferon therapy in juvenile laryngeal papillomatosis. Arch Otolaryngol 107(6):327–332

27. Hammermann H, Glanz H, Kleinsasser O (1997) Lipomas of the larynx and hypopharynx: possible transformation into well-differentiated liposarcomas. In: Kelinsasser O, Glanz H, Olofsson J (eds) Advances of laryngology in Europe. Elsevier, Amsterdam, pp. 87–90

28. Healy GB, Gelber RD, Trowbridge AL, et al (1988) Treatment of recurrent respiratory papillomatosis with human leukocyte interferon. Results of a multicenter randomized clinical trial. N Eng J Med 319(7):401–417

29. Hinni ML (2000) Giant cell tumor of the larynx. Ann Otol Rhinol Laryngol 109:63–66

30. Holinger PH, Johnston KC (1951) Benign tumors of the larynx. Ann Otol Rhinol Laryngol 60(2):496–509

31. Jensen K, Swartz K (2006) A rare case of rhabdomyoma of the larynx causing airway obstruction. Ear Nose Throat J 85(2):116–118

32. Jines DA, Dillard SC, Bradford CR, et al (2003) Cartilage tumors of the larynx. J Otolaryngol 32(5):332–337

33. Johansen EC, Illum P (1995) Rhabdomyoma of the larynx: a review of the literature with a summary of previously described cases of rhabdomyoma of the larynx and a report of a new case. J Laryngol Otol 109(2):147–153

34. Jungehulsing M, Fishbach R, Pototschnig C, et al (2000) Rare benign tumors: laryngeal and hypopharyngeal lipomata. Ann Otol Rhinol Laryngol 109:301–305

35. Kapur TR (1968) Recurrent lipomata of the larynx and the Pharynx with late malignant change. J Laryngol Otol 82:761–768

36. Kawakami M, Hayashi I, Yoshimura K, et al (2006) Adult giant hemangioma of the larynx. Auris, Nasus Larynx 33:479–482

37. LaBagnara J, Hitchcock E, Spitzer T (1999) Rhabdomyoma of the true vocal fold. J Voice 13(2):289–293

38. Leventhal BG, Kashima HK, Mounts P. et al (1991) Long-term response of recurrent respiratory papillomatosis to treatment with lymphoblastoid interferon alfa-N1. Papilloma Study Group. N Eng J Med 325(9):613–617

39. Liang GS, Loevner LA, Kumar P (2000) Laryngeal rhabdomyoma involving the paraglottic space. Am J Radiol 174:1285–1387

40. Liess BD, Zitsch RP, Lane R, et al (2005) Multifocal adult rhabdomyoma: a case report and literature review. Am J Otolaryngol 26:214–217

41. Lucioni M, Marioni G, Libera DD, et al (2006) Adult laryngeal hemangioma CO_2 laser excision. Acta Otolaryngol 126:621–626

42. MacGregor AR, Batsakis JG, El-Naggar AK (2003) Myofibroblastoma of the larynx: a study of two cases. Head Neck 25:606–611

43. Martines F, Martines E, Caamitjana CF, et al (2007) Inflammatory myofibroblastic tumor of the larynx: Case report. An Otorhinolaringol Ibero Am. 34(2):210–208

44. Michaels L, Hellquist HB (2001) Textbook: ear nose and throat histopathology. Springer, London

45. Milford CA, Mulgliston TA, O'Flynn P, et al (1989). Carcinoma arising in a pleomorphic adenoma of the epiglottis. J Laryngol Otol 103:324–327

46. Motta G, Salzano FA, Motta S, et al (2003) CO_2 - laser treatment of laryngeal amyloidosis. J Laryngol Otol 117:647–650

47. Myer CM, 3rd, Willging JP, McMurray S, et al (1999) Use of a laryngeal micro resector system. Laryngoscope 109(7 Pt 1): 1165–1166

48. Myssiorek D, Rinaldo A, Barnes L, et al (2004). Laryngeal paraganglioma: an update critical review. Acat Otolaryngol 124:995–999

49. Nappi O, Ritter JH, Pettinato G, et al (1995) Haemangiopericytoma: histopathological pattern or clinicopathologic entity? Semin Diagn Pathol 12(3):221–232

50. Narozny WB, Mikaszewski B, Stankiewicz C (1995) Benign neoplasms of the larynx. Auris Nasus Larynx 22(1):38–42

51. New GB, Erich JB (1938) Benign tumors of the larynx: a study of 722 cases. Arch Otolaryngol Head Neck Surg 28:841

52. Newton JR, Ruckley EW, Earl UM (2006) Laryngeal neurilemmoma: a case report. Ear, Nose Throat J 85:448–449

53. Pelucchi, S, Amoroso C, Grandi E, et al (2002) Granular cell tumor of the larynx: Literature review and case report. J Laryngol 31:234–235

54. Pontes P, Avelino M, Pignatari S, et al (2006) Effect of local application of cidofovir on the control of recurrences in recurrent laryngeal papillomatosis. Otolaryngol Head Neck Surg 135(1):22–27

55. Popella C, Glanz H, Kelinsasser O, et al (1997) Various clinical and pathomorphological appearances on amyloid deposits in the larynx. In: Kelinsasser O, Glanz H, Olofsson J (eds) Advances of laryngology in Europe. Elsevier, Amsterdam, pp. 53–55

56. Reeves WC, Ruparelia SS, Swanson KI et al (2003) National registry for juvenile-onset recurrent respiratory papillomatosis. Arch Otolaryngol Head Neck Surg 129(9):976–982

57. Reidy PM, Dedo HH, Rabah R, et al (2004) Integration of human papillomavirus type 11 in recurrent respiratory papilloma-associated cancer. Laryngoscope 114(11):1906–1909

58. Rihkanen H, Aaltonen LM, Syrjanen SM (1993) Human papillomavirus in laryngeal papillomas and in adjacent normal epithelium Clin Otolaryngol 18(6):470–474

59. Rinaldo A, Fisher C, Mannara GM, et al (1998) Hamartoma of the larynx: a critical review of the literature. Ann Otol Rhinol Laryngol 107:264–267

60. Rinaldo A, Howard DJ, Ferlito AA (2000) Laryngeal chondrosarcoma: a 24 year experience at the Royal National Throat, Nose and Ear Hospital. Acta Otolaryngol 120:680–688

61. Sabri JA, Hajjar MA (1967) Malignant mixed tumor of the vocal cord. Arch Otolaryngol 85:118–120

62. Sanders KW, Abreo F, Rivera E (2001) A diagnostic and therapeutic approach to paragangliomas of the larynx. Arch Otolaryngol Head Neck Surg 127(5):565–569

63. Sanghvi V, Lala M, Borges A, Rodrigues G, Pathak KA, Parikh D (1999). Lateral thyrotomy for neurilemmoma of the larynx. J Laryngol Otol 113:346–348

64. Sawatsubashi M, Tuda K, Tokunaga O, et al (1997). Pleomorphic adenoma of the larynx: a case report and a review of the literature in Japan. Otolaryngol Head Neck Surg 117(4):415–417

65. Schraff S, Derkay CS, Burke B, et al (2004). American Society of Paediatric Otolaryngology members' experience with recurrent respiratory papillomatosis and the use of adjuvant therapy. Arch Otolaryngol Head Neck Surg130(9): 1039–1042

66. Sesterhenn AM, Folz BJ, Lippert BM, et al (2003). Laser surgery treatment of laryngeal paraganglioma. J Laryngol Otol 117(5):641–646

67. Shehab N, Sweet BV, Hogikyan ND (2005) Cidofovir for the treatment of recurrent respiratory papillomatosis: a review of the literature. Pharmacotherapy 25(7):977–989

68. Snoeck R,Wellens W, Desloovere C, et al (1998). Treatment of severe laryngeal papillomatosis with intralesional injections of cidofovir [(S)-1-(3-hydroxy-2-phosphonylmethoxypropyl) cytosine]. J Med Virol 54(3):219–225

69. Syeda F, Hussain A (2005) Schwannoma of the larynx: A case report. Ear, Nose Throat J 84(11):732–734

70. Taylor J, Stiefel M, Park SY (2006) Schwannoma of the true vocal fold: A rare diagnosis. Ear, Nose Throat J 85(1): 52–53, 59

71. Toprak M, Oz F, Oktem F, Acioglu E, et al (2003). Granular cell tumor of the larynx. J Otolaryngol 34:363–365

72. Van Cutsem E, Snoeck R, Van Ranst M, et al (1995) Successful treatment of a squamous papilloma of the hypopharynx-esophagus by local injections of (S)-1-(3-hydroxy-2-phosphonylmethoxypropyl)cytosine. J Med Virol 45(2):230–235

73. Wenig BM (1995) Necrotising sialometaplasia of the larynx. Am J Clin Pathol 103(5):609–613

74. Wenig BM, Devaney K, Bisceglia M (1995) Inflammatory myofibroblastic tumor of the larynx. Cancer 76(11): 2217–2229

75. Wenig BM, Devaney K, Wenig BL (1995). Pseudoneoplastic lesions of the oropharynx and larynx simulating cancer. Pathol Annu 30(pt 1):143–187

76. Wiatrak BJ, Wiatrak DW, Broker TR et al (2004). Recurrent respiratory papillomatosis: a longitudinal study comparing severity associated with human papilloma viral types 6 and 11 and other risk factors in a large pediatric population. Laryngoscope 114(11 Pt 2 Suppl 104):1–23

77. Windfuhr JP (2003). Pitfalls in the diagnosis and management of laryngeal chondrosarcoma. J Laryngol Otol 117: 651–655

78. World Health Organisation (1991). Histological typing of tumors of the upper respiratory tract and ear. Springer-Verlag, Berlin

79. Yilmaz MD, Aktepe F, Altuntas A (2004). Cavernous hemangioma of the left vocal cord. Eur Arch Otorhinolaryngol 261: 310–311

80. Yellin S, LaBruna A, Ananol VK et al (1996). Nd: YAG laser treatment for laryngeal and hypopharyngeal hemangiomas: A new technique. Ann Otol Rhinol Laryngol 105:510–515

81. Zeitels SM, Akst LM, Burns JA, et al (2006) Office-based 532-nm pulsed KTP laser treatment of glottal papillomatosis and dysplasia. Ann Otol Rhinol Laryngol 115(9):679–685

Laryngotracheal Blunt Trauma

8

Ferhan Öz and Barış Karakullukçu

Core Messages

> Laryngotracheal trauma is probably underestimated but the consequence of such trauma can range from mild hoarseness to complete airway compromise

> Narrowing of the airway results in breathing difficulty. We find this by looking through the patients registered in emergency archives. Complication rates among these patients are as high as 15–25%. The team in charge of the patient must keep in mind that the airway compromise will become worse with time as the edema increases.

> The elasticity of the cartilage framework contributes to airway's recoil, saving the airway even if the external pressure or the blow is strong enough to exceed the resistance of this structure.

> The larynx and trachea are vulnerable only to direct blows to the anterior neck. For damage to occur the object of contact has to approach the larynx in a horizontal manner. If the object is in vertical position relative to the body, the impact is blocked by the facial skeleton and/or sternum and clavicle heads.

> Fiberoptic laryngoscopy has become the initial evaluation tool for laryngeal injury. In case the endolarynx cannot be assessed with flexible laryngoscopy due to laryngeal edema, direct laryngoscopy should be carried out under general anesthesia. All of the upper aerodigestive tract mucosa should be examined

> Cartilage frame fractures are rare in the pediatric group, but soft tissue edema and hematoma are more common. In elderly people, the cartilage framework is usually calcified and has undergone osseous transformation. The laryngotracheal fractures in this age group are more common and usually more severe.

> Posterior or lateral dislocations of the arytenoids may occur at this stage when the thyroid cartilage is pressed against the vertebra by external pressure. Posterior dislocation of the arytenoids is reported to be more common. It is usually associated with traumatic orotracheal intubation rather than external trauma. Arytenoid dislocations can be confused with vocal cord paralysis during examination. Electromyography is an important tool to differentiate the two conditions.

> In the rare case of complete disruption between the cricoid cartilage and the trachea, the strap muscles and the surrounding fascia can serve as a temporary airway until the patient is managed by intubation or tracheotomy.

> Once the injuries are addressed and the patient is stabilized and assessed, the larynx and cervical trauma should be repaired surgically as soon as possible. A patient with minimal soft tissue edema, mobile vocal cords, and no difficulty with breathing can be observed closely without any surgical intervention.

F. Öz (✉)
Valikonagi cad.No:161/12 Nisantasi, 80200 Istanbul, Turkey
e-mail: ferhanoz@tkbbv.org.tr

Laryngotracheal trauma, including blunt and penetrating trauma, is one of the common causes of airway compromise. This type of injury is probably underestimated but the consequence of a laryngotracheal trauma

M. Remacle, H. E. Eckel (eds.), *Surgery of Larynx and Trachea,*
DOI: 10.1007/978-3-540-79136-2_8, © Springer-Verlag Berlin Heidelberg 2010

can range from mild hoarseness to complete airway compromise. In the United States 1 in 14,000 to 1 in 30,000 emergency room visits is due to laryngotracheal trauma [1, 2]. Many more go undiagnosed because the injured person does not take mild hoarseness seriously and does not go to the emergency department.

The most common causes of laryngotracheal trauma are motor vehicle accidents and sports injuries [3, 4]. A decrease in the incidence of laryngotracheal injury was observed after the automobile safety belt use was mandatory and other safety features of motor vehicles were developed. The presence of airbags should eliminate sudden, savage blows to the anterior neck due to collision with the steering wheel or other hardware on the dashboard as well as injuries caused by misplaced safety belts. However, there is no objective study demonstrating this beneficial effect. Laryngotracheal trauma due to sports injuries are common in contact sports such as football, basketball, baseball, and soccer.

The degree of injury may vary from mild soft tissue edema to severe laryngeal framework fractures and to complete separation between the larynx and trachea. Mild injuries that result in temporary voice changes or throat pain probably go unregistered in medical archives. This degree of injury is temporary due to the extreme flexibility and resistance of the laryngotracheal framework. More severe trauma may cause injury to the framework and severe soft tissue edema or hematoma. Narrowing of the airway results in breathing difficulty. These are the cases that are registered in emergency department archives. Among these patients complication rates are as high as 15–25% [5, 6].

Complications include chronic airway obstruction and chronic voice changes. Injury to the laryngotracheal structure can be lethal because of airway compromise. Severe injuries with complete airway obstruction necessitate immediate airway management with orotracheal intubation or, more commonly, emergent tracheotomy. Many of these patients may not survive the time interval between the accident and arrival of medical assistance. Mortality rates are reported to be 2–35% among those with severe laryngotracheal injury [5, 6]. The principles of immediate airway management and long-term management of complications are discussed in this chapter.

8.1 Injury of the Cartilage Framework of the Larynx and Cervical Trachea

The airway is well protected as it passes through the neck. Thyroid cartilage and tracheal rings provide a framework that protects the airway from external compression. The elasticity of the cartilage framework contributes to its recoil, saving the airway even if the external pressure or the blow is strong enough to exceed the resistance of this structure. The larynx, and more pronouncedly the trachea, can be almost completely compressed and can recoil back to the original structure once the external pressure subsides. The optimal balance of strength and elasticity of the cartilage network is achieved by the time of early adulthood. During childhood the cartilage is much more elastic and lacks structural strength. At this period in life the airway is more vulnerable to external pressure that results in complete airway obstruction. However, the recoil effect is more pronounced as well. Once the external pressure is removed, the recoil is almost complete. Therefore, cartilage frame fractures are rare in the pediatric age group, whereas soft tissue edema and hematoma are more common [7, 8]. In elderly people the cartilage framework is usually calcified and has undergone osseous transformation. The airway is more resistant to external pressure. This increased resistance does not necessarily serve as airway protection. Loss of elasticity results in fractures with less forceful blows. Laryngotracheal fractures in this age group are more common and usually more severe [6, 8].

Surrounding the cartilage framework are the strap muscles, subcutaneous fat, and skin. These extralaryngeal soft tissues offer a buffer between the impact and the laryngotracheal cartilage framework. Sternocleidomastoid muscles protect the larynx from lateral blows. The mandible often blocks the impact that comes from the superior to inferior angle. Likewise, the clavicles and sternum may block an impact that comes from the inferior direction. The larynx and trachea are vulnerable only to direct blows to the anterior neck for damage to occur. The object of contact—whether a bat, a steering wheel, a dashboard, or a rope—must approach the larynx in a horizontal manner. If the object is in a vertical position relative to the body, the impact is blocked by the facial skeleton and/or sternum and clavicle heads [8].

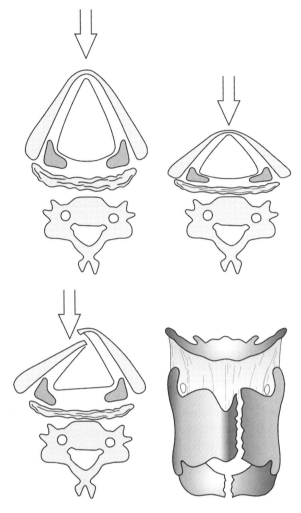

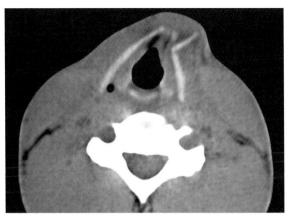

Fig. 8.2. Computed tomography (CT) image of a patient with a paramedian fracture of the thyroid cartilage. A fragment of cartilage is displaced laterally. The airway appears to be patent

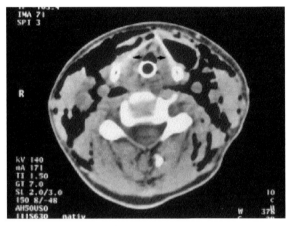

Fig. 8.1. The first impact is taken by the thyroid prominence, and thyroid cartilage is compressed against the vertebra, displacing the thyroid alas laterally. When the point of maximum compressibility is reached, the thyroid cartilage fractures in the vertical axis either medially or more commonly paramedially

Fig. 8.3. CT image of a patient with a median fracture of the thyroid cartilage. There is extensive subcutaneous emphysema in the neck, suggesting soft tissue injury to the larynx. There is an endotracheal tube in the larynx

The most common blunt trauma to the larynx and cervical trachea is caused by motor vehicle accidents. The steering wheel and dashboards are located at the correct angle to produce an injury to the larynx and trachea. Collision of the vehicle causes sudden deceleration, throwing the body into the steering wheel and dashboards. Safety belts help slow the velocity of the impact, and airbags help prevent the contact totally. In the case where no seatbelt or airbag is present, the upper body is thrown violently against the steering wheel and dashboard. Even in this situation the head is usually flexed, and the mandible serves to protect the larynx. If the larynx comes into contact with hardware,

the first impact is taken by the thyroid prominence; in this case the thyroid cartilage is compressed against the vertebra, displacing the thyroid alas laterally. When the point of maximum compressibility is reached, the thyroid cartilage fractures in the vertical axis either medially or more commonly paramedially [8, 9] (Figs. 8.1, 8.2, and 8.3). The point of maximum compressibility varies greatly with age and from person to person. Young victims may experience a single line of fracture, whereas older people may have multiple fractures.

If the impact is more inferior, the cricoid cartilage may be affected (Fig. 8.4). The cricoid cartilage is a complete cartilage ring with more rigidity than tracheal

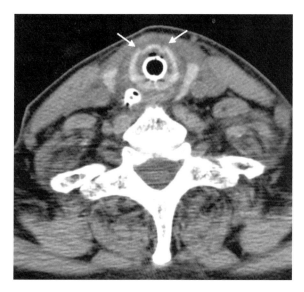

Fig. 8.4. CT image of a patient with a cricoid fracture. The cricoid cartilage is fractured in two places. There is an endotracheal tube in the airway

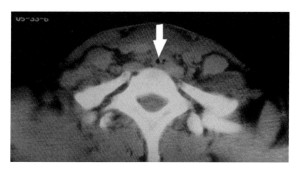

Fig. 8.5. CT image of a patient with almost complete collapse of the airway

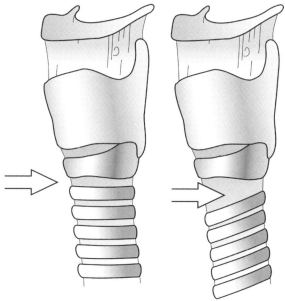

Fig. 8.6. Horizontal trauma at the level of the cricoid and first thyroid cartilage usually results in cricotracheal separation. The posterior tracheal wall may still be attached

rings or thyroid cartilage. Whereas the thyroid ala can spread laterally with the advantage of being an incomplete circular structure, the cricoid cartilage cannot displace laterally but, is rather, compressed into an oval shape [8]. This can result in a median fracture. More severe blows can cause fragmentation of the cricoid cartilage and loss of the airway (Fig. 8.5). This fragmentation can also cause the injury to one or both recurrent laryngeal nerves at the region of the cricothyroid joint, with subsequent vocal cord paralysis and further narrowing of the airway.

If the impact is on an area lower than the cricoid cartilage, complete separation of the larynx and trachea may occur. The usual site of separation is between the cricoid cartilage and the first tracheal ring [10] (Fig. 8.6). The separation may be accompanied by cricoid cartilage

fracture or may occur without a fracture. This type of injury is more commonly associated with the neck coming into contact with a fixed cable or rope while riding a motorbike, jet ski, snowmobile, or a similar vehicle where the neck is not protected against outside objects.

Two vectors of force cause laryngotracheal separation. The first is compression of the cricoid cartilage and the trachea against the vertebral bodies, as described above. The second vector is the "telescoping effect." When the neck comes into contact with a fixed wire or a rope while traveling fast, it comes to a complete stop while the body still moves forward. This pulls the trachea from the fixed larynx, causing separation [11]. The separation can be complete or incomplete. The posterior membranous portion of the trachea may remain attached while the anterior cartilaginous trachea is separated from the larynx. In that case, the trachea does not retract completely into the chest. An intubation or a tracheotomy are easier in case of incomplete separation of the airway, the posterior wall serving as a guide for airway management.

If the trachea is completely separated from the larynx, it retracts into the chest. This most often results in complete and sudden loss of airway, which is fatal. Rarely, the strap muscles and surrounding fascia serve as a temporary airway until the patient is managed by intubation or tracheotomy.

Another mechanism of injury is falling onto the handlebar of a bicycle or onto any horizontally positioned hard object. This kind of impact may cause the cricoid cartilage to be displaced superiorly under the thyroid cartilage [12, 13], resulting in the soft tissues doubling onto themselves and severe soft tissue edema. Frequently, this injury is seen in young children with flexible cartilage. Fractures do not occur with this kind of trauma in young children, whereas adults who experience this sort of impact present with cricoid fractures. This displacement may cause injury to one or both of the recurrent laryngeal nerves with subsequent vocal cord paralysis [11–14].

8.2 Injury of the Cricoarytenoid Joint

Arytenoid cartilages are in relation with the cricoid cartilage via a joint, and with the thyroid cartilage via the vocal ligament and the thyroarytenoid muscle. Arytenoid cartilages are located deep to the thyroid cartilage and the hyoid bone. In case of external laryngeal trauma, fracture of arytenoid cartilages is prevented by the thyroid cartilage but, most importantly, by the extreme mobility of the cricoarytenoid joint [15]. When the thyroid cartilage is pressed against the vertebra by external pressure, the arytenoid cartilages are displaced laterally and posteriorly. Posterior or lateral dislocation of the arytenoids may occur at this stage. With the sudden release of pressure, the thyroid cartilage springs back to its original shape. This sudden springing motion pulls the arytenoid cartilage by its muscular attachments anteriorly to the thyroid cartilage [9, 16]. This motion may result in anterior luxation or subluxation of the arytenoid cartilage. Posterior dislocation of the arytenoids is reported to be more common, but it is usually associated with traumatic orotracheal intubation trauma rather than external trauma [16]. Dislocation of the arytenoid cartilages is usually associated with severe soft tissue trauma, which can cause edema, masking the larynx and making the diagnosis of dislocation difficult [17]. Dislocation of the cricoarytenoid joint impairs vocal cord movement. Arytenoid dislocations can be confused with vocal cord paralysis. Electromyography (EMG) is an important tool to use to differentiate the two conditions. EMG would detect muscle contraction potentials in case of arytenoid dislocation. These potentials would be absent in the case of vocal cord paralysis.

8.3 Laryngeal Soft Tissue Injury

External blunt trauma to the larynx almost always results in soft tissue injury. The loose submucosal connective tissue is prone to fluid collection and edema. Even the mildest trauma results in some degree of swelling of the endolarynx. This may manifest as a change in voice or more seriously as breathing difficulty. As the impact of the trauma increases, the likelihood of having a mucosal laceration increases as well. Lacerations may cause bleeding and contribute to airway problems. Laryngeal framework fractures are usually associated with mucosal injuries [9]. Mucosal injury may range from mild tissue edema to large lacerations. The mucosa can be crushed or caught between cartilage fragments. In the case of laryngotracheal separation, the mucosa cannot withstand the pulling forces and is separated as well. Large lacerations of the mucosa may cause emphysema due to air leakage into the soft tissues of the neck. Air can accumulate around the strap muscles as well as in the subcutaneous plane. Extensive ecchymosis and crepitation of the skin makes the diagnosis of emphysema easily recognizable. Soft tissue emphysema may contribute to airway compromise (Figs. 8.7 and 8.8). After repair of the larynx, air in the soft tissues is gradually resorbed.

A distinct soft tissue injury is rupture of the thyroarytenoid muscle and ligament. As the thyroid cartilage is pressed against the vertebra and springs back, the muscle and the ligament relax and undergo

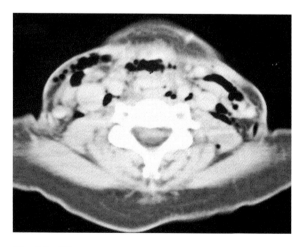

Fig. 8.7. CT scan shows that there is extensive subcutaneous emphysema, and the airway cannot be identified

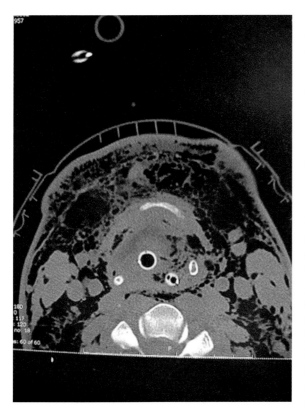

Fig. 8.8. CT scan at the level of the hyoid bone demonstrates subcutaneous emphysema. The airway can be identified only by the presence of an endotracheal tube

tension within a short period of time. This may result in rupture or detachment of the ligament from the thyroid cartilage at the level of the anterior commissure. As the ligament detaches from the anterior commissure, usually a small piece of cartilage also detaches. Rupture or detachment results in bunching of the vocal cord and narrowing of the airway. The injury is always accompanied by severe edema of the Reinke's space. Dislocation of the arytenoid cartilage may also accompany the injury [15].

Suicidal or accidental hanging causes trauma to the supraglottic larynx. The rope around the neck tightens at the level of the thyrohyoid membrane [18]. The external pressure causes the preepiglottic space to move posteriorly, pushing the epiglottis against the arytenoid cartilages. This causes complete obstruction of the airway. If the person survives the impact, the subsequent injury is severe supraglottic edema. The thyrohyoid membrane may rupture, and the preepiglottic fat tissue may herniate into the airway. Hyoid bone fractures occur rarely if the rope tightens

at the level of the hyoid bone [19]. Hyoid bone fractures do not have any clinical implications unless a fragment tears through the airway mucosa. Thyroid and cricoid cartilage can also be fractured. Laryngotracheal separation has been reported to occur due to hanging injuries [20].

8.4 Emergency Management of Laryngotracheal Blunt Trauma

Blunt trauma to the laryngotracheal area can cause an airway emergency. All cases should be managed according to the emergency airway management protocol of the managing (??? manageing yerine başka bir gelime gelebilir mi?) institution regardless of the degree and the place of trauma. Loss of critical time can be lethal in case of laryngotracheal injuries. Elaborate examination and imaging should be left for later. Management of the airway is the primary objective. If the patient is not breathing at the time of initial management, cardiopulmonary resuscitation (CPR) should be carried out immediately. Many of these patients have accompanying cervical spine injuries. Care should be taken not to move the cervical spine. Unless proven otherwise, all patients should be assumed to have cervical spine injury.

Endolaryngeal edema develops immediately after laryngotracheal trauma. If the emergency team arrives soon after the trauma, orotracheal intubation may be successful. After a certain period of time edema would be present, and intubation could be extremely difficult, necessitating a tracheotomy [21, 22]. The team in charge of the patient must keep in mind that the airway will become worse in time as the edema increases. In case of extensive laryngotracheal trauma, intubation should be considered even if the patient is able to breathe sufficiently. As mentioned, intubation could be difficult if not impossible as time passes. Orotracheal intubation can be achieved even in case of laryngotracheal separation. Laryngotracheal separation usually occurs in the anterior wall of the trachea between the cricoid and the first tracheal rings, with the posterior wall of the trachea staying intact. If the endotracheal tube is advanced following the tract of the posterior tracheal wall, intubation of the separated tracheal segment can be achieved. Even if complete separation occurs, the surrounding soft tissues would not collapse immediately and can

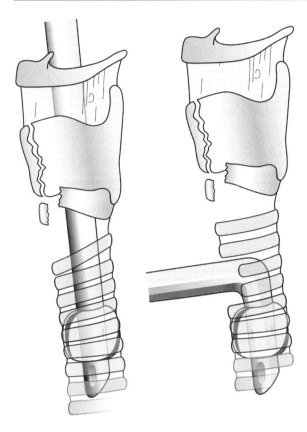

Fig. 8.9. The first option for airway management is endotracheal intubation. The posterior tracheal wall can guide the endotracheal tube in the airway even if the distant airway cannot be visualized. The second option is to perform a tracheotomy. The best place to perform a tracheotomy is two tracheal rings below the site of injury

serve as a guide for intubation [21, 22] (Fig. 8.9). If orotracheal intubation can be achieved, the endotracheal tube serves as a stent, preventing possible synechia of the endolaryngeal mucosa thus making further airway management easier. If intubation cannot be achieved after a few trials, no time should be wasted before attempting the tracheotomy.

The level of tracheotomy should be chosen according to the level of the place of the trauma. For a high positioned laryngeal injury, such as a hanging case, the fastest and easiest method would be a cricothyrotomy. However, if the thyroid cartilage and/or the cricoid cartilage is fractured, a lower tracheotomy would be necessary. The level of the place of the injury can be determined by palpating the neck under emergency conditions. Fragments of cartilage and/or depressions in the laryngotracheal framework indicate the site of injury. Sometimes edema and hematomas developing

in the soft tissues of the neck make this examination difficult. In such a case, the mechanism of injury gives clues about the injury site. As already noted, the most common laryngotracheal injuries are caused by steering wheel and dashboard impacts in motor vehicle accidents, inducing injuries at the level of the thyroid and cricoid cartilages. Bicycle and sports accidents also cause injuries at the same level. In this case, the best level for tracheotomy is two tracheal rings below the injury site [21, 22] (Fig. 8.9). Tracheotomy should be performed below the third tracheal ring.

Laryngotracheal separation is likely to occur in case of a jet-ski or snowmobile accident, where the neck comes in contact with a fixed object such as a rope. Laryngotracheal separation is the most difficult injury to manage in terms of the airway. The airway can be secured by neck exploration and identification of the separated tracheal segment low in the neck or thorax. The endotracheal tube can be passed through the separated trachea. The tracheal segment should be secured to the skin incision and to the head of the clavicle with nonabsorbable sutures. This step facilitates reintubation in case of accidental extubation. Once the airway is secured, other life-threatening injuries should be addressed before any attempt is made to repair the laryngotracheal damage.

8.5 Evaluation of Laryngotracheal Injury

Once the patient is stabilized, evaluation of the laryngotracheal damage should be done. Endoscopic assessment is the next step. Today, fiberoptic laryngoscopy has become the initial evaluation tool. It is less traumatic and more comfortable for the patient than the methods mentioned previously. Checking airway patency and any potential causes that might impair the airway is the priority. Tracheotomy should be performed in case of increasing edema or hematoma. If the airway patency is adequate, the site and degree of damage are then evaluated. Mucosal lacerations, location of arytenoids, and vocal cord mobility must be assessed.

Supraglottic edema may prevent examination of glottic and subglottic areas [23]. In case the endolarynx cannot be assessed with flexible laryngoscopy due to laryngeal edema, direct laryngoscopy can be carried out under general anesthesia. During direct laryngoscopy all of the upper aerodigestive tract mucosa is examined. Mobility of the arytenoid cartilages is tested with a blunt instrument, such as a velvet tipped suction or cup forceps with the tip in closed position. Additional trauma to the laryngeal mucosa should be avoided.

Bronchoscopy is performed to assess the trachea. Esophagoscopy should be carried out as well because esophageal trauma as a result of an impact to the neck can be infrequent.

The downside of direct laryngoscopy is the inability to assess function properly. Videostroboscopy is a valuable tool for assessing vocal cord injuries. It can even reveal subtle injuries to the vocal cords. If the patient is already intubated, direct laryngoscopy is indicated.

Imaging of the laryngotracheal framework can precede direct laryngoscopy. Computed tomography (CT) scans of the neck should be performed if flexible laryngoscopy reveals extensive soft tissue injury, vocal cord paralysis, bare cartilage or if there are palpable cartilage fractures and crepitations in the neck. The CT scan should include fine cuts through the larynx. Special attention should be given to thyroid, cricoid, and tracheal cartilages as well as the localization of arytenoid cartilages. Magnetic resonance imaging (MRI) is better for assessing soft tissue injuries, but CT remains to be the first method of choice for imaging while assessing the laryngotracheal framework.

Laryngeal EMG is important for assessing nerve injuries. The superior laryngeal nerve is usually not injured by external trauma to the larynx. However, the recurrent laryngeal nerve is frequently affected by injury involving the cricoid cartilage and laryngotracheal separation. EMG can detect contraction potentials and resting potentials even in unconscious patients.

If observation is chosen, repeated fiberoscopy or direct laryngoscopy can be performed at 24, 48, and 72 hours after surgery to monitor the endolaryngeal edema.

8.6 Laryngotracheal Trauma Repair

Once the lethal injuries are addressed and the patient is stabilized and assessed, surgical repair of the larynx and cervical trauma should be done as soon as possible. Early repair has more favorable results than late repair [24].

The decision to repair the laryngotracheal injury should be based on the presence and the severity of cartilage fragmentation, the degree of airway obstruction, and

Table 8.1. Indications for open surgery

Displaced single fracture of the laryngotracheal framework
Multiple fractures of the laryngotracheal framework (including nondisplaced fractures)
Laryngotracheal separation
Thyroarytenoid muscle and ligament tear or detachment
Esophageal tears
Arytenoid dislocation that cannot be reduced endoscopically
Hematoma that is obstructing the airway
Denuded cartilage

Table 8.2. Endoscopic findings that require surgery

Exposed cartilage
Depressions in the airway that suggest cartilage fracture
Laryngotracheal separation
Mucosal fragments that obstruct the airway
Injury to the free edge of vocal cords
Cricoarytenoid dislocation
Displacement of the epiglottis
Herniation of preepiglottic contents
Thyroarytenoid muscle or ligament injury

a recurrent laryngeal nerve injury (Table 8.1). A patient with minimal soft tissue edema, mobile vocal cords, and no difficulty breathing can be observed closely without any surgical intervention. The managing team should remember that soft tissue edema may get worse with time. Close observation is necessary. Extensive soft tissue injuries necessitate either endoscopic or open repair. Table 8.2 is a list of endoscopic findings that indicate laryngeal repair. If an arytenoid dislocation is observed, the best results are obtained with early endoscopic reduction.

Cartilage fractures usually require open exploration, repair, and fixation. Although there is no displacement some cartilage fractures can be detected by CT. Single median or paramedian vertical thyroid cartilage fractures are the most common. Close observation is an option if the fracture is single and not displaced and if there is no extensive soft tissue injury or detachment of the thyroarytenoid muscle. However, fixation of the framework by an external approach is a safe alternative because the fragments of cartilage can be displaced afterwards, obstructing the airway.

Penetrating tears of the esophagus should be addressed with an open neck exploration.

If there is no indication for the open approach (see Table 8.1), repair can be carried out with rigid laryngoscopy. Mucosal flaps that obstruct the airway or interfere with phonation should be removed. Obtaining straight, free edges of vocal cords is essential. Mucosal flaps on the free edges of the vocal cords should be positioned back in place or removed. Cold steel instruments, powered instruments, or laser can be used for removal. If the preepiglottic space contents are herniated into the airway without accompanying fractures, these tissues should be removed. In case of the epiglottis obstructing the airway, the entire epiglottis or a part of it can be resected. This can be achieved with laser or powered instruments.

In case of cricoarytenoid luxation, repositioning the arytenoid cartilage should be attempted. Early reduction has better results because ankylosis becomes apparent within about a week. Posterior dislocation can be reduced by applying a medial and anterior force with an instrument placed posterior to the dislocated arytenoid. The laryngoscope can be used to force the arytenoids anteriorly. Anterior dislocations can be reduced by placing the rigid laryngoscope just anterior to the displaced arytenoids and applying posterior pressure. With anterior dislocations there is a tendency of the arytenoid to be displaced inferiorly. In that case, a blunt right-angle instrument such as a blunt hook can be placed anteriorly and inferiorly to the arytenoid, and the arytenoid can be lifted and pushed posteriorly. The maneuvers must be gentle. These vocal process can be fractured with forceful movements, resulting in poor quality of the voice after the reduction.

On some occasions, endoscopic repair can be combined with an open neck approach. Open surgery is done through a horizontal incision in a skin crease or close to the thyroid cartilage. Subplatysmal flaps are elevated, and strap muscles are divided in two through the midline and retracted laterally. Adequate exposure of the thyroid and cricoid cartilages is essential. Care should be taken not to injure the external branches of the superior laryngeal nerves or the recurrent nerves. If there is a vertical thyroid cartilage fracture, entry to the larynx can be through the fracture line. The mucosal incision is preferentially made through the midline across the anterior commissure to prevent further mucosal injury. If there is a horizontal fracture, the opening can be achieved with a laryngofissure vertical to the midline.

Mucosal injury should be assessed when exposure is achieved. Reconstruction of the deep structures is the first step. Arytenoid cartilages are restored to their original positions, and thyroarytenoid muscle or ligament tears are repaired with sutures. If there is a thyroarytenoid muscle detachment, a strong suture can be passed through the vocal ligament and fixed to the cartilage

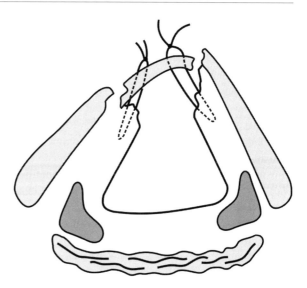

Fig. 8.10. In the case of detachment of the anterior commissure, the vocal ligaments should be suspended to the cartilage fragment that corresponds to the cartilage portion of the anterior commissure with nonabsorbable sutures

segment corresponding to the original position of the anterior commissure (???) (Fig. 8.10). Incorrect positioning of the vocal ligament results in poor vocal quality. Once the deeper architecture is restored, the mucosal tears can be considered. The goal is to cover the entire endolaryngeal surface with mucosa to facilitate wound healing and to prevent granuloma formation. Irreparable mucosal fragments are removed. Remaining mucosa is then aligned and sutured with fine absorbable sutures. If there is not enough mucosa to cover the entire larynx, priority is given to the glottic area and especially the anterior commissure, which is the most common site of scar and synechia formation. Keels can be used to prevent web formation as well. The second important area is the arytenoid cartilage. Adequate covering of the arytenoids prevents ankylosis of the joint by scar formation. Local mucosal flaps can be raised to facilitate mucosal redraping. Laterally based piriform sinus flaps and posteriorly based postcricoid flaps can be used to cover the arytenoid region. Epiglottic flaps can be used to cover the anterior commissure. If there is extensive mucosal and cartilage fragmentation in the anterior commissure, the epiglottic cartilage can be mobilized from its anterior attachments and pulled inferiorly to cover both the mucosa and the cartilage defects.

In case of epiglottis displacement and herniation of the preepiglottic contents, the is epiglottic contents are removed and the epiglottis is pulled anteriorly and fixed to the hyoid bone with strong absorbable sutures. Removal of part of the epiglottis should be considered if traction cannot be achieved.

When the endolaryngeal repairing is achieved, it must be decided whether to place a stent or not. Stents are useful for preventing synechiae. If the mucosal injury is extensive and synechia formation is likely to happen, a stent should be placed. There are several commercially available stents. A custom-made stent can be constructed from a finger of a surgical glove or a Penrose drain filled with sponge and tied at both ends with silk sutures. Stents should be fixed to the neck skin to prevent dislocation. Strong silk sutures are passed through the stent and brought to the neck skin; they are then tied on a button to prevent pulling on the sutures and irritating the neck skin. Stents can be taken out endoscopically after 3–5 weeks. In case of anterior commissure injury, a keel should be placed and secured to the skin (see Chapter 12b).

The next step is the reconstruction of the laryngotracheal framework. Each cartilage fragment has to be identified and positioned in correct alignment. Perfusion of the cartilage is through the perichondrium. Free cartilage fragments can still be used as free grafts as long as they are covered with well perfused tissue. Comminuted pieces that cannot be fixed are removed. Complete reconstruction of the cartilage frame is not necessary as long as the three-dimensional shape of the larynx can be achieved. Miniplates and recently introduced absorbable plates are the best materials to use for joining the cartilage fragments (Fig. 8.11). Single fractures that resemble their natural shape once brought together can be repaired with wire or sutures, but miniplates should be used if they are available. Miniplates of 1.0–1.4 mm thickness are preferred because they are easy to shape and their thinner profile is not visible through the skin. If the remaining cartilage is not sufficient to reconstruct the framework, free cartilage grafts (e.g., nasal septal cartilage or costal cartilage) can be used. The epiglottis is another source of cartilage and has the advantage of providing a pedicled flap. Correct placement of the vocal ligaments is essential to obtain a good vocal-quality after reconstruction. The cartilage fragment attached to the vocal ligaments must be exactly positioned at the level of the normal anterior commissure. If one of the vocal ligaments is detached, it must be reattached at exactly the same level of the contralateral ligament with a sturdy suture. If the vocal ligament cannot be attached to a cartilage fragment, the suture can be tied on a plate. In this case, nonabsorbable suture and plate are preferred to avoid detachment.

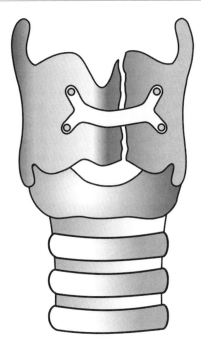

Fig. 8.11. External fixation of the tracheal cartilage with miniplates gives excellent reconstructive results

Laryngotracheal separation is repaired by end-to-end anastomosis. If the tracheotomy tube is placed in the tracheal segment, it must be removed and placed through a tracheotomy incision two or three rings below the avulsed site as the first step of reconstruction. If the tracheal ring is severed, it should be removed.

The tracheal ring is suspended to the cricoid ring with sturdy absorbable sutures that are outside (???) as much as possible. Ideally, the stitches are also placed extramucosally. These precautions are taken to prevent granulomas and stenosis. If the end-to-end anastomosis cannot be performed perfectly and the laryngeal reconstruction is not stable, a T-tube is put in place to serve as a stent, allowing voice production and breathing. According to the trauma and reconstruction, this tube can stay in place 3 weeks to 3–4 months.

All additional neck injuries are addressed as the neck is being explored. Esophageal tears should be repaired as soon as possible. Leaks from the esophagus may have life-threatening consequences, such as mediastinitis. Tears should be closed in a watertight fashion. Today absorbable sutures placed in a running mattress style are preferred. A second layer of muscle should be closed over the suture line. A nasogastric feeding tube can be placed in during surgery to allow postoperative feeding.

If a recurrent nerve injury is observed, the separated segments should be sought. It is sometimes difficult to find both ends of the recurrent laryngeal nerve in the trauma field. The nerve may part intralaryngeally or, more frequently, right where it enters the larynx. If both ends of the nerve are found, end-to-end anastomosis should be done. Primary repair of the recurrent laryngeal nerve does not have favorable results. Abduction and adduction functions of the vocal cords may not return. However, if tonus to the vocal cord can be achieved, voice rehabilitation is easier.

Additional repair may be necessary after the initial surgical repair. Laryngotracheal separation causes a high rate of stenosis after primary anastomosis. Anterior commissure injuries are associated with anterior web formation. Synechiae and granulomas may develop after extensive soft tissue injuries. Secondary repairs are beyond the scope of this chapter and are addressed in the other chapters of this book. Unilateral vocal cord paralysis can be treated by applying vocal cord injection or medialization thyroplasty.

8.7 Postoperative Management

Last but not least, (??? daha profesyonel bir ifade kullanılabilir mi?) postoperative care is crucial. Voice rest and adequate humidification helps the healing process. Antibiotics are administered to prevent chondritis. Antireflux medications should also be given Steroids may be used to limit endolaryngeal edema for patients without tracheotomy. Patients with tracheotomy, however, should not receive steroids, as steroids may impair tissue healing. Stents and keels are usually removed 3–5 weeks after placement.

Closing the tracheotomy should be delayed until the tissue edema is resolved and the patient is able to clear secretions adequately. Permanent tracheotomy may be necessary for some patients—in case of severe stenosis or bilateral vocal cord paralysis. Speech therapy is an important part of postoperative care. Speech therapy should be initiated as soon as the tissue edema is resolved.

8.8 Tips and Pearls

- The level of injury can be determined by palpating the neck under emergency conditions. Fragments of cartilage and/or depressions in the laryngotra-cheal framework indicate the site of injury. Edema and hematomas developing in the soft tissue of the neck can make this examination difficult. In this case, the mechanism of injury gives clues about the injury site.
- Suicidal or accidental hanging causes trauma to the supraglottic larynx. The most common laryngotracheal injuries are caused by steering wheel and dashboard impacts in motor vehicle accidents, inducing injury at the level of the thyroid and cricoid cartilages. Bicycle and sports accidents also cause injury at that level. Laryngotracheal separation is likely in case of jet-ski or snowmobile accidents where the neck comes in contact with a fixed object such as a rope.
- Large lacerations of the mucosa may cause emphysema by air leakage into the soft tissues of the neck. Extensive ecchymosis and crepitation of the skin makes the diagnosis of emphysema easily recognizable (???).
- Intubation or tracheotomy is easier to apply in cases of incomplete separation airway, the posterior wall serving as a guide for airway management.
- On some occasions, endoscopic repair can be combined with open neck approach.
- If there is a vertical thyroid cartilage fracture, entry to the larynx can be through the fracture line. If there is a horizontal fracture, the opening can be achieved with a midline vertical laryngofissure. Mucosal incision is preferentially made through the midline across the anterior commissure to prevent further mucosal injury.
- If there is not enough mucosa to cover the entire larynx, priority is given to the glottic area and especially the anterior commissure.
- Complete reconstruction of the cartilage frame is not necessary as long as the three-dimensional shape of the larynx can be achieved.
- Miniplates and recently introduced absorbable plates are the best materials to use for joining cartilage fragments.
- If the reconstruction is not stable, a T-tube is put in place to serve as a stent, allowing voice production and breathing.

References

1. Bent JP, Silver JR, Porubsky ES (1993) Acute laryngeal trauma: a review of 77 patients. Otolryngol Head Neck Surg 109:441–449

2. Schafer SD (1991) The treatment of acute external laryngeal injuries. Arch Otolaryngol Head Neck Surg 117:35–39

3. Komisar A, Blaugrund SM, Camins M (1991) Head and neck trauma in taxicabs. Arch Otolaryngol Head Neck Surg 117:442–445

4. Angood PB, Attia EL, Brown RA, Mudder DS. Extrinsic civilian trauma to the larynx and cervical trachea- important predictors of long term morbidity

5. Minard G, Kudsk KA, Croce MA, Butts JA (1992) Laryngotracheal trauma. Am Surg 58:181–187

6. Jewett BS, Schocley WW, Rutledge R (1999) External laryngeal trauma: analysis of 392 patients. Arch Otolaryngol Head Neck Surg 125:877–880

7. Hollinger PH, Schild JA (1972) Pharyngeal,tracheal and laryngeal injuries in the pediatric age group. Ann Otol Rhinol Laryngol 81:538–545

8. Travis LW, Olson NR, Melvin JW, Snyder RG (1975) Static and dynamic impact trauma of the human larynx. Am Acad Ophthalmol Otolaryngol 80:382–390

9. Pennington CL (1972) External trauma of the larynx and trachea: immediate treatment and management. Ann Otol Rhinol Laryngol 81:546–554

10. Ashbaugh DG, Gordon JH (1975) Traumatic avulsion of the trachea associated with cricoid fracture. Thor Cardiovasc Surg 69:800–803

11. Ford HR, Gardner MJ, Lynch JM (1995) Laryngotracheal disruption from blunt pediatric neck injuries: impact of early recognition and intervention on outcome. J Pediatr Surg 30:331–334

12. Gold SM, Gerber MF, Shott SR, Myer CM III (1997) Blunt laryngotracheal trauma in children. Arch Otolaryngol Head Neck Surg 123:83–87

13. Alonso WA, Caruso VG, Roncace EA (1973) Minibkes, a new factor in laryngotracheal trauma. AnnOtol Rhinol Laryngol 82:800–804

14. Myer CM, Orobello P, Cottor RT, Bratcher GO (1987) Blunt laryngeal trauma in children. Laryngoscope 97:1043–1048

15. Dillon JP, Gallagher R, Smyth D (2003) Arytenoid subluxation. Ir J Med Sci 172(4):206

16. Bryce DP (1983) Current management of laryngotracheal injury. Adv Otorhinolaryngol 29:27 38

17. Rubin AD, Hawkshaw MJ, Moyer CA, Dean CM, Sataloff RT (2005) Arytenoid cartilage dislocation: a 20-year experience. J Voice 19(4):687–701

18. Khokhlov VD (1997) Injuries to the hyoid bone and laryngeal cartilages: effectiveness of different methods of medico-legal investigation. Forensic Sci Int 88(3):173–183

19. DiMaio VJ (2000) Homicidal asphyxia. Am J Forensic Med Pathol 21(1):1–4

20. Borowski DW, Mehrotra P, Tennant D, El Badawey MR, Cameron DS (2004) Unusual presentation of blunt laryngeal injury with cricotracheal disruption by attempted hanging: a case report. Am J Otolaryngol 25(3):195–198

21. Bent JP III, Silver JR, Porubsky ES (1993) Acute laryngeal trauma: a review of 77 patients. Otolaryngol Head and Neck Surg 109:441–449

22. Schaeffer SD (1991) The treatment of acute external laryngeal injuries. Arch Otolaryngol Head Neck Surg 117:35–39

23. Schaefer SD, Close LG (1989) Acute management of laryngeal trauma. Ann Otol Rhinol Laryngol 98:98–104

24. Leopold DA (1983) Laryngeal trauma: a historical comparison of treatment methods. Arch Otolaryngol 109:106–112

Glottic Airway Stenosis

Hans Edmund Eckel and György Lichtenberger[†]

9

Core Messages

> The larynx forms the narrowest part of the central respiratory tract. As a result, anatomical or neurogenic changes can easily lead to clinically significant airway narrowing.

> Glottic airway stenosis most frequently arises from bilateral vocal cord immobility caused by recurrent laryngeal nerve injury.

> Previous surgery, mostly thyroid surgery, is the most common cause of laryngeal nerve paralysis.

> The diagnostic protocol includes detailed history-taking, inspection, palpation, zoom laryngoscopy and/or transnasal flexible laryngoscopy, thyroid gland workup, stroboscopy, microlaryngoscopy, pharyngoesophagoscopy, tracheobronchoscopy, and suspension laryngoscopy with tactile assessment of arytenoid cartilage mobility. Ultrasonography of the neck, video-fluoroscopy, magnetic resonance imaging studies of the brain, computed tomography scans of the thorax and lateral skull base, and specific laboratory tests should be performed when needed. The flow–volume curve, peak expiratory flow (PEF), peak inspiratory flow (PIF), and total airway resistance are the standard function tests for diagnosing central airway obstruction. PEF and PIF seem to be the best suitable follow-up parameters to assess airway mechanics before and after surgical procedures.

> A variety of endoscopic procedures are available for treatment. The most important ones are arytenoidectomy, cordectomy, posterior cordectomy, temporary lateral fixation of the vocal cord, and definitive lateralization of the vocal.

9.1 Anatomical Background

Because of its dual functions in preventing aspiration and producing speech, the larynx must be able to close the airway temporarily during deglutition. Disturbances of this physiological process can lead to permanent narrowing of the airway lumen. Inflammatory swelling, scarring, movement disorders of the vocal cords, and tumor masses can narrow or obstruct the airway. The larynx forms the narrowest part of the central respiratory tract. As a result, anatomical or neurogenic changes can easily lead to clinically significant airway narrowing. The relative narrowness of the respiratory tract at this level is based on the physiological function of the larynx as a safety valve between the upper respiratory and alimentary tracts. In adults, the airway lumen at the level of the trachea is 300–500 mm^2, the subglottic airway measures approximately 200–300 mm^2. and the glottic airway (with abducted vocal cords) 150–200 mm^2. With bilateral vocal cord paralysis, the glottic airway is reduced to 30–60 mm^2, measuring only some 20–30% of the glottic airway in healthy individuals (Fig. 9.1) [1, 2].

H. E. Eckel (✉)
Department of Oto-Rhino-Laryngology,
A.ö. Landeskrankenhaus Klagenfurt, HNO, St. Veiter Str. 47,
A-9020 Klagenfurt, Austria
e-mail: hans.eckel@kabeg.at

M. Remacle, H. E. Eckel (eds.), *Surgery of Larynx and Trachea,*
DOI: 10.1007/978-3-540-79136-2_9, © Springer-Verlag Berlin Heidelberg 2010

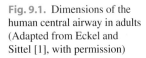

Fig. 9.1. Dimensions of the human central airway in adults (Adapted from Eckel and Sittel [1], with permission)

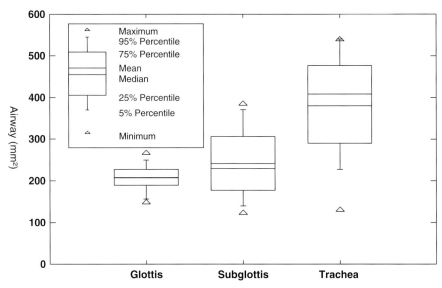

9.2 Classification

Glottic airway stenosis most frequently arises from bilateral vocal cord immobility caused by recurrent laryngeal nerve injury. Paralysis of the vagus nerve or, more commonly, of the inferior laryngeal nerve most frequently occurs after surgical procedures in the neck (especially in the thyroid gland) and upper mediastinum. It may also be caused by malignant tumors invading the larynx, hypopharynx, esophagus, thyroid, or tracheobronchial tree and other malignant neoplasms in the lower neck or upper mediastinum. Neurogenic laryngeal stenosis may also develop during the course of viral inflammation or as a result of central nervous system processes (cerebral or skull-base tumors, injuries, surgical procedures on the lateral skull base). The recognition of concomitant superior laryngeal nerve paralysis on one side is important because it may be relevant for planning surgical measures (especially arytenoidectomy) that could result in increased aspiration [3].

Previous surgery, mostly thyroid surgery, is the most common cause of laryngeal nerve paralysis (Table 9.1). Revision thyroidectomy bears a particularly high risk for inferior and superior laryngeal nerve trauma. The rate of immediate postoperative unilateral recurrent laryngeal nerve paresis following primary thyroid surgery for benign disease is approximately 2–7%; the rate of permanent paralysis has been reported to be 0.5–4.0%. During revision surgery and operations for malignant conditions of the thyroid gland, unilateral recurrent

laryngeal nerve paresis occurs in some 10–20% of all interventions. Bilateral vocal fold paralysis is obviously seen far less frequently. Surgery of the cervical spine via an anterior approach and surgery of the larynx, pharynx, cervical esophagus, upper mediastinum, and carotid artery surgery can typically result in laryngeal nerve or even vagus nerve injury. Other conditions causing laryngeal nerve palsies include the following.

- Lesions of the brain stem
- Neurovascular disorders (stroke) and other central nervous system disorders
- Demyelinating disorders of the peripheral nervous system (Guillain-Barré syndrome)
- Lateral skull base lesions (trauma, tumor)
- Sequel of skull base surgery
- Cervical spine injury or surgery
- Degenerative motor unit disorders (e.g., amyotrophic lateral sclerosis)
- Infectious diseases of the affected nerves
- Neurotoxins (e.g., lead)
- Primary neurogenic tumors (e.g., schwannoma)
- Malignant tumors of the thyroid, larynx, pharynx, trachea, esophagus, bronchus, thymus, neck, and mediastinum
- Traumatic lesions of the neck
- Aortic aneurysm

Bilateral recurrent nerve paralysis frequently leads to functional glottic stenosis, with the vocal folds in a fixed paramedian position. The predominant symptom

Table 9.1. Etiology of bilateral vocal cord immobility in 218 patients

	Bilateral vocal cord paralysis	Bilateral arytenoid cartilage fixation	Total
Previous surgery	**154 (82.8%)**	**1 (3.1%)**	**155 (71.1%)**
Thyroid surgery (revision surgery)	141 (75.8%)	0	141 (91.0%)
Thyroid surgery (primary intervention)	4 (2.2%)	0	4 (2.6%)
Esophageal surgery	4 (2.2%)	0	4 (2.6%)
Other surgery	5 (2.7%)	1 (100%)	6 (3.8%)
Long-term intubation (> 24 hours)	**0**	**22 (68.8%)**	**22 (10.1%)**
Malignant tumors	**16 (8.6%)**	**0**	**16 (7.3%)**
Esophageal carcinoma	9 (56.2%)	0	9 (56.2)
Bronchogenic carcinoma	4 (25.0%)	0	4 (25.0%)
Other	3 (18.8%)	0	3 (18.8%)
Short term intubation	**5 (2.7%)**	**3 (9.4%)**	**8 (3.7%)**
Neurogenic	**7 (3.8%)**	**0**	**7 (3.2%)**
Wegener's granulomatosis	**0**	**3 (9.4%)**	**3 (1.4%)**
Rheumatoid arthritis	**0**	**2 (6.2%)**	**2 (0.9%)**
Caustic ingestion	**0**	**1 (3.1%)**	**1 (0.5%)**
Other/unknown	**4 (2.2%)**	**0**	**4 (1.8%)**
Total	**186 (100%)**	**32 (100%)**	**218 (100%)**

Modified from Eckel et al. [3], with permission

is airway compromise. It ranges from unnoticeable to mild dyspnea to inspiratory stridor and respiratory distress, even without physical effort. Acute airway obstruction resulting from bilateral vocal fold immobility (e.g., following thyroidectomy) frequently requires immediate surgical or medical intervention (e.g., tracheotomy) to maintain an adequate airway and prevent acute asphyxiation or pulmonary consequences of chronic central airway obstruction. In contrast to unilateral vocal cord paralysis, voice quality is not the primary concern in these patients. Voice quality is usually only mildly affected (if just the recurrent laryngeal nerves are involved). For idiopathic palsies, a less than 50% rate of partial and complete recovery can be expected [4].

Congenital malformations, including aerodynamically relevant synechiae of the ligamentous glottis and laryngeal atresia, are rare.

Inflammatory laryngeal stenosis is rare in adults (exceptions: epiglottitis and glottic stenosis due to severe Reinke's edema) but is a frequent and dreaded condition in children [5]. Acute infections of the larynx and trachea are particularly ominous in children owing to the small size of their airways [6]. Swelling of the mucosa or an accumulation of tracheal secretions can cause considerably greater obstruction of the anatomically smaller airways than that in adult patients. Acute obstructive airway inflammation in children is seen in a heterogeneous group of infectious diseases with a

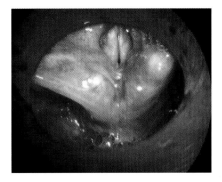

Fig. 9.2. Arytenoid cartilage fixation. Both arytenoid cartilages are fixed and cannot be abducted passively during microlaryngoscopy

common presentation marked by a typical barking cough (croup), inspiratory stridor, hoarseness, and airway obstruction. Generally, these cases are managed by endoscopy, endolaryngeal intubation, or tracheotomy, specific high-dose antibiotic therapy, or intensive care of the affected child. Further surgical measures are not required.

The most common laryngeal injuries, which generally resolve spontaneously, are caused by intubation. Long-term intubation can cause permanent trauma-related changes in the larynx, particularly interarytenoid synechiae and arytenoid cartilage fixation (Fig. 9.2–9.4). With the latter condition, the arytenoid cartilage is fixed

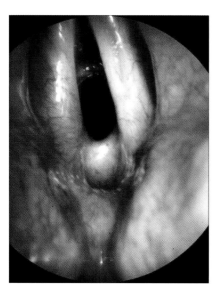

Fig. 9.3. Interarytenoid scarring following long-term intubation, causing paramedian immobility of the vocal cords

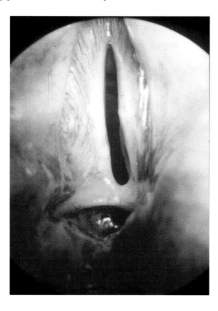

Fig. 9.4. Posterior synechia following intubation, causing paramedian immobility of the vocal cords

in the cricoarytenoid joint, causing vocal cord immobility. Some of these cases are clinically indistinguishable from recurrent nerve paralysis, but the correct diagnosis is suggested by the history, passive mobility of the arytenoid cartilage during microlaryngoscopic examination under anesthesia, and electromyography to record summation action potentials from the muscle groups supplied by the inferior laryngeal nerve [4, 7]. In patients with bilateral immobility of the vocal cords,

bilateral recurrent laryngeal nerve paralysis is usually suspected, but various causes of arytenoid cartilage fixation may produce a clinical image that is indiscernible from recurrent laryngeal nerve paralysis during routine office laryngoscopy or videostroboscopy. Impaired movement of the cricoarytenoid cartilage with immobility of the vocal cord and airway obstruction may occur as a consequence of disorders of the cricoarytenoid articulation, interarytenoid fibrous adhesion, or both. Immobility of the cricoarytenoid joint may arise from arytenoid cartilage dislocation during laryngotracheal intubation and consequent ankylosis, arthritis, or tumorous infiltration of laryngeal or hypopharyngeal carcinoma. Interarytenoid fibrous adhesion most commonly results from prolonged or traumatic endotracheal intubation. The tube causes a decubitus with chondritis and consequent scar tissue formation involving the arytenoid cartilages and the interarytenoid area resulting in severe impairment of both cricoarytenoid joints' motility and laryngeal stenosis. Table 9.1 gives the frequency of various etiological factors in recurrent nerve paralysis and arytenoid cartilage fixation.

Benign or malignant tumours (laryngeal or tracheal carcinoma, esophageal carcinoma invading the cervical trachea, central bronchial carcinoma, locally advanced thyroid carcinoma, malignant tumours of the upper mediastinum) occasionally lead to malignant central airway stenosis. This type of stenosis may be caused by extrinsic airway compression, tumor invasion of the tracheal wall with subsequent malacia, or intraluminal tumor growth in the trachea and larynx. Tumor infiltration of the recurrent nerve with subsequent vocal cord paralysis in a paramedian position can also lead to functional airway stenosis. In all of these situations, endolaryngeal surgery with CO_2 laser (or occasionally Nd:YAG laser for larger tumor masses) provides an excellent tool for airway recanalization. The enlarged airway can be maintained in the intermediate term by implanting stents in the carina, thoracic trachea, and cervical trachea as far as the laryngotracheal junction [8, 9].

9.3 Diagnostic Procedures and Preoperative Assessment

In most patients presenting with glottic airway stenosis, the underlying condition is obvious from the patient's history (e.g., recurrent laryngeal nerve paresis following thyroidectomy). In patients with unclear etiology of the underlying condition, a complete diagnostic workup is compulsory. The diagnostic protocol for these patients includes detailed history taking (particularly regarding previous surgery), inspection, palpation, zoom laryngoscopy and/or transnasal flexible laryngoscopy, thyroid gland workup, stroboscopy, microlaryngoscopy, pharyngoesophagoscopy, tracheobronchoscopy, and suspension laryngoscopy with tactile assessment of arytenoid cartilage mobility. Ultrasonography of the neck, video-fluoroscopy, magnetic resonance imaging (MRI) studies of the brain, computed tomography (CT) scans of the thorax and lateral skull base, and specific laboratory tests should be conducted if needed [7]. Pulmonary function tests should be obtained to clarify the resulting airway compromise. The flow-volume curve, peak expiratory flow (PEF), peak inspiratory flow (PIF), and total airway resistance are the standard function tests for diagnosing central airway obstruction. Among all conventional lung function values, PEF and to a certain degree PIF seem to be the most suitable follow-up parameters to assess airway mechanics before and after surgical/endoscopic procedures [10–13].

Upper airway stenosis involving surface areas of no more than 50 mm^2 can be overcome using adequate respiratory compensation, but any narrowing beyond this limit results in hypoventilation, inappropriate oxygen uptake, and retention of CO_2. Experimental evidence indicates that laryngotracheal obstruction within a critical range of < 50 mm^2 surface area compromises respiratory efforts enough to be of clinical importance [12–14]. Glottic stenosis alters the flow–volume curve by causing increased airway resistance, turbulence (at high flow rates), and a decrease in luminal cross section. Unlike an anatomically fixed cicatricial stenosis of the subglottis or trachea, the airway stenosis associated with bilateral recurrent nerve paralysis is characterized by passive abduction of the vocal cords during expiration and adduction (medialization) of the cords through a suction effect (Bernoulli) during inspiration. This produces a characteristic curve with extreme inspiratory flattening, often accompanied by an essentially normal expiratory pattern.

Voice analysis should be done prior to airway-restoring surgery. Laryngeal electromyography may be helpful for assessing the prognosis in patients with vocal cord paresis.

9.4 Indications for Surgery

Surgical correction is not appropriate for every central airway stenosis. The need for surgery depends in part on whether the stenosis is acute or chronic, the resulting adaptation of the respiratory muscles to the increased central airway resistance (conditioning), and especially the degree to which the respiratory compromise restricts normal levels of physical activity. Studies by the author indicate that an inspiratory resistance of more than 2.5 kPa × s/L is a good empirical cutoff point for selecting patients who require surgical correction [12–14]. Ultimately, however, the decision to operate depends on the level of physical exertion at which the patient can still compensate for the stenosis through increased respiration.

Acute bilateral recurrent nerve paralysis generally presents as severe inspiratory airway obstruction with inspiratory stridor. Occasionally, tracheotomy is required to overcome airway distress.

Once the acute respiratory compromise caused by bilateral recurrent nerve paralysis of recent onset has been overcome, most patients can breathe well at rest and during mild physical exertion. High-dose intravenous steroids are used during the early phase of this disorder. Once the patient has adjusted to the glottic narrowing, mild physical training should be encouraged to adapt the thoracic muscles to overcome increase inspiratory airway resistance. Upper airway stenosis involving surface areas of no more than 50 mm^2 can be overcome using adequate respiratory compensation, but any narrowing beyond this limit results in hypoventilation, inappropriate oxygen uptake, and retention of CO_2.

Conservative treatment for airway improvement in bilateral vocal cord paralysis includes the following.

- Nasotracheal intubation for acute airway distress due to bilateral vocal cord paralysis is not recommended, or only for a very short term so long as the patient is in an institution where immediate reversible lateralization can be performed after extubation in the operating theater and introducing jet-anesthesia for glottis-dilating surgery.
- High-dose intravenous steroids and nonsteroidal antiphlogistics.
- Antiviral or antibiotic agents if an infection is suspected.
- Mild physical training once the patient has adjusted to the glottic narrowing.

The indication for glottis-expanding surgery is mainly based on the following conditions.

- Inspiratory stridor at rest and/or inspiratory resistance of more than 2.5 kPa × s/L
- A lack of exercise tolerance
- Potential risk to the patient from sporadic respiratory inflammations (flu-like infections) that may cause swelling of the already-tight glottis

So long as the degree of respiratory compromise is acceptable to the patient at rest and during mild exercise, it is reasonable to wait for approximately 9 months after the onset of paralysis to watch for spontaneous recovery of nerve function.

Occasionally, the prognosis of recurrent nerve paralysis can be based on the clinical situation, as in the case of a thyroidectomy for thyroid carcinoma in which a recurrent nerve had to be deliberately sacrificed. It is rarely possible, however, to make such a confident prognosis based on clinical status alone. Electromyography is useful for making a prognostic assessment, although it cannot be done with certainty in patients with neurapraxic paralysis [4, 15, 16]. A confident prognosis can be made only by waiting and watching for the return of normal vocal cord mobility over a period of 6–9 (up to 12) months. It should be noted that in patients with bilateral paralysis the prognosis may be different for each of the affected sides. It is not unusual for the paralysis on one side to regress over time whereas that on the opposite side persists indefinitely. Once the acute respiratory compromise caused by bilateral recurrent nerve paralysis of recent onset has been overcome by adaptation of the respiratory muscles, most patients can breathe well at rest and during mild physical exertion.

Bilateral recurrent nerve paralysis must be differentiated mainly from arytenoid cartilage fixation (rare cases may also involve paralysis on one side and cartilage fixation on the other) [3]. Ankylosis of the arytenoid cartilage or fibrosis of the connective tissue capsule of the cricoarytenoid joint most commonly develops as a result of previous intubation. Therefore, it is difficult to differentiate cartilage fixation (ankylosis) from paralysis based on the history alone. Accordingly, arytenoid cartilage fixation or posttraumatic fibrosis of the joint capsule should be considered in each patient who presents with limited vocal cord motion and a prior history of intubation. Mechanical restriction of joint motion can be differentiated from paralysis by means of laryngeal electromyography and also by testing the passive mobility of the arytenoid cartilage during microlaryngoscopic

examination of the larynx under general anesthesia. It is important to distinguish between paralysis and ankylosis because treatment options are not the same for these two disorders.

Apart from paralysis or arytenoid cartilage fixation, glottic stenoses are occasionally caused by congenital malformations (webs), synechiae (postoperative or postinflammatory), or tumors. Synechiae can be divided by laser surgery. In patients with synechiae of the anterior commissure, the intervention should include insertion of a keel and, if necessary, a free mucosal graft, but even then the vocal results are usually unsatisfactory.

9.5 Surgical Procedures

Whereas extralaryngeal surgical procedures (lateral fixation with its numerous variants) were once the standard treatment for bilateral vocal cord paralysis, endoscopic techniques have advanced considerably since the advent of endolaryngeal laser surgery. Today, endoscopic procedures have largely replaced open laryngeal surgery in the treatment of this disorder.

- Arytenoidectomy [15, 17–19] is highly effective for expanding the airway if the surgeon can completely remove the arytenoid cartilage and completely divide the conus elasticus as far as the cricoid cartilage. Even partial arytenoidectomy is believed to provide satisfactory airway enlargement. The disadvantages of this technique include frequent transient aspiration, the risk of cricoid chondritis and necrosis in patients who have previously had radiation to the neck, scarring, and granuloma formation.
- Cordectomy [17] is as effective as arytenoidectomy for airway restoration. However the resected vocal cord is eventually replaced by scar tissue, similarly to that seen after cordectomy performed for removal of vocal cord carcinoma. There is no risk of aspiration with this procedure, but the voice may more severely deteriorate compared to that after arytenoidectomy.
- The procedure is carried out with a surgical CO_2 laser coupled to an operating microscope with a 400-mm objective lens. The laser is set to an output power of 4 W in the continuous beam delivery mode at a spot size of approximately 0.8 mm². Patients are usually intubated transorally for surgery. Following transsection of the vocal process of the arytenoid cartilage, the vocal ligament, vocalis muscle, and much of the

lateral thyroarytenoid muscle are resected. The most anterior portion of the vocal cord, however, is not included in the resection, as its removal would contribute little to the desired airway enlargement.

- Posterior cordectomy [20, 21], in which the vocal cord is divided in the area of the vocal process of the arytenoid cartilage combined with division of the conus elasticus, is considered by many laryngologists to be the best compromise between expanding the airway and preserving voice quality (Fig. 9.5a, b).

- Temporary lateral fixation of the vocal cord as described by Lichtenberger [15, 22–24] is the only potentially reversible procedure for glottic airway enlargement (Fig. 9.6a–e). It is indicated if the vocal

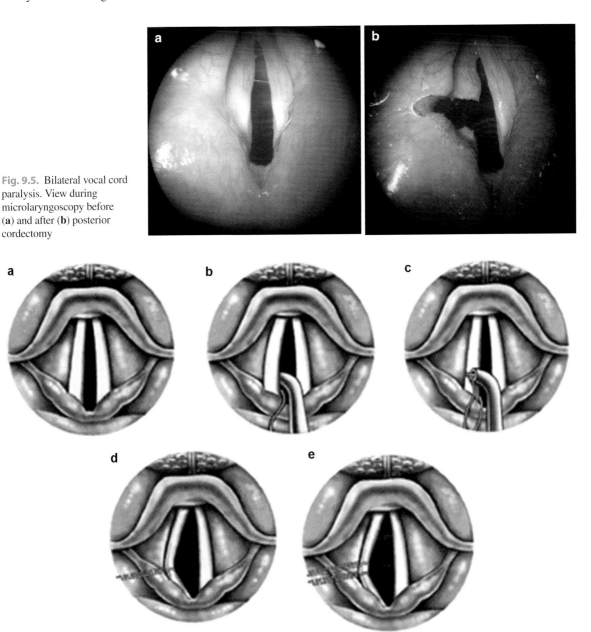

Fig. 9.5. Bilateral vocal cord paralysis. View during microlaryngoscopy before (**a**) and after (**b**) posterior cordectomy

Fig. 9.6. Temporary lateral fixation of the vocal cord as described by Lichtenberger. (**a**) Paralyzed vocal cords. (**b**) One end of the lateral fixation suture was pushed through the larynx below the posterior third of the vocal cord. (**c**) The other end of the lateral fixation suture was pushed through the larynx above the posterior third of the vocal cord. (**d**) The ends of the fixation suture were pulled and knotted over a small silicone sheet placed on the thyroid cartilage or on the sternohyoid muscle. (**e**) The second lateral fixation suture was placed in a similar fashion 1–2 mm anterior to the first suture

cords are in a paramedian position, functional recovery of at least one vocal cord is anticipated, and there is no scar formation in the lumen of the larynx. It can be performed correctly only with jet anesthesia or apnea. Once recurrent nerve function has recovered, the endoscopically performed lateral fixation of the vocal cord can be reversed.

- To achieve laterofixation of one vocal cord, fixation sutures are placed through the larynx with the help of the endoextralaryngeal needle carrier. The skin is cut in the same line as the previous incision for thyroidectomy. Only the skin and platysma flap are identified and retracted. The laryngoscope is then introduced. The paralyzed vocal cords are brought into the field of vision (Fig. 9.6a). One end of the lateral fixation suture is pushed through the larynx below the posterior third of the vocal cord (Fig. 9.6b). A similar stitch is made, this time above the posterior third of the vocal cord (Fig. 9.6c). The ends of the fixation suture are pulled and knotted over a small silicone sheet placed on the thyroid cartilage or on the sternohyoid muscles (Fig. 9.6d). Formerly, we used the silicone sheet only if the sternohyoid muscle had been damaged during thyroid surgery. The second lateral fixation suture is placed in a similar fashion 1–2 mm anterior to the first suture (Fig. 9.6e). The knotted suture over the sternohyoid muscle is then left subcutaneously, and the wound is closed. As a surgical alternative, the assistant surgeon can make an approximately 10 mm long incision between the two ends of the thread, which were pushed through the larynx and neck skin; then, both ends are pulled back under the skin and tied above the prelaryngeal muscles. Finally, the skin incision is closed with sutures. The patients are discharged from the hospital within a few days when it is thought that the airway is stable.

- Definitive lateralization of the vocal cord as described by Lichtenberger (partial laser arytenoidectomy with submucosal cordectomy covering the defect with the spared mucosa of the arytenoid and vocal cord using endoextralaryngeal suture technique) [22, 24–26] (Fig. 9.7a–f). This operation is indicated if the vocal cords are in a paramedian position and there is no chance for recovery. This operation also can be performed without tracheostomy with Jet ventilation during surgery. A triangular incision is made laryngoscopically under microscopic magnification with a microscalpel and scissors or with laser. The incision begins a few millimeters in front of the vocal process and extends posteriorly over the vocal process 1.0–1.5 mm from the edge of the vocal cord to the area above the arytenoid cartilage. Another incision is made from the vocal process to the muscular process of the arytenoid. The two incisions are then connected with a transverse incision at the height of the muscular process (Fig. 9.7a). The arytenoid cartilage is dissected and removed, usually only partially. A submucous cordectomy is performed on the thyroarytenoid muscle as previously described, again sparing the mucous membrane (Fig. 9.7b). The suture then is fixed again in the neck as described for the previous procedure (Fig. 9.7c–f).

As a rule, modern endoscopic laser operations to expand the glottis are considered reliable techniques for airway restoration. Generally, they can be performed without a temporary tracheotomy, making them easier for patients to tolerate. However, any surgical widening of the glottis trades voice for airway. Therefore, a compromise must be found between retaining voice quality and restoring an adequate airway. These considerations should be discussed with the patient preoperatively to weigh the physical activity needs of the patient against anticipated voice deterioration and strive for a compromise that is best for the individual situation, although the phonatory outcome of a glottis-expanding operation cannot be predicted accurately.

Additional sites of stenosis are more frequently identified in patients with glottic stenosis due to arytenoid cartilage fixation. Although stenosis due to recurrent laryngeal nerve paralysis can be managed endoscopically without a preliminary tracheotomy, patients with arytenoid cartilage fixation frequently require total arytenoidectomy or open surgery with a temporary tracheotomy [3, 27].

9.6 Postoperative Care

Extubation is usually performed 30–60 minutes after the end of the intervention, and patients are observed for 4–24 hours in an intensive or intermediate care unit after extubation. Patients are usually kept in hospital for 3–5 days after surgery. With procedures exposing the cartilaginous structures of the larynx, preoperative antibiotic prophylaxis is indicated to prevent wound infection. Antibiotics should be given 30 minutes before surgery.

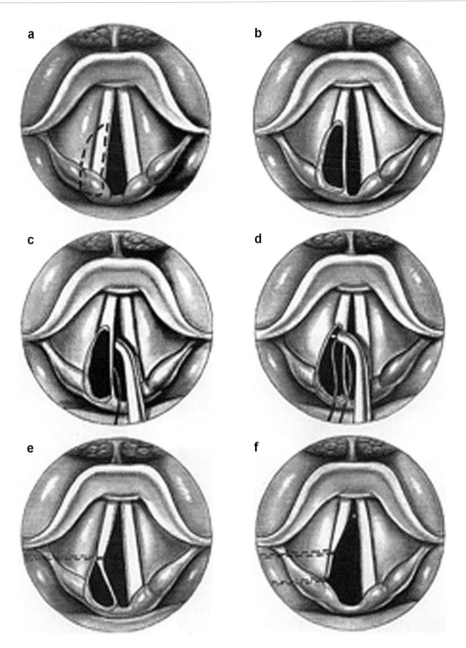

Fig. 9.7. Definitive vocal cord lateralization as described by Lichtenberger. (**a**) Triangular incision using CO_2 laser with microscopic magnification. (**b**) The arytenoid cartilage and the medial and lateral thyroarytenoid muscles were removed endoscopically, preserving the medial mucous membrane part of the vocal cord. (**c**) One end of the thread was pushed through the larynx with the help of the needle carrier below the posterior third of the residual vocal cord. (**d**) The other end of the thread was pushed through the larynx above the posterior third of the residual vocal cord. (**e**) The ends of the thread were pulled. (**f**) The ends of both threads were pulled

The agents of choice are first- or second-generation cephalosporins, a combination of penicillins and penicillinase inhibitors, or clindamycin. The efficacy of steroids is a controversial issue. High steroid doses (e.g., 250 mg methylprednisolone) during the immediate postoperative period have a number of beneficial effects, most notably the prevention of surgery-related tissue swelling and reduced surgical trauma. Occasionally, steroids are given for a prolonged period after surgery to prevent new connective tissue formation and undesired new scarring. It is the authors' opinion, however, that this therapy is of uncertain benefit. Delaying or reducing new connective tissue formation ultimately means a delay in wound healing. The authors do not routinely prescribe steroids during the initial days after surgical correction of airway stenoses. Recently, several reports have been published on the local application of mitomycin C for the prevention and treatment of undesired scarring of the larynx and trachea. Mitomycin C is an antibiotic first isolated from *Streptomyces caespitosus* in 1958. It inhibits DNA synthesis due to alkylation and is a potent inhibitor of connective tissue formation. Mitomycin C is an effective antineoplastic cytostatic drug that is used systemically and locally for the treatment of carcinoma at various sites. High local concentrations and low plasma levels are achieved following local application. In laryngology, the use of this agent has been described following endoscopic laser treatment of airway stenosis and after open operations to reduce granuloma and scar formation but with very different effects [28].

9.6.1 Tips and Pearls to Avoid Complications

- Before a final decision is made regarding the type of surgery for the individual patient, a comprehensive endoscopic evaluation of the airway, including tracheobronchoscopy with flexible endoscopes, should be undertaken.
- Temporary tracheotomy can usually be avoided in patients undergoing endoscopic airway surgery for glottic stenosis. However, all patients must be informed that tracheotomy may become necessary during or shortly after surgery.
- Patients should receive 250 mg of methylprednisolone prior to surgery and during the first days thereafter. Antibiotic prophylaxis is recommended.
- Patients should be extubated immediately after surgery and need to be monitored at an intermediate care or intensive care unit for one night.
- In patients with a history of previous radiotherapy to the neck, there is considerable risk for chondritis, chondronecrosis, and severe laryngeal edema.
- The endoextralaryngeal needle carrier is mandatory for temporary end definitive endoscopic laterofixation.

References

1. Eckel HE, Sittel C (1994) [morphometric studies at the level of the glottis as a principle in larynx enlarging microlaryngoscopic surgical procedures in bilateral recurrent nerve paralysis] morphometrische untersuchungen der glottisebene als grundlage kehlkopferweiternder mikrolaryngoskopischer operationsverfahren bei beidseitiger rekurrenslahmung. Laryngorhinootologie 73:417
2. Eckel HE, Vossing M (1996) [endolaryngeal surgical procedures in glottis expansion in bilateral recurrent nerve paralysis]. Laryngorhinootologie 75:215–222
3. Eckel HE, Wittekindt C, Klussmann JP, Schroeder U, Sittel C (2003) Management of bilateral arytenoid cartilage fixation versus recurrent laryngeal nerve paralysis. Ann Otol Rhinol Laryngol 112:103–108
4. Sittel C, Stennert E, Thumfart WF, Dapunt U, Eckel HE (2001) Prognostic value of laryngeal electromyography in vocal fold paralysis. Arch Otolaryngol Head Neck Surg 127:155–160
5. Damm M, Eckel HE, Jungehulsing M, Roth B (1999) Management of acute inflammatory childhood stridor. Otolaryngol Head Neck Surg 121:633
6. Eckel HE, Koebke J, Sittel C, Sprinzl GM, Pototschnig C, Stennert E (1999) Morphology of the human larynx during the first five years of life studied on whole organ serial sections. Ann Otol Rhinol Laryngol 108:232–238
7. Eckel HE, Sittel C (2001) [bilateral recurrent laryngeal nerve paralysis]. Hno 49:166–179
8. Wassermann K, Mathen F, Eckel HE (2001) Concurrent glottic and tracheal stenoses: Restoration of airway continuity in end-stage malignant disease. Ann Otol Rhinol Laryngol 110:349–355
9. Wassermann K, Mathen F, Eckel HE (2000) Malignant laryngotracheal obstruction: a way to treat serial stenoses of the upper airways. Ann Thorac Surg 70:1197
10. Leitersdorfer S, Lichtenberger G, Bihari A, Kovacs I (2005) Evaluation of the lung test in reversible glottis-dilating operations. Eur Arch Otorhinolaryngol 262:289–293
11. Leitersdorfer S, Lichtenberger G, Kovacs I (2002) Assessment of the results of glottis-dilating operations using lung function tests. Eur Arch Otorhinolaryngol 259:57–59
12. Wassermann K, Gitt A, Weyde J, Eckel HE (1995) Lung function changes and exercise-induced ventilatory responses to external resistive loads in normal subjects. Respiration 62:177
13. Wassermann K, Koch A, Warschkow A, Mathen F, Muller-Ehmsen J, Eckel HE (1999) Measuring in situ central airway resistance in patients with laryngotracheal stenosis. Laryngoscope 109:1516–1520
14. Wassermann K, Eckel HE (1999) [stenoses of the upper airways. Lung function, local resistance and load compensation. A review] funktionsdiagnostik zentraler atemwegsstenosen. HNO 47:947
15. Lichtenberger G (1999) Reversible immediate and definitive lateralization of paralyzed vocal cords. Eur Arch Otorhinolaryngol 256:407
16. Werner JA, Lippert BM (2002) [lateral fixation of the vocal cord instead of tracheotomy in acute bilateral vocal cord paralysis]. Dtsch Med Wochenschr 127:917–922

17. Eckel HE, Thumfart M, Wassermann K, Vossing M, Thumfart WF (1994) Cordectomy versus arytenoidectomy in the management of bilateral vocal cord paralysis. Ann Otol Rhinol Laryngol 103:852–857
18. Eskew JR, Bailey BJ (1983) Laser arytenoidectomy for bilateral vocal cord paralysis. Otolaryngol Head Neck Surg 91:294–298
19. Kleinsasser O (1968) [endolaryngeal arytenoidectomy and submucous hemichordectomy for the widening of the glottis in bilateral abductor paralysis]. Monatsschr Ohrenheilkd Laryngorhinol 102:443–446
20. Dennis DP, Kashima H (1989) Carbon dioxide laser posterior cordectomy for treatment of bilateral vocal cord paralysis. Ann Otol Rhinol Laryngol 98:930
21. Kashima HK (1991) Bilateral vocal fold motion impairment: pathophysiology and management by transverse cordotomy. Ann Otol Rhinol Laryngol 100:717
22. Lichtenberger G (1989) [laryngeal microsurgical laterofixation of paralyzed vocal cords using a new suture instrument]. Laryngorhinootologie 68:678–682
23. Lichtenberger G (2002) Reversible lateralization of the paralyzed vocal cord without tracheostomy. Ann Otol Rhinol Laryngol 111:21–26
24. Lichtenberger G, Toohill RJ (1997) Technique of endo-extralaryngeal suture lateralization for bilateral abductor vocal cord paralysis. Laryngoscope 107:1281–1283
25. Lichtenberger G (1983) Endo-extralaryngeal needle carrier instrument. Laryngoscope 93:1348–1350
26. Lichtenberger G, Toohill RJ (1991) The endo-extralaryngeal needle carrier. Otolaryngol Head Neck Surg 105:755–756
27. Lichtenberger G (1999) Endoscopic microsurgical management of scars in the posterior commissure and interarytenoid region resulting in vocal cord pseudoparalysis. Eur Arch Otorhinolaryngol 256:412
28. Rahbar R, Shapshay SM, Healy GB (2001) Mitomycin: effects on laryngeal and tracheal stenosis, benefits, and complications. Ann Otol Rhinol Laryngol 110:1

Subglottic and Tracheal Stenosis

Philippe Monnier

Core Messages

> Train yourself adequately in laryngotracheal surgery and upper airway endoscopy before addressing the challenging surgery of laryngotracheal stenosis (LTS).

> Remember that inappropriate initial management of LTS may lead to permanent intractable sequelae and that the best chance for the patient lies in the first operation.

> Perform a thorough preoperative assessment of the patient's medical condition and of the stenosis to choose the best surgical option and timing.

> Address only mature cicatricial stenosis for a definitive endoscopic or open surgical repair.

> Perform a bacteriologic aspirate of the trachea prior to any treatment.

> Treat gastro-oesophageal reflux.

> Master all types of surgeries starting from appropriate use of CO_2 laser for minor stenosis to laryngotracheal reconstruction with cartilage expansion and partial cricotracheal resection for the most severe grades of stenosis.

10.1 Introduction

The management of laryngotracheal stenosis (LTS) remains a challenging problem for the otolaryngologist, especially in the pediatric age group. The complexity of the various preoperative situations implies that no single treatment modality can solve the problem. One has to take into consideration the type of the stenosis (congenital or acquired), its location (supraglottic, glottic, subglottic, combined), its degree of obstruction and length in the craniocaudal axis, and finally its association with vocal cord ankylosis or neurogenic paralysis. Furthermore, the presence of tracheal damage (stenosis or localized malacia) related to the tracheostoma or to the tracheotomy cannula can further complicate the surgical management. According to the nature and severity of the condition, a variety of treatments exists. They range from endoscopic laser sessions with or without dilatation or stenting [13, 14, 36, 51] to laryngotracheal reconstruction (LTR) with anterior, posterior, or combined costal cartilage grafts [8, 43, 44], to partial cricotracheal resection (PCTR) for the most severe grades of stenosis, and to extended PCTR for combined glotto-subglottic stenosis (SGS) [37, 55].

Needless to say, thorough preoperative endoscopic assessment is prerequisite to selecting the best surgical option for a given condition.

10.2 Etiology

10.2.1 Infants and Children

10.2.1.1 Subglottis

In the pediatric age group, the most common reason for SGS is prolonged intubation. In newborns, however,

P. Monnier
Professor and Chairman, Otolaryngology, Head & Neck Surgery Department, Centre Hospitalier Universitaire Vaudois, Rue du Bugnon 46, CH-1011 Lausanne, Switzerland
e-mail: philippe.monnier@chuv.ch

M. Remacle, H. E. Eckel (eds.), *Surgery of Larynx and Trachea*,
DOI: 10.1007/978-3-540-79136-2_10, © Springer-Verlag Berlin Heidelberg 2010

congenital SGS represents the third most common laryngeal anomaly after laryngomalacia and bilateral vocal fold paralysis [24]. According to Holinger, congenital SGS is classified into cartilaginous and soft tissue stenoses [25]. It is present when the lumen of the cricoid region measures less than 4 mm in diameter in a full-term infant or 3 mm in a premature infant. The cartilaginous type results from failure of complete recanalization of the laryngeal lumen after the eighth week of gestation. The cricoid may have a normal shape but is too small for the infant's size, or it may show different abnormalities, such as general thickening, a large anterior or posterior lamina, or an elliptical shape. Sometimes a trapped first tracheal ring is responsible for the small size of the subglottis.

In approximately 50% of cases, congenital SGS is associated with mediastinal malformations including cardiovascular, tracheobronchial, or esophageal anomalies [41]. For the otolaryngologist, thoracic surgeon, and anesthetist, this implies that any mediastinal malformation warrants bronchoesophagoscopy before treatment to rule out minor asymptomatic congenital SGS.

Injuries leading to acquired SGS in infants and children are more likely to occur after traumatic intubation for resuscitation, after intubation for severe cranial injuries, when laryngoscopy is difficult because of anatomical problems, or when mild congenital subglottic stenosis has been overlooked. Any systemic condition that diminishes capillary perfusion (i.e., shock, anemia) or that increases the susceptibility to infection (i.e., diabetes, immunosuppression) aggravates the subglottic damage caused by the indwelling endotracheal (ET) tube, as does gastroesophageal reflux [29]. The evolution of acute lesions of intubation into cicatricial sequelae of the glottis and subglottis were clearly described by Benjamin in 1993 [3]. They are similar in adults and children but with more prominent involvement of the glottis in children.

Grading System

In the pediatric community, the Myer-Cotton grading system is routinely used. This system classifies SGS into four grades (Table 10.1) [42].

10.2.1.2 Trachea

In infants, tracheal stenosis is most commonly related to congenital anomalies of the trachea itself (tracheomalacia, web, long-segment stenosis with circular

Table 10.1. Myer-Cotton grading system for pediatric subglottic stenosis

Grade	Obstruction (%)
I	0–50
II	51–70
III	71–99
IV	No lumen

From Myer et al. [42]

rings) or to extrinsic compressions from cardiovascular malformations. Even after correcting the vascular anomaly, localized tracheomalacia may necessitate further specific tracheal surgery. These entities have been clearly described in textbooks [26]. Their detailed description is beyond the scope of this chapter.

In older children, the etiology of benign tracheal stenoses is similar to that seen in the adult population (see Sect. 3.2.2).

10.2.2 Adults

10.2.2.1 Subglottis

Although several conditions—e.g., blunt trauma, inhalation injuries, high tracheotomy or cricothyroidotomy, Wegener's granulomatosis—and idiopathic causes can lead to benign SGS, postintubation injury remains by far the most common cause of SGS that is amenable to resection and primary reconstruction [35].

In the supraglottic region, sequelae of endotracheal intubation are usually absent or minimal. At the level of the glottis, they predominantly appear as bands of scar tissue tethering the vocal cords posteriorly, with or without cricoarytenoid ankylosis. This is the so-called posterior glottic stenosis (PGS). More seldomly, fusion of the vocal cords is also encountered. In the subglottis, circumferential ulcerations can induce granulation tissue formation which matures into contracting scars leading to SGS (Fig. 10.1).

Grading System

In adults where cricotracheal resection is now routinely used for the cure of laryngotracheal stenosis, Mc Caffrey's grading system of SGS helps predict the rate of success of the operation (Table 10.2) [32].

Fig. 10.1. Cicatricial sequelae of endotracheal intubation. (**a**) Interarytenoid adhesion. (**b**) Posterior glottic stenosis. (**c**) Cicatricial fusion of the vocal cords. (**d**) Subglottic stenosis

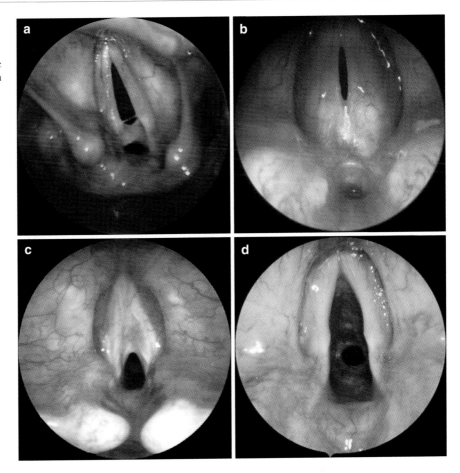

Table 10.2. Grading system for adult laryngotracheal stenosis according to McCaffrey [32]

Stage	Location of stenosis
I	Subglottis or trachea < 1 cm long
II	Subglottis within cricoid ring > 1 cm long
III	Subglottis + upper trachea
IV	Subglottis + glottic involvement

10.2.2.2 Trachea

Benign tracheal stenoses result from cuff lesions induced by endotracheal or tracheotomy tubes or from the sequelae of tracheotomy (i.e., triangular deformation at the site of the former stoma, tip of cannula anterior stenosis, or suprastomal granuloma and collapse) (Fig. 10.2) [35].

10.3 Indications

10.3.1 Primary Endoscopic Treatment

Cautious carbon dioxide (CO_2) laser incision combined with dilatation may be effective in thin, web-like cicatricial stenoses of the subglottis, but extensive laser resection is liable to make an acquired stenosis worse [36].

The indications set down by Simpson et al. (Table 10.3) [52] are still valuable today as a basis for the endoscopic treatment of LTS. CO_2 laser should be set to superpulse or ultrapulse mode and the laser beam directed to the target with a microspot manipulator (250 μm spot size at 400 mm focal distance) to minimize heat diffusion into the surrounding tissue. Radial incisions in the stenosis are made using Shapsay's technique [51], and gentle

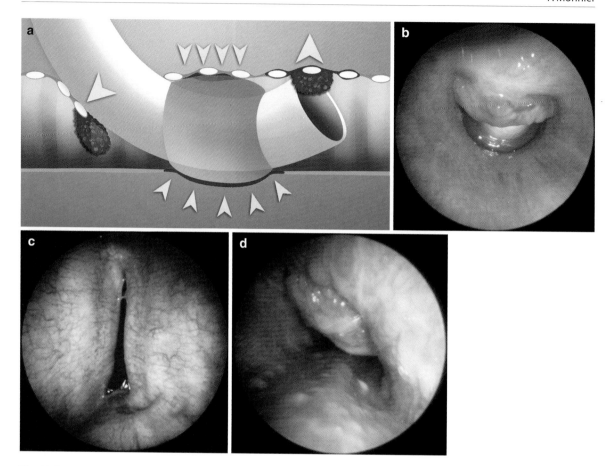

Fig. 10.2. Tracheal stenosis resulting of sequelae of tracheotomy. (**a**) Potential complications (i.e., suprastomal collapse, ostial or cuff-induced stenosis, tip of cannula stenosis). (**b**) Suprastomal collapse with granulation tissue. (**c**) Severe triangular narrowing of the trachea at the site of the former stoma. (**d**) Tip of cannula stenosis with granulation tissue

Table 10.3. Contraindications to CO_2 laser treatment of laryngeal stenosis

- Circumferential scarring
- Vertical scar > 1 cm
- Posterior scarring with arytenoid fixation
- Loss of cartilage support

From Simpson et al. [52]

dilatation is done with tapered bougies or angioplasty balloons. Then, a cotton swab soaked in a solution of 2 mg/ml mitomycin C may be topically applied to the subglottis for 2 minutes. Repeated mitomycin C application should probably be avoided, however, owing to uncertainty regarding possible late adverse effects [16, 48].

Finally, if the primary endoscopic treatment (CO_2 laser/dilatation/stenting) leads to a recurrence of the stenosis to its initial grade, any further endoscopic treatment is strictly contraindicated. Open surgery should be considered instead. The expected result is superior if the stenosis does not involve the posterior wall of the airway, especially at the level of the membranous trachea.

10.3.2 Laryngotracheal Reconstruction with Cartilage Expansion

Laryngotracheal reconstruction with cartilage expansion is almost exclusively reserved for mild grades of pediatric SGS or for combined glotto-subglottic stenoses. Although in adults LTR has been replaced by cricotracheal resection it is still used when further resection of the subglottis and trachea is impossible because of previous failed surgeries.

In children, LTR with an anterior graft alone is used as a single-stage operation to cure grade II stenosis [9, 33]. Mild grade III stenosis is likely to need an anterior graft with posterior cricoid split supported by an endoluminal stent, and severe grade III stenosis requires both anterior and posterior grafts with stenting [7, 43–55]. However, over the last decade, PCTR has shown to be superior to LTR for curing grade III and IV SGS [27].

In case of congenital stenosis, the LTR may be combined with submucosal resection of cartilage to increase the size of a thickened anterior lamina of the cricoid ring. Posterior glottic stenosis presents particular difficulties in children. A posterior cartilage graft is needed, but overexpansion of the posterior commissure should be avoided as it impairs voice quality and induces potential aspiration. Stenting is essential until the glottis and subglottis are completely healed.

10.3.3 Partial Cricotracheal Resection

In infants and children, PCTR is the procedure of choice for the treatment of severe (> 70% luminal obstruction) SGS of congenital or acquired etiology, but it is generally advisable to wait until the child reaches 10 kg body weight before surgery is undertaken [2, 38, 53–55]. The latter is performed as a single-stage operation (with concomitant resection of the tracheostoma during the surgery) when the stenosis is purely subglottic and the child is otherwise healthy. The only exception to this rule is a very distal location of the tracheostoma (fifth or sixth tracheal ring) with normal, steady tracheal rings available for the anastomosis between the subglottic stenosis and the upper margin of the tracheostoma. The latter is then closed in a second stage.

In children with multiple congenital anomalies or impaired neurological or cardiopulmonary function, a double-stage PCTR (with postoperative maintenance of the tracheostoma) is preferable. In adults, PCTR is almost exclusively performed as a single-stage operation for simple SGS or SGS combined with posterior glottic stenosis if cricoarytenoid joint mobility can be restored during the surgery and there is no bilateral neurogenic vocal cord paralysis [10, 23, 30, 31, 46].

10.3.4 Extended PCTR

In the pediatric age group, when SGS is combined with glottic involvement (e.g., posterior glottic stenosis), cicatricial fusion of the vocal cords, or distortion of the laryngeal framework resulting from failed LTRs, the PCTR is supplemented with posterior cricoid split and costal cartilage graft that needs stenting with an LT-Mold (see Sect. 4.5) for about 3 weeks until the subglottic area is completely healed. The tracheostoma is then closed in a second stage [37, 50]. The alternative to this treatment is an LTR with anterior and posterior costal cartilage grafts with stenting [8, 43, 44].

In adults, a posterior cricoid split and costal cartilage graft is rarely necessary. Resection of the scar tissue constituting the interarytenoid aspect of the stenosis suffices in most cases, although sometimes stenting with an LT-Mold is necessary with maintenance of the tracheostoma until complete healing has occurred.

10.3.5 Stenting

Laryngeal stents are mainly used to keep the airway expanded after surgical reconstruction (LTR with costal cartilage grafts or extended PCTR). They provide support for cartilage grafts, allow approximation and immobilization of mucosal grafts to the recipient site, and maintain the lumen in a reconstructed area that lacks adequate support. Unfortunately, laryngeal stents can also act as foreign bodies in a reconstructed airway and induce mucosal injuries, ulcerations, granulation tissue formation, and subsequent restenosis if their anatomical conformity to the inner laryngeal contours is not perfect or if their consistency is too hard.

Several laryngeal stents are currently available on the market, but none truly meets the requirements for safe use without potential damage to the reconstructed airway. The simplest ones—the finger cot and the rolled Silastic sheet—are custom-made [18]). They are quite primitive, however, and have now been largely replaced by the Aboulker stent [1], Montgomery T-tube [39], Healy pediatric T-tube, and Montgomery or Eliachar laryngotracheal stents [17].

Unfortunately, none of these stents is devoid of potential severe complications [6, 19, 57]. To overcome this problem, the LT-Mold has been designed for temporary stenting of the airway after surgical treatment of cicatricial stenoses of the larynx. Its design was created after molding cadaver larynges and increasing the interarytenoid distance to obtain the intralaryngeal contours of a fully abducted larynx (Fig. 10.3) [34]. Made of silicone at a strength of 50 Shore-A, it is soft and thus prevents pressure necrosis at the medial aspect of the arytenoids. To avoid possible granulation tissue formation at the distal extremity of the LT-Mold, a dedicated silicone cap is manufactured for each prosthesis. The prosthesis comes in 10 sizes, from 6 to 15 mm in outer diameter, and can be used in pediatric and adult populations. Moreover, the prosthesis can be used during open surgery (intraoperative use) or after endoscopic resection of a laryngotracheal stenosis (endoscopic use) with temporary maintenance of the tracheostoma.

The current experience in 28 patients shows excellent tolerance of the stent, without erosion or granulation tissue formation in the supraglottis or glottis or in the vicinity of the tracheostoma when the prosthesis is used with a distal cap.

10.3.6 Tracheal Resection

For simple tracheal stenosis amenable to segmental resection, end-to-end anastomosis with immediate postoperative extubation is the preferred method of treatment in adults and children. In the latter group. a short-time intubation may be necessary. For multilevel stenoses (SGS + cuff tracheal stenoses), a two-stage approach is sometimes necessary if the tracheal segment to be resected is too long (cf. specific recommendations to the technique).

10.4 Preoperative Workup

10.4.1 Basic Assessment

Thorough endoscopic evaluation usually provides all the information needed for carefully planned surgery.

If precise description and measurement of the stenosis are obtained via endoscopy, radiography adds little to the preoperative workup. However, lateral soft tissue and anteroposterior high-kilovoltage radiography or computed tomography scans with three-dimensional reconstructions are useful for documenting the length of the segment to be resected. When malformation of the mediastinum is suspected, CT or magnetic resonance imaging (MRI) are the examinations of choice.

Finally, pulmonary, cardiac, and neurological evaluations should be considered in children with congenital anomalies or previous long-term intubation for neonatal dyspnea of various etiologies. In adults, the same investigations should be undertaken on an individual basis depending on the patient's medical condition.

Last but not least, gastroesophageal reflux should be systematically ruled out or actively treated, if present.

10.4.2 Endoscopic Evaluation

Considering the potential dramatic consequences of failed PCTR or LTR, careful attention should be given to the preoperative endoscopic workup. It should comprise transnasal flexible laryngoscopy (TNFL) with spontaneous respiration or direct laryngotracheoscopy under general anesthesia with suspension microlaryngoscopy (if needed) and bronchoesophagoscopy.

10.4.2.1 Transnasal Flexible Laryngoscopy

In adults, neonates, and cooperative children, TNFL is done in the awake patient without sedation. For noncooperative children, TNFL under deep sevoflurane anesthesia with mask ventilation and spontaneous respiration is the preferred method (Fig. 10.4). This examination should not only give information on the mobility of the vocal cords but also on the patency of the nose, choanae, nasopharynx, and oropharynx. However, it provides only adequate visualization of the supraglottis and is unhelpful in the assessment of SGS. If there is any doubt regarding the mobility of the vocal cords, additional investigation by suspension microlaryngoscopy is mandatory [38].

Fig. 10.3. LT-Mold stent.
(**a**) Made of soft silicone at a strength of 50 Shore-A, the LT-mold was designed after molding adult and pediatric cadaver larynges and increasing the interarytenoid distance to obtain the intralaryngeal contours of a fully abducted larynx.
(**b**) The LT-Mold comes in 10 sizes, from 6 to 15 mm in outer diameter. To avoid possible granulation tissue formation at its distal extremity, a dedicated silicone cap has been manufactured for each prosthesis.
(**c**) Retrograde view of the stent through the tracheostoma : absence of granulation tissue at the stent-mucosal interface

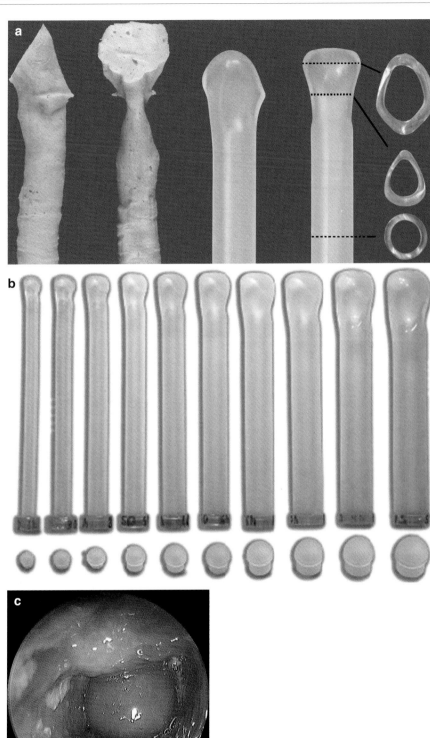

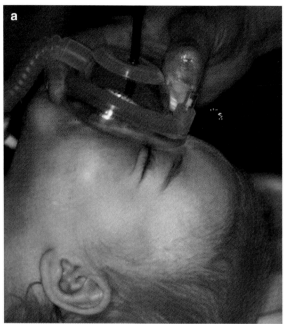

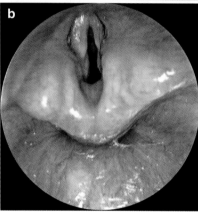

Fig. 10.4. Transnasal fiberoptic laryngoscopy (TNFL). (**a**) External view. In small children, this technique allows thorough evaluation of extralaryngeal sites of obstruction, vocal fold mobility, and tracheal dynamics with spontaneous respiration. (**b**) Internal view. Bilateral vocal cord paralysis

10.4.2.2 Direct Laryngotracheoscopy and Suspension Microlaryngoscopy

The location, extent, and degree of stenosis are assessed using a bare magnifying telescope and an intubation laryngoscope while the patient is under general anesthesia and fully relaxed (Fig. 10.5). The exact location of the stenosis with respect to the vocal folds, the tracheostoma, and the carina are measured in millimeters. The degree of the stenosis is measured by passing telescopes, endotracheal tubes, or bougies of different given sizes through the stricture. In the pediatric community, the Myer-Cotton airway grading system is routinely used [42]. This system classifies SGS into four grades and helps predict the rate of success after laryngotracheal reconstruction: The less severe grades (I and II) have a far better outcome than do severe grades (III and IV), which correspond to subtotal or total obstruction. This grading system is not useful as a predictor of success or failure for partial cricotracheal resection because the stenotic segment is fully resected.

Differentiating vocal fold immobility due to a neurogenic cause from an interarytenoid fibrous adhesion is done by carefully inspecting the posterior commissure of the larynx using a 30°, angled telescope and by direct palpation the arytenoid cartilages during suspension microlaryngoscopy [15, 36]. The systematic use of Lindholm's self-retaining vocal cord retractor (Storz no. 8654B) helps differentiate bilateral vocal fold paralysis from posterior glottic stenosis. A fixed arytenoid raises the suspicion of fibrous ankylosis of the joint; but in the most difficult cases, this diagnosis is safely made only during open surgery (Fig. 10.6).

The endoscopy report should also mention the presence of any localized tracheomalacia as well as a possible infection of the airway. A bacteriological smear is routinely taken and submitted to the laboratory.

10.4.2.3 Bronchoesophagoscopy

In infants and children, this additional examination is mandatory in all cases of congenital SGS to rule out an associated mediastinal malformation (i.e., tracheoesophageal fistula, tracheobronchial anomalies, extrinsic vascular compression of the airway), gastroesophageal reflux, and eosinophilic esophagitis [28, 41, 56].

For adult acquired SGS, a bronchoesophagoscopic examination is undertaken based on individual criteria. A systematic workup for gastroesophageal reflux is routinely done in patients with a positive medical history.

10.5 Operative Technique

10.5.1 Primary Endoscopic Treatment

Strict adherence to proper indications as described in Sect. 4.1 is a prerequisite if one wishes to avoid the

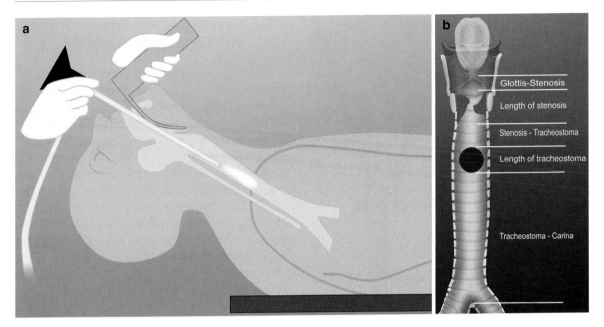

Fig. 10.5. Endoscopic assessment of laryngotracheal stenosis. (**a**) Direct laryngotracheoscopy with a 0° bare telescope. Examination down to the carina is possible without mucosal trauma in nontracheostomized patients. (**b**) Endoscopy report for subglottic stenosis. Precise measurements with reference to the vocal folds, tracheostoma, and carina should be given in all cases, including the number of residual normal tracheal rings. A precise surgical strategy is chosen at that time, taking all parameters into account: vocal fold mobility, extension and degree of stenosis, location of tracheostoma, length of residual normal trachea, and segments of tracheomalacia

dramatic consequences of overuse of laser [36]. In many cases, cold instruments, such as the sickle knife, can be used to incise a web-like cicatricial SGS. However, preference must be given to the use of CO_2 laser, which offers more precision and a bloodless field. Proper selection of CO_2 laser parameters is essential (Table 10.4) to obtain a char-free resection bed. Radial incisions of the cicatricial SGS according to Shapsay's technique [51] preserve mucosal bridges for better, faster reepithelialization of the subglottis. In addition to laser incisions, gentle dilatation with tapered Savary-Gilliard bougies or angioplasty balloons blown up to a pressure of 8 atm optimally enlarges the subglottic lumen. Then, topical application with a cotton swab soaked in a solution of mitomycin at a concentration of 1–2 mg/ml for 2 minutes gives satisfactory clinical results, although no experimental study has yet set up the optimal dosage or duration of topical application of the drug (Fig. 10.7) [16, 48]. However, if the SGS recurs at its initial grade after the first endoscopic treatment, open surgery should be considered without delay. [36].

The management of posterior glottic stenosis (PGS) requires expertise in selecting the appropriate candidate for the right type of treatment. Interarytenoid adhesion with a residual posterior opening is usually not associated with cricoarytenoid (CA) joint fixation. Dividing the scar with CO_2 laser is thus the first appropriate choice of treatment with a potentially high success rate [13, 14]. True PGS without residual posterior opening deserves first-try endoscopic treatment with CO_2 laser and adjuvant topical application of mitomycin C. Postoperative intubation with a soft blue-line Portex tube for 5–7 days helps obtain a satisfactory result. If CA joint mobility is restored, the abductive force of both posterior cricoarytenoid muscles prevents recurrence of the PGS at least to some degree. In tracheostomized patients, 2–3 weeks of stenting with an Easy LT-Mold [34] ensures reepithelialization of the posterior commissure in abduction, thus re-creating an adequate airway for breathing. In the case of true fixation of the CA joints, laser arytenoidectomy, posterior cordotomy, or posterior costal cartilage grafting should be envisaged. When PGS is combined with a subglottic stenosis, open surgery is mandatory in most cases.

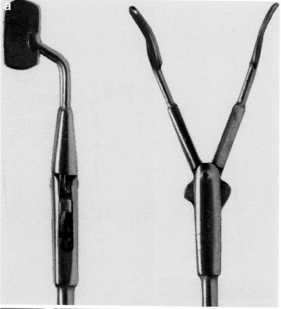

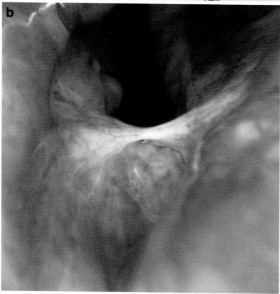

Fig. 10.6. Use of Lindholm's self-retaining vocal fold retractor. (**a**) Vocal fold retractor. (**b**) Spreading of posterior commissure with the self-retaining vocal fold retractor displays the scar tissue of the posterior glottic stenosis

Table 10.4. CO_2 laser parameters for treating laryngotracheal stenosis

- Ultrapulse mode
- 150 mJ/cm^2
- 50 Hz repetition rate
- 250 μm microspot at 400 mm focal distance

10.5.2 Laryngotracheal Reconstruction with Cartilage Expansion

The LTR with cartilage expansion is performed through a small collar incision placed at the superior edge of the tracheostoma (Fig. 10.8). The strap muscles are separated from the midline to expose the anterior portion of the larynx and upper trachea. For simple LTR with an anterior cartilage graft only, the incision typically extends through the lower third of the thyroid cartilage, the thyrocricoid membrane, the cricoid, and the first two tracheal rings. The costal cartilage harvested from the fifth, sixth, or seventh rib is boat-shaped and placed with the perichondrium intraluminally, serving as a lattice for reepithelialization. Lateral flanges of cartilage to the inset portion of the graft are secured to the thyroid, cricoid, and tracheal rings with 4.0 Vicryl sutures, thus preventing the graft from prolapsing into the airway.

The treatment of an associated PGS or a grade III SGS requires both anterior and posterior grafts with stenting. Placement of the posterior cartilage graft requires that the anterior thyrotracheal incision be extended into a full laryngofissure. The cricoid plate is then divided in the midline, and interarytenoid scarring is accurately resected. A rectangular costal cartilage graft is then inserted between the two parts of the posterior cricoid plate with the perichondrium facing the lumen. The graft must fit flush between the divided posterior cricoid laminae. It is sutured into place with 4.0 Vicryl sutures. An LT-Mold of appropriate diameter is placed at that stage and securely fixed with two 3.0 Prolene sutures, one placed exactly at the anterior commissure of the larynx and the other craniocaudally on one lateral side of the trachea. Depending on the individual situation, the vertical incision of the trachea is closed over the stent with or without additional anterior costal cartilage grafting (Fig. 10.9).

10.5.2.1 Single-Stage Versus Double-Stage LTR

The decision of whether to perform single-stage versus double-state LTR is based on the severity of the initial stenosis, the type of LTR that was performed (anterior graft only versus anterior and posterior costal cartilage grafts), and the patient's medical condition. Poor cardiopulmonary function and neurological impairment are contraindications to a single-stage LTR, even for a grade II or mild grade III SGS. Depending on the

Fig. 10.7. Combined supraglottic, glottic, and subglottic stenosis. (**a**) Anteriorly displaced right arytenoid combined with posterior and subglottic stenosis. (**b**) Endoscopic view after CO$_2$ laser resection. (**c**) Final endoscopic result at 3 months

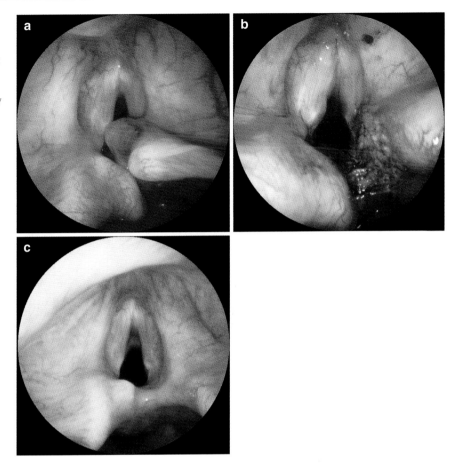

stability of the reconstructed airway, an LT-Mold stent is secured in place and left in the airway for a period of 3 weeks to 6 months [34].

10.5.3 Partial Cricotracheal Resection for Subglottic Stenosis

PCTR for SGS is performed with the neck fully extended. A collar incision is usually made at the level that will best expose the stenotic segment of the airway (Fig. 10.10). In tracheotomized patients, a horizontal crescent-shaped excision of the skin is made around the stoma. This is necessary for upward mobilization of the trachea even if the tracheostoma is kept at the end of the operation. The subplatysmal skin flaps are elevated, and the strap muscles are separated from the midline to provide exposure from the hyoid bone to the suprasternal notch. At that stage, the use of a Denys-Brown retractor (Lone Star Medical Products, Stafford TX, USA) is extremely useful. As the dissection progresses, the surgeon advances the position of stays into deeper tissue (i.e., strap muscles and thyroid lobes reflected aside). As a consequence, the larynx and trachea are almost at the level of the skin, which markedly facilitates the dissection and resection–anastomosis. With benign stenosis, the trachea is dissected anteriorly and laterally without identifying the recurrent laryngeal nerves by staying in close contact with the underlying cartilaginous rings. With neoplastic stenosis, one or the other recurrent laryngeal nerve is usually identified to determine the extent of the disease. The vascular supply coming laterally from the tracheoesophageal grooves should always be carefully preserved, especially during extensive mobilization of the distal trachea. Prior to any incision of the trachea or subglottis, this mobilization gives an idea on how much of the trachea can safely be resected without a laryngeal release procedure.

Fig. 10.8. Laryngotracheal reconstruction with cartilage expansion. (**a**) Costal cartilage harvested from the seventh rib. (**b**) Anterior costal cartilage graft. (**c**) Laryngofissure and posterior cricoid split for the treatment of posterior glottic stenosis (PGS) combined with subglottic stenosis (SGS). (**d**) Posterior costal cartilage graft. Note that the flanges of cartilage are wedged between the divided cricoid laminae. (**e**) Combined anterior and posterior cartilage grafts for grade III SGS

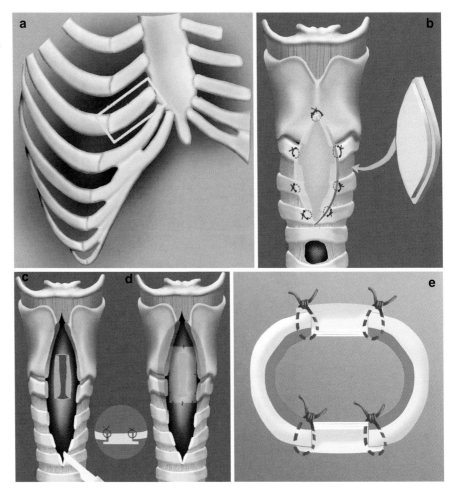

At the level of the cricoid arch, the cricothyroid muscles are sharply dissected off the underlying cartilage and reflected laterally over the cricothyroid joint. This maneuver protects the recurrent laryngeal nerves, which run posteriorly to the cricothyroid joint. After having placed stay sutures to the distal normal tracheal wall, the inferior resection line is made first at the lower end of the stenosis or at the level of the tracheostoma if the latter is to be resected during the same surgical procedure. This allows a view of the stenosis from below and affords a good distal airway for ventilation. The membranous trachea is then dissected and separated from the anterior wall of the esophagus over a distance that corresponds to the height of the cricoid plate. Unnecessary extensive separation of the trachea from the esophagus should be avoided to preserve an optimal vascular supply. Advancement of the distal tracheal stump upward is achieved by freeing the cartilaginous rings from the mediastinal structures anteriorly and laterally only.

Owing to its elasticity, the esophagus shortens spontaneously without anterior bulging. The superior incision is started at the inferior margin of the thyroid cartilage in front and is passed laterally just anterior to the cricothyroid joints. This results in complete resection of the anterior cricoid arch while avoiding injury to the recurrent laryngeal nerves that run posterior to the joint. In the subglottis, the uppermost incision of the posterior mucosa is made just below the cricoarytenoid joints; and the submucosal fibrosis, constituting the posterior aspect of the subglottic stenosis, is fully resected, thereby exposing the cricoid plate completely. As the luminal diameter of the distal airway is always larger than that of the subglottis, the first normal tracheal ring used for the anastomosis must be adapted to the size of the subglottic lumen. In adults, this is best achieved by plicating the membranous trachea to accommodate the differences in diameter. In children, the discrepancy in luminal diameter between the

Fig. 10.9. Peroperative use of the LT-Mold. (**a**) The LT-Mold is cut at the appropriate length, and the distal cap is glued to the prosthesis with silicone glue. (**b**) Diagram showing proper LT-Mold placement in the larynx. (**c**) Endoscopic view of the LT-Mold in the larynx. (**d**) View of the larynx immediately after stent removal

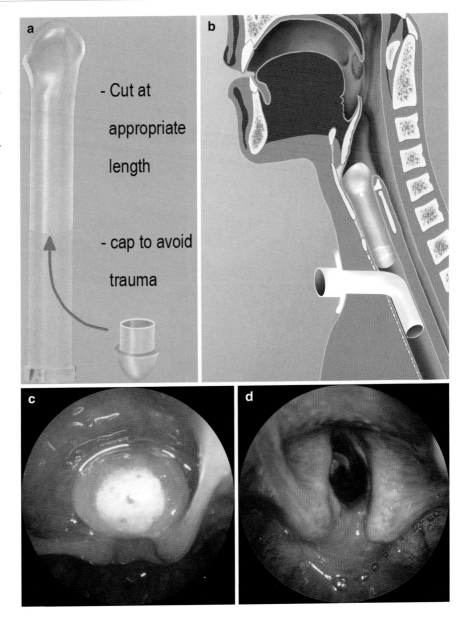

subglottic space and the tracheal stump is even more pronounced than it is in adults. Any attempt to reduce the caliber of the trachea should be avoided. Instead, one should enlarge the subglottic lumen as much as possible without compromising voice quality. This is best achieved by widening the cricoid plate posteriorly and laterally with a diamond burr and by performing an inferior midline thyrotomy up to the level of the anterior commissure of the larynx without transecting it. Because the thyroid cartilage is usually soft and pliable in infants and children, the inferior margins of both thyroid alae are easily spread apart. In this way, the subglottic lumen is enlarged considerably while the anterior commissure is kept intact, thus preserving a good voice. The triangular defect is filled in with a mucosa-lined cartilaginous wedge that is obtained from the first normal tracheal ring below the resected stricture. This requires additional resection of the lateral portion of the first normal tracheal ring used for the anastomosis.

Unfortunately, this technique is not feasible in adults, whose thyroid cartilage is often calcified or even ossified.

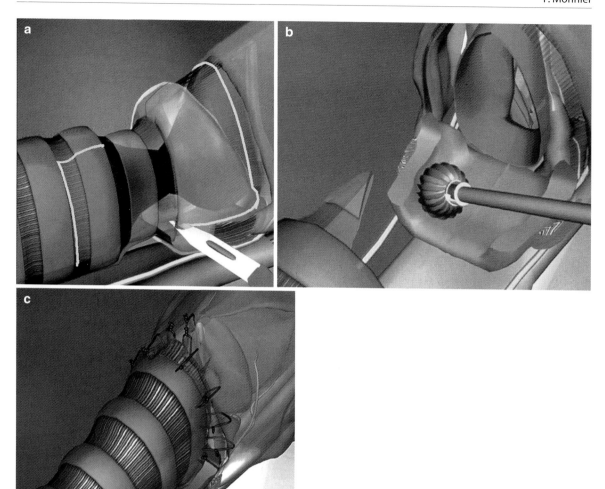

Fig. 10.10. Partial cricotracheal resection. (**a**) After careful preparation and mobilization of the trachea and larynx, the superior resection line is made at the inferior margin of the thyroid cartilage. The inferior resection line is carried out one ring below the first normal tracheal ring to harvest an anterior pedicled wedge of cartilage that will be used to enlarge the subglottic lumen. The lateral resection line is made just anterior to the cricothyroid joint on both sides. The recurrent laryngeal nerve is shown here for anatomical purposes only; it is deliberately not identified during the surgery. (**b**) After resection of the anterior arch of the cricoid, the fibrous tissue constituting the posterior aspect of the stenosis is fully resected. The uppermost posterior section of the mucosa passes immediately below the cricoarytenoid joints. The denuded cricoid plate is then flattened with a diamond burr. This allows better adaptation of the tracheal stump to the subglottis. The cartilaginous wedge of the anterior trachea will be used to enlarge the subglottic lumen. (**c**) Except for the most posterolateral suture, which is placed between the trachea and the cricoid plate, all lateral and anterior stitches are passed between the tracheal ring and the thyroid cartilage. The adaptation of the large tracheal ring to the narrower subglottic space is facilitated by enlargement of the subglottic lumen with the partial inferior midline thyrotomy. The triangular defect is then filled in with the cartilaginous wedge pedicled to the tracheal ring used for the anastomosis

The denuded cricoid plate is covered with the membranous trachea after its upward mobilization. Interrupted Vicryl sutures (4.0 or 3.0 in adults, 6.0 or 5.0 in children) are used for the posterior anastomosis, with the knots tied inside the lumen. The disadvantage of having a few sutures tied inside the lumen posteriorly is largely compensated for by the optimal approximation of the mucosa, which is difficult to obtain with the knots tied outside the lumen. At this stage, tension-releasing sutures are also placed bilaterally between the third or fourth tracheal ring laterally and the inferior border of the cricoid plate. Fibrin glue is used to secure the membranous trachea to the cricoid plate. Vicryl sutures (2.0 in adults, 3.0 or 4.0 in children) are used for the anterior and lateral anastomosis. The first stitch is passed through the posterolateral aspect of the first normal tracheal ring and through the cricoid plate laterally. It should emerge in a subperichondrial plane from the outer surface of the cricoid plate to avoid any lesion to the recurrent laryngeal nerves. This stitch is extremely important and should be placed as meticulously as possible to bring the mucosa of the subglottis in close contact with the mucosa of the trachea. The thyrotracheal anastomosis is then completed by placing the Vicryl sutures between the tracheal ring and the thyroid cartilage anteriorly, with the knots tied on the outside.

At the end of the procedure, the neck is maintained in a flexed position. It is not necessary to place sutures from the chin to the chest to limit extension of the neck during the postoperative period. Motivated patients receiving clear explanations maintain their neck flexed for a period of 10 days without any difficulty.

10.5.3.1 Single-Stage Versus Double-Stage PCTR

If the patient is fit for single-stage surgery, two options usually exist, depending on the location of the tracheostoma. Single-stage PCTR with preoperative resection of the tracheostoma is chosen if no more than five tracheal rings must be resected with the subglottic stenosis. The absence of a postoperative tracheostoma is highly favorable for healing of the anastomosis, but longer tracheal resections carry greater risk of anastomotic dehiscence.

If the location of the tracheostoma requires resection of six or more tracheal rings, or if for anatomical reasons mobilization of the tracheal stump is difficult, it is preferable to use a steady, normal ring (situated between the SGS and the upper margin of the tracheostoma) for the anastomosis and to close the tracheostoma separately or keep it into the postoperative period. In some cases, owing to proximal damage of the trachea, insufficient steadiness of the upper tracheal rings prevents their use for the anastomosis. A longer tracheal resection must then be envisaged with a laryngeal and/or hilar release procedure.

10.5.4 Extended PCTR for Subglottic Stenosis Combined with Glottic Pathologies

Initially used for purely subglottic stenosis, partial cricotracheal resection with primary thyrotracheal anastomosis has proved to be efficient also for the cure of combined subglottic and glottic pathologies: posterior glottic stenosis, cicatricial fusion of the vocal cords, anterior glottic web extending into the subglottis, combined supraglottic, glottic, and suglottic scarring, and distortion of the larynx after failed LTR (Fig. 10.11). The surgical procedure (extended PCTR) is then modified as follows. A complete laryngofissure is created. In adults, the scar tissue constituting the posterior glottic stenosis is removed; and, if necessary, the transverse interarytenoid muscle is sectioned in the midline. Most often, a posterior cricoid split with costal cartilage grafting is not necessary because the interarytenoid distance is large enough in adults. On the contrary, the latter procedure is almost always necessary in children. The two parts of the posterior cricoid plate are then sufficiently distracted to allow correct positioning of the costal cartilage harvested from the sixth or seventh rib. The graft must fit flush between the divided posterior cricoid laminae with the perichondrium facing the lumen. Lateral flanges of perichondrium on the luminal side and small cartilaginous extensions of the graft under the cricoid plate stabilize the graft, which is fixed in place with 4.0 Vicryl sutures. In both adults and children, a pedicled flap of membranous trachea is created by resecting one or two additional rings of the tracheal stump distally.

The trachea is then advanced upward, and its membranous portion is sutured with 5.0 Vicryl stitches to the mucosa of the posterior commissure of the larynx. The lateral and anterior anastomosis is completed as for conventional PCTR using 3.0 or 4.0 Vicryl sutures. A fully mucosalized anastomosis is thus obtained. Closure of the laryngofissure over a nasotracheal tube or a stent is performed meticulously by placing a Vicryl suture exactly at the level of the vocal cords to restore a sharp anterior commissure. In adults, stenting is not usually necessary. In children, we currently use an LT-Mold that conforms to the inner laryngeal contours to restore it as close to a normal laryngotracheal airway as possible.

The cartilaginous wedge pedicled to the tracheal ring used for the anastomosis is inserted between the alae of the thyroid cartilage inferiorly to enlarge the subglottic lumen without compromising voice quality in children. Next, the isthmus of the thyroid gland is resutured in the midline, over the anastomosis, to optimize the vascular supply.

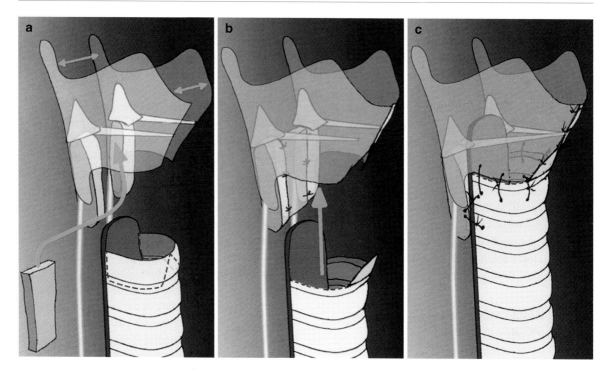

Fig. 10.11. Extended PCTR. (**a**) PCTR is performed according to the conventional technique. A temporary midline thyrotomy gives access to the cricoid plate. A posterior midline incision of the cricoid plate is made, and a costal cartilage graft is interposed between the divided cricoid laminae (*blue arrow*). (**b**) A pedicled flap of membranous trachea is obtained by removing one or two more rings of the tracheal stump distally. This allows delineation of the anterior cartilaginous wedge that will be used to fill in the triangular defect resulting from the inferior midline thyrotomy. (**c**) The trachea is advanced upward, and its membranous portion is sutured to the mucosa of the posterior commissure of the larynx. The lateral and anterior anastomosis is completed as in conventional PCTR with a pedicled wedge of tracheal cartilage filling in the triangular defect of the inferior midline thyrotomy. Precise repositioning of the anterior commissure is essential to preserve a good voice when suturing the alae of the thyroid cartilage together

10.5.5 Tracheal Resection with End-to-End Anastomosis

Tracheal resection with an end-to-end anastomosis is basically identical to that described for PCTR, but the initial dissection is carried out only up to the level of the cricoid cartilage unless a laryngeal release procedure is envisaged during the course of the surgery [22].

When a tracheostoma is present, hemostats are placed for traction on either side of the ellipse of skin that has been left around the stoma. This helps mobilize the mediastinal portion of the trachea cranially while its dissection is carried out anteriorly and laterally only and in close contact with the cartilaginous rings. At that stage, all the vascular supply coming bilaterally from the tracheal esophageal grooves should be preserved. Before resecting the stenotic segment, pulling on the mediastinal trachea gives a good idea on how much cranial mobilization can be achieved without a laryngeal release procedure. If there is any doubt about the exact location of the upper and lower edges of the intrinsic portion of the stenosis, it is best to incise the trachea transversally through the narrowest portion of the airway and to progress cranially and caudally by slicing the trachea until normal rings are found. The steadiness and quality of the tracheal rings are essential to the success of the surgery. No compromise should be made at this point. If necessary, a laryngeal and/or hilar and pericardial release procedure should be performed with the help of a thoracic surgeon, instead of using unstable tracheal rings for the anastomosis.

Once appropriate tension-free approximation of the trachea has been achieved, only minimal separation of the membranous trachea from the anterior esophageal wall should be performed in order to preserve an optimal vascular supply. The esophagus shortens spontaneously without anterior bulging.

Because the proximal and distal stumps of the trachea are usually well matched, performing the anastomosis is much easier than with PCTR. It is done with 3.0

interrupted Vicryl sutures for the membranous trachea and 2.0 Vicryl sutures for the lateral and anterior anastomosis. All inverted stitches should emerge in a submucosal plane with the knots tied on the outer surface of the trachea. At that stage, lifting the head of the patient helps obtain a tension-free anastomosis. A Penrose drain is placed distal to the site of the anastomosis, after which the thyroid isthmus and strap muscles are resutured on the midline and the skin is closed in two layers.

10.6 Specific Recommendations

This section essentially focuses on resections and anastomoses for subglottic or tracheal stenosis.

10.6.1 Primary Location of the Tracheostoma

Although the primary location of the tracheostoma at the time of acute lesions of intubation may seem straightforward, it is of significant importance for delayed reconstructive surgery.

In case of incipient SGS, the tracheostoma should be placed either between the cricoid and the first tracheal ring or as low as possible in the neck. In the former situation, this allows single-stage PCTR with limited resection of the trachea or single-stage LTR and easy closure of the tracheostoma with the same cartilage graft. In the latter situation, the tracheostoma located at the fifth or sixth tracheal ring always preserves a sufficient number of normal tracheal rings between the inferior border of the SGS and the upper rim of the tracheostoma, thus allowing double-stage PCTR with a short tracheal resection. In case of LTR, the SGS can be treated without too much proximity to the tracheostoma, thus allowing better healing and closure of the tracheostoma during a second stage procedure.

Knowing that the risk of anastomotic dehiscence is proportional to the length of the tracheal resection, correct placement of the tracheostoma is of utmost importance for the future success of reconstructive surgery. In case of incipient tracheal stenosis, the tracheostoma should always be placed through the stenosis, thus avoiding further damage to the normal trachea.

If these basic principles were respected by all surgeons, the outcome of surgery for subglottic and tracheal stenoses would certainly be much better. Improved medical education is of key importance in this field.

10.6.2 Extensive Airway Resection

The usual question that arises is how much trachea can be resected and the anastomosis still safely accomplished. There is no straightforward answer. The permissible length varies with patient's age, body build, and height and any prior surgery performed. A young adult with a long, supple neck and cranial location of the larynx differs completely from an old, kyphotic patient with the cricoid ring situated at the level of the sternal notch. In the former, 50% of the trachea can certainly be resected and reanastomosed safely, whereas in the latter only a short (less than one-fourth) segment of trachea is amenable to safe reconstruction. Furthermore, cranial mobilization of the mediastinal tracheal stump is unpredictable and varies significantly from one patient to another, even without previous surgery.

Although experimental studies on dogs and human cadavers have been conducted, no clear answer has yet emerged. For the time being, surgical experience shows that approximately one-half of the pediatric or adult trachea may be removed and reconstruction safely made. However, this is where the surgeon's experience and judgment contribute to the final decision of what is likely to be safely possible in each patient, with or without laryngeal and/or hilar and pericardial release.

10.6.3 Recapture of Tracheal Length

Various techniques of tracheal and supralaryngeal release may be used to diminish the tension on the suture line for PCTR and segmental resection of the trachea [4, 12, 40, 58] (Fig. 10.12). It depends on the length of the tracheal segment to be resected and the individual anatomy. Usually, advancement of the distal tracheal stump upward is much easier in children than it is in adults. If a laryngeal release procedure is necessary, however, it is best performed by sectioning the

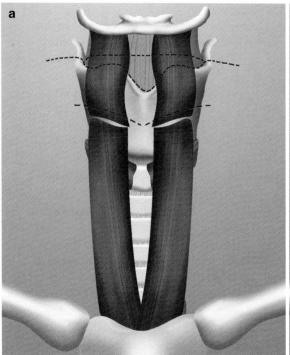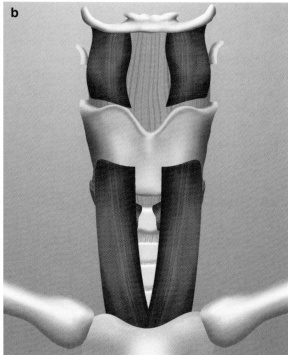

Fig. 10.12. Laryngeal release procedure. (**a**) At the level of the second layer of the strap muscles. The sternohyoid muscle is preserved. The thyrohyoid muscle is cut bilaterally just above its insertion on the thyroid cartilage. Then, the thyrohyoid membrane is cut in the midline and along the upper edge of the thyroid cartilage, leading laterally to the upper cornu, which is cut bilaterally with a pair of straight Mayo scissors. (**b**) Result of the laryngeal drop: a distance of 1.5–2.0 cm has been obtained

thyrohyoid muscle at the level of its insertion line on the thyroid cartilage. Then, by pulling the cartilage caudally with a laryngeal hook placed at the thyroid notch, the thyrohyoid membrane can be cut along the upper border of the thyroid cartilage. This leads laterally to its upper cornu, which is then sectioned with a pair of straight Mayo scissors. A laryngeal drop of 1.5–2.0 cm can thus be obtained. A hilar and pericardial release procedure, performed through a sternotomy and a T incision into the left fourth interspace is sometimes necessary in adults but not in children. However, it hugely increases the extent of surgery otherwise planned as a cervicomediastinal procedure. It does provide another 2 cm of length for a tension-free thyrotracheal anastomosis though. It is best to plan this additional surgery with the thoracic surgeon prior to the day of cricotracheal resection. It can be anticipated by a thorough preoperative endoscopic and radiological workup.

10.7 Postoperative Care and Follow-Up

10.7.1 Laryngotracheal Reconstruction

Patients with long-standing tracheotomies may be colonized with *Pseudomonas aeruginosa* or *Staphylococcus aureus*— hence the importance of the preoperative bacteriological smear.

Appropriate antibiotics are given until the subglottic airway is fully healed. If reflux is present, proton pump inhibitors are continued for up to 6 months postoperatively.

Patients with single-stage LTRs are kept intubated without paralysis for 7–14 days, depending on the type of reconstruction (anterior graft versus posterior graft). Control endoscopy is mandatory on the day of extubation to ensure proper incipient healing of the reconstructed airway and again at 3 months if clinically the patient shows no sign of upper airway obstruction.

With double-stage LTRs, tracheotomized patients may return to the ward on the first operative day as the parents are already familiar with care of the tracheotomy cannula. The first control endoscopy is done at the time of stent removal and then 3 weeks later. Plugging the cannula early after stent removal gives information on the patency of the reconstructed airway above the tracheostoma. If for some reason (e.g., suprastomal collapse) this is not possible, a control endoscopy should be scheduled after 10 days to ensure that no incipient subglottic stenosis is redeveloping. When the subglottis is fully healed and stable, downsizing the cannula over a period of several days facilitates eventual closure of the tracheostoma.

10.7.2 Partial Cricotracheal Resection and Segmental Tracheal Resection

Postoperative management after single-stage PCTR or segmental tracheal resection is more challenging in children, whose airways are much smaller than those of adults.

Nontracheotomized children stay under close supervision in the intensive care unit until extubation is achieved. Broad-spectrum antibiotics and antireflux medication are given to all patients until a mucosalized anastomosis is obtained. Proton pump inhibitors are continued postoperatively over a period of up to 6 months. Corticosteroids are started on the day prior to extubation and are continued for the following days if necessary. Depending on the child's age, a first control endoscopy is performed at 5, 7, or 10 days postoperatively. If there is only slight to moderate edema of the vocal folds and subglottis, the child is tentatively extubated. Because of its very low viscosity, heliox (a mixture of helium and oxygen) is sometimes used to diminish the inspiratory stridor resulting from postoperative laryngeal edema. In the case of significant edema, the child is reintubated with a one-size-smaller tube, and a plug of corticosteroid-gentamicin ointment is applied to the endolarynx. The next tentative extubation is planned for 2 days later. Additional endoscopic controls are routinely performed at 3 weeks and 3 months. The final result may then be optimized at 3 months by gentle bougienage with Savary-Gilliard dilators.

If a double-stage PCTR is performed without stenting, no clinical information on subglottic airway patency is available as the child breathes through the tracheostoma. A control endoscopy at the third postoperative week is then mandatory to assess the quality of healing at the site of the anastomosis. To salvage a suboptimal result (i.e., incipient restenosis), a laryngeal stent (LT-Mold) should be placed endoscopically.

With extended PCTRs and double-stage PCTRs with stenting, the treacheostoma is left in place until the subglottic anastomosis is completely healed. Stenting is usually necessary for about 3 weeks. However, depending on the complexity of the reconstruction after LTR or extended PCTR, stenting is sometimes maintained for up to 6 months or longer, especially after reconstruction of distorted larynges resulting from previous failed LTRs.

10.8 Results

10.8.1 Pediatric LTR and PCTR

Results from the most experienced centers [8, 43, 44] show a decannulation rate of just under 90% for grades I and II SGS following LTR. However, it drops to around 80% for grade III and to 50% or less for grade IV SGS, implying the need for revision surgery in a significant number of cases [8, 43, 44]. From the six international centers that published their results on pediatric PCTR for severe (grades III and IV) SGS, a global decannulation rate of 96% (258/269 cases) was achieved [2, 37, 49, 53–55]. Looking at these results in a more detailed manner, the two centers with the largest experience in PCTR [37, 55] showed a decannulation rate of 98% (56/57 cases) for primary surgery and 93% (70/75 cases) for salvage surgery after failed previous airway reconstruction (unpublished results on 86 cases from Lausanne).

Extended PCTRs for SGS with glottic involvement showed an interesting decannulation rate of 91% (42/46 cases), but 11 of 25 (44%) patients in the Cincinnati group and 6 of 21 (29%) patients in the Lausanne group required more than one open procedure to achieve

Table 10.5. Results of PCTR for severe pediatric SGS from the two largest series

Type of surgery	Decannulation	
	Cincinnati [55]	Lausanne (unpublished series)
Primary PCTR	13/13 (100%)	43/44 (98%)
Salvage PCTR	51/55 (93%)	20/21 (95%)
Extended PCTR	23/25 (92%)	19/21 (90%)
Total	87/93 (94%)	81/86 (95%)

PCTR, part cricotracheal resection; SGS, subglottic stenosis

these results (Table 10.5). This reflects the challenge of treating some of these extremely complex cases that have undergone several prior open surgeries.

In a recent publication on the long-term outcome of 57 PCTRs with a median follow-up of 5.1 year (minimum follow-up of 1 year), 55 of the 57 (96%) patients were decannulated [27]. Only one patient had moderate exertional dyspnea, and all other patients could participate in sports without restriction. Voice quality was found to improve after PCTR of 1.0 ± 1.34 grade, according to the GRBAS grading system.

10.8.2 Adult PCTR

The overall results in the international literature published from 1972 to 2000 [10, 20, 21, 31, 45] on 249 patients in the adult age group were similar to those of the pediatric population, with a 95% (237/249 cases) success rate and a 1% (2/249 cases) mortality rate.

10.8.3 Segmental Tracheal Resection

Grillo's large series of 503 patients who underwent segmental tracheal resection for postintubation stenosis shows a 94% (471/503 cases) good to satisfactory postoperative result [22]. The latter was classified as good if the patient could play sports without exertional dyspnea, and satisfactory if the patient could perform normal activities but was stressed on exercise. These results are in accordance with smaller reported series of tracheal resections with end-to-end anastomosis in adults [5, 11, 47]. Failure occurred in 20 (3.9%) and death in 12 (2.4%) of the cases.

10.9 Tips and Pearls to Avoid Complications

- Perform a thorough preoperative assessment of the patient's medical condition.
- Establish a precise endoscopy report on extralaryngeal sites of obstruction, vocal fold mobility and site, extent, and degree of airway stenosis.
- Address only mature cicatricial stenosis for a definitive endoscopic or open surgical treatment.
- Do workup studies for gastroesophageal reflux.
- Carefully respect the indications for the management of each type of stenosis and for single-stage or double-stage procedures.
- Use meticulous technique for LTR, PCTR, and segmental tracheal resection.
- Follow up your patient carefully during the postoperative period.
- Remember that inappropriate initial management of LTS may lead to permanent intractable sequelae and that the best chance for the patient lies in the first operation.

References

1. Aboulker P, Sterkers JM, Demaldent JE, Sauton P (1966) Modifications apportées à l'intervention de Rethi. Intérêt dans les sténoses laryngo-trachéales et trachéales. Ann Otolaryngol Paris 83:98–106
2. Alvarez-Neri H, Penchyna-Grub J, Porras-Hernandez JD, Blanco-Rodriguez G, Gonzalez R, Rutter MJ (2005) Primary cricotracheal resection with thyrotracheal anastomosis for the treatment of severe subglottic stenosis in children and adolescents. Ann Otol Rhinol Laryngol 114:2–6
3. Benjamin B (1993) Prolonged intubation injuries of the larynx: endoscopic diagnosis, classification and treatment. Ann Otol Rhinol Laryngol 160:S1–15
4. Biller HF, Munier MA (1992) Combined infrahyoid and inferior constrictor muscle release for tension-free anastomosis during primary tracheal repair. Otolaryngol Head Neck Surg 107:430–433
5. Bisson A, Bonnette P, El Kadi B (1992) Tracheal sleeve resection for iatrogenic stenoses. J Thorac Cardiovasc Surg 104:882–887
6. Calhoun KH, Deskin RW, Bailey BJ (1988) Near-fatal complication of tracheal T-tube use. Ann Otol Rhinol Laryngol 97:542–544
7. Cotton RT (2000) Management of subglottic stenosis. Otolaryngol Clin North Am 33:111–130
8. Cotton RT, Gray SD, Miller RP (1989) Update of the Cincinnati experience in laryngotracheal reconstruction. Laryngoscope 99:1111–1116

9. Cotton RT, Myer CM 3rd, O'Connor DM, Smith ME (1995) Pediatric laryngotracheal reconstruction with cartilage grafts and endotracheal tube stenting: the single stage approach. Laryngoscope 105:818–821

10. Couraud L, Brichon PY, Velly JF (1988) The surgical management of inflammatory and fibrous laryngotracheal stenosis. Eur J Cardiothorac Surg 2:410–415

11. Couraud L, Jongon JB, Velly JF (1995) Surgical treatment of non tumoral stenosis of the upper airway. Ann Thorac Surg 60:250–260

12. Dedo HH, Fishman NH (1969) Laryngeal release and sleeve resection for tracheal stenosis. Ann Otol Rhinol Laryngol 78:285–296

13. Dedo HH, Sooy CD (1984) Endoscopic laser repair of posterior glottic, subglottic and tracheal stenosis by division or micro-trapdoor flap. Laryngoscope 94:445–450

14. Duncavage JA, Ossoff RH, Toohill RJ (1985) Carbon dioxide laser management of laryngeal stenosis. Ann Otol Rhinol Laryngol 94:565–569

15. Eckel HE, Wittekindt C, Klussmann JP, Schroeder U, Sittel C (2003) Management of bilateral cricoarytenoid cartilage fixation versus recurrent laryngeal nerve paralysis. Ann Otol Rhinol Laryngol 112:103–108

16. Eliachar R, Eliachar I, Esclamado R, Gramlich T, Strome M (1999) Can topical mitomycin prevent laryngotracheal stenosis? Laryngoscope 109:1594–1600

17. Eliachar I, Nguyen D (1990) Laryngotracheal stent for internal support and control of aspiration without loss of phonation. Otolaryngol Head Neck Surg 103:837–840

18. Evans JNG, Todd GB (1974) Laryngotracheoplasty. J Laryngol Otol 87:589–597

19. Froehlich P, Truy E, Stamm D (1993) Role of long-term stenting in treatment of pediatric subglottic stenosis. Int J Pediatr Otorhinolaryngol 27(3):273–280

20. George M, Lang F, Pasche Ph, Monnier P (2005) Surgical management of laryngotracheal stenosis in adults. Eur Arch Otorhinolaryngol 262:609–615

21. Gerwat J, Bryce DP (1974) The management of subglottic stenosis by resection and direct anastomosis. Laryngoscope 84:940–947

22. Grillo HC, Donahue DM, Mathisen DJ (1995) Postintubation tracheal stenosis. Treatment and result. J Thorac Cardiovasc Surg 109:486–493

23. Grillo HC, Mathisen Dj, Wain JC (1992) Laryngotracheal resection and reconstruction for subglottic stenosis. Ann Thorac Surg 53:54–63

24. Holinger LD (1980) Etiology of stridor in the neonate, infant, and child. Ann Otol Rhinol Laryngol 89:397

25. Holinger LD. Congenital laryngeal anomalies. In: Pediatric laryngology and bronchoesophagology,. Philadelphia, PA/New York: Lippincott-Raven; 1997

26. Holinger LD, Green CG, Benjamin B, Shorp JK (1997) Tracheobronchial tree. In: Holinger LD, Lusk RP, Green CG (eds) Pediatric laryngology and bronchoesophagology. Lippincott-Raven, Philadelphia, PA/New York

27. Jaquet Y, Lang F, Pilloud R, Savary M, Monnier P (2005) Partial cricotracheal resection for pediatric subglottic stenosis: long-term outcome in 57 patients. J Thorac Cardiovasc Surg 130(3):726–732

28. Johnson L, Cotton RT, Rutter MJ (2003) Airway stenosis and eosinophilic esophagitis. Abstract presented at Annual Meeting of the American Academy, May 3, Nashville, TN

29. Lang F, Pasche P, Monnier P (2001) Sténoses laryngotrachéales. Encycl Med Chir Pneumologie 6-035-A-20:1–20. Elsevier, Paris

30. Macchiarini P, Verhoye JP, Chapelier A, Fadel E, Dartevelle P (2001) Partial cricoidectomy with primary thyrotracheal anastomosis for postintubation subglottic stenosis. J Thorac Cardiovasc Surg 121:68–76

31. Maddaus MA, Toth JL, Gullane PJ, Pearson FG (1992) Subglottic tracheal resection and synchronous laryngeal reconstruction. J Thorac Cardiovasc Surg 104:1443–1450

32. McCaffrey TV (1992) Classification of laryngotracheal stenosis. Laryngoscope 102:1335–1340

33. McQueen CT, Shapiro NL, Leighton S, Guo XG, Albert DM (1999) Single-stage laryngotracheal reconstruction: the Great Ormond Street experience and guidelines for patient selection. Arch Otolaryngol Head Neck Surg 125:320–322

34. Monnier Ph (2003) A new stent for the management of adult and pediatric laryngotracheal stenosis. Laryngoscope 113: 1418–1422

35. Monnier Ph (1999) Complications laryngées et trachéales après intubation et trachéotomie. In: Cros AM, Bourgain JL, Ravussin P (eds) Les voies aériennes: leur contrôle en anesthésie - réanimation. Pradel Revil-Malmaison, France

36. Monnier Ph, George M, Monod ML, Lang F (2005) The role of the CO_2 laser in the management of laryngotracheal stenosis: a survey of 100 cases. Eur Arch Otorhinolaryngol 262: 602–608

37. Monnier P, Lang F, Savary M (2003) Partial cricotracheal resection for pediatric subglottic stenosis: a single institution's experience in 60 cases. Eur Arch Otorhinolaryngol 260:295–297

38. Monnier P, Savary M, Chappuis G (1993) Partial cricoid resection with primary tracheal anastomosis for subglottic stenosis in infants and children. Laryngoscope 103:1273–1283

39. Montgomery W (1965) T-tube tracheal stent. Arch Otolaryngol 82:320–321

40. Montgomery WW (1974) Suprahyoid release for tracheal anastomosis. Arch Otolaryngol 99:255–260

41. Morimitsu T, Matsumoto I, Okada S, Takahashi M, Kosugi T (1981) Congenital cricoid stenosis. Laryngoscope 91:1356–1364

42. Myer CM, O'Connor DM, Cotton RT (1994) Proposed grading system for subglottic stenosis based on endotracheal tube sizes. Ann Otol Rhinol Laryngol 103:319–323

43. Ndiaye I, Van de Abbeele T, François M, Viala P, Tanon-Anoh MJ, Narcy P (1999) Traitement chirurgical des sténoses laryngées de l'enfant. Ann Otolaryngol Chir Cervicofac 116: 143–148

44. Ochi JW, Evans JNG, Bailey CM (1992) Pediatric airway reconstruction at Great Ormond Street: a 10-year review. Ann Otol Rhino Laryngol 101:465–468

45. Ogura JH, Roper CL (1972) Surgical correction of traumatic stenosis of the larynx and pharynx. Laryngoscope 72:468–470

46. Pearson FG, Gullane P (1996) Subglottic resection with primary tracheal anastomosis including synchronous laryngotracheal reconstruction. Semin Thorac Cardiovasc Surg 4: 381–391

47. Pearson FG, Andrews MJ (1971) Detection and management of tracheal stenosis following cuffed tube tracheostomy. Ann Thorac Surg 12:359–374

48. Rahbar R, Shapsay SM, Healy GB (2001) Mitomycin: effects on laryngeal and tracheal stenosis, benefits and complications. Ann Otol Rhinol Laryngol 110:1–6

49. Ranne RD, Lindley S, Holder TM, Ashcraft KW, Sharp RJ, Amoury RA (1991) Relief of subglottic stenosis by anterior cricoid resection: an operation for the difficult case. J Pediatr Surg 26:255–259

50. Rutter MJ, Hartley BEJ, Cotton RT (2001) Cricotracheal resection in children. Arch Otolaryngol Head Neck Surg 127:289–292

51. Shapshay SM, Beamis JF, Hybels RL (1987) Endoscopic treatment of subglottic and tracheal stenosis by radial laser incision and dilation. Ann Otol Rhinol Laryngol 96: 661–664

52. Simpson GT, Strong MS, Healy GB, Shapshay SM, Vaughan CW (1982) Predictive factors of success or failure in the endoscopic management of laryngeal and tracheal stenosis. Ann Otol Rhinol Laryngol 91:384–388

53. Triglia JM, Nicollas R, Roman S (2001) Primary cricotracheal resection in children: indications, technique and outcome. Int J Pediatr Otorhinolaryngol 58:17–25

54. Vollrath M, Freihorst J, von der Hardt H (1999) Die Chirurgie der erworbenen laryngotrachealen Stenosen im Kindesalter. Erfahrungen und Ergebnisse von 1988–1998. Teil II: Die cricotracheale Resektion. HNO 47:611–622

55. White DR, Cotton RT, Bean JA, Rutter MJ (2005) Pediatric cricotracheal resection. Surgical outcomes and risk factor analysis. Arch Otolaryngol Head Neck Surg 131:896–899

56. Yellon RF, Szeremeta W, Grandis JR, Diguisseppe F, Dickman PS (1997) Role of subglottic injury, gastric juice and peptide growth factors in a porcine model. Int Anesthesiol Clin 35:115–125

57. Zalzal GH (1988) Use of stents in laryngotracheal reconstruction in children: indications, technical considerations, and complications. Laryngoscope 98:849–854

58. Zitch RP III, Mullins JB, Tampler J, Davis WE (1995) Suprahyoid and inferior constrictor release for laryngeal lowering. Arch Otolaryngol Head Neck Surg 121: 1310–1313

Tracheotomy

Georges Lawson

Core Messages

> The tracheal wall is incised between the second and third tracheal ring. The cricoid should be palpated before tracheal incision to determine the correct level at which to enter the trachea.

> Opening of the trachea with an inferiorly based flap is recommended.

> To avoid subcutaneous emphysema, pneumothorax, and infection, a tracheotomy wound is never closed tightly around the tube.

> Setting of threads is useful for stoma opening and tracheostomy tube introduction in children helpful for the stoma opening and tracheostomy tube reinsertion.

> Percutaneous dilatation tracheostomy (PCDT), when performed by experienced surgerons is safe and easy to perform with a low complication rate.

> PCDT is suitable only in adult patients without a midline neck mass and if cricoids cartilage can be palpated above the sternal notch.

> We strongly recommend this technique with good airway control by anesthetists or intensivists, under direct vision with fiberscopy during the procedure.

G. Lawson
Department of ORL Head & Neck Surgery, Cliniques Universitaires UCL de Mont-Godinne, Therasse avenue 1, 5530 Yvoir, Belgium
e-mail: george.lawson@uclouvain.be

11.1 Introduction

Tracheostomy is one of the oldest surgical procedures in the history of head and neck surgery. The evolution of tracheotomy stretches back over many centuries. It has been performed for more than 2000 years, but the first successful well documented tracheotomy is attributed to Antonio Musa Brasavolo in 1546. In 1932, Chevalier Jackson [1, 2] standardized the technique and taught the medical community about a well performed tracheotomy and routine surgical care; more specifically, he pointed out the side effects of "the high tracheotomy." The procedure is described as a potential lifesaving surgery performed sometimes in emergency situations but more often as a planned surgery in the operating room or intensive care unit.

Tracheotomy is a surgical opening into the trachea. It is performed for the purpose of ventilation or/and pulmonary toilet. Today, in the English-language literature the term tracheotomy and tracheostomy are used interchangeably. To clarify, *tracheotomy* is used here for the procedure of opening the trachea and *tracheostomy* as a permanent opening and exteriorizing the trachea to the cervical skin until the opening has become epithelialized. Performed under ideal circumstances (in an operating room, as an elective procedure, on a patient with a slender neck without airway obstruction), tracheotomy is a simple, safe, easy procedure.

Successful management of the airway requires a complete understanding of the structure and function of the upper aerodigestive tract. The goal is to apply the appropriate solution for each specific case to avoid complications and a life-threatening situation.

M. Remacle, H. E. Eckel (eds.), *Surgery of Larynx and Trachea*,
DOI: 10.1007/978-3-540-79136-2_11, © Springer-Verlag Berlin Heidelberg 2009

This chapter is design to provide information about the following.

- Indications for tracheotomy
- Decision making for open neck tracheotomy versus percutaneous tracheotomy
- Surgical technique
- Management of the tracheostomy

11.2 Indications for Tracheotomy

Tracheotomy means "making a stoma into the trachea." This temporary or permanent opening of the trachea may be necessary when circumstances exist that compromise adequate respiration. There are several situations in which tracheotomy is needed.

- Upper airway obstruction
  - Inflammatory disease
  - Benign laryngeal pathology
  - Malignant laryngeal tumors
  - Benign and malignant tracheal tumors
  - Laryngeal trauma or stenosis
  - Tracheal stenosis
- Need for assisted ventilation over a prolonged period of time
- Deficit of lower airway protection against aspiration of oral or gastric secretions
- Clearance of lower respiratory tract secretions

There is no fixed list of circumstances and morphological or pathological situations for tracheotomy. However, there are a variety of alternatives to tracheotomy.

- Noninvasive positive-pressure ventilation with a face mask or a laryngeal mask
- Endotracheal intubation
- Endoscopic procedure to remove some foreign bodies

An appropriate decision should be made for each patient, taking in account the following facts.

- The laryngeal mask airway is not suitable for all patients, particularly for patients at risk for aspiration, and it requires close intensive care monitoring.
- Endotracheal intubation is not always possible, depending on the patient's anatomy or pathological situation. In case of difficult airway management, tracheotomy should be considered according to the "Practice Guidelines for Management of the Difficult Airway" [3].
- Prolonged intubation for more than a week can induce laryngeal and tracheal damage [4].

11.3 Decision Making for Open Neck Tracheotomy Versus Percutaneous Tracheotomy

Conventional surgical tracheotomy reported as open neck tracheotomy is a safe, less easy procedure when performed under ideal circumstances. However, many complications following the operation have been reported [5]. Since the report by Ciaglia et al. [6] in 1985 on percutaneous dilatation tracheostomy (PCDT), several studies demonstrated that this technique is safe and easy with a low complication rate; furthermore, it is superior to the conventional surgical tracheostomy as immediate complications as well as complications with the tracheostomy tube in situ are fewer and of less severity [7].

It must be stressed that PCDT is suitable only in adult patients without a midline neck mass and if cricoid cartilage can be palpated above the sternal notch. All patients below the age of 18 years or with a neck deformity or/and unidentifiable anatomy of the neck represent a group for whom PCDT is contraindicated.

During PCDT the surgeon is sharing the airway with the anesthetist from the start of the procedure. The endotracheal tube is deflated and withdrawn above the vocal cord. In emergency cases or in patients with difficult airway management, this maneuver can result in a nonfunctional airway. In such a situation, conventional tracheostomy is more advisable.

11.4 Tracheotomy Techniques

11.4.1 Conventional or Open Neck Tracheotomy

Convention, open neck tracheotomy can be performed in various situations: in an emergency or as an elective

Fig. 11.1. The patient is placed on supine position, with the head extended

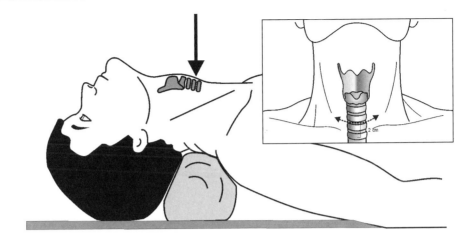

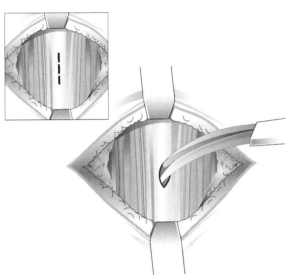

Fig. 11.2. The strap muscles are identified, and then the dissection is changed to the vertical plane

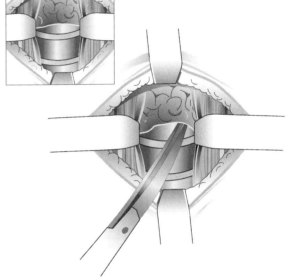

Fig. 11.3. Identification of the trachea anterior wall

operation, under general or local anesthesia, in the operating room or by the bedside.

Elective tracheotomy is best carried out in the operating room under general anesthesia, where efficient assistance is available with adequate equipment (light, suction, electrocautery, different size and shape tracheostomy tubes). The patient is placed on supine position, with the head extended using a shoulder roll (Fig. 11.1). A horizontal incision is made midway between the sternal notch and the cricoid cartilage. A sharp dissection is carried down through subcutaneous tissue and platysma. The strap muscles are

identified, and then the dissection is changed to the vertical plane (Fig. 11.2). The strap muscles are separated in the midline with a retractor until the thyroid isthmus is encountered and the anterior wall of the trachea is identified (Fig. 11.3). Inferior and median thyroid blood vessels are ligated; the thyroid isthmus is transected, and each side is suture-ligated to prevent bleeding (Fig. 11.4). The anterior wall of the trachea is incised between the second and third tracheal ring. The cricoid should be palpated before tracheal incision to determine the correct level at which to enter the trachea. To secure the opening of the stoma, an

Fig. 11.4. Section of the thyroid isthmus

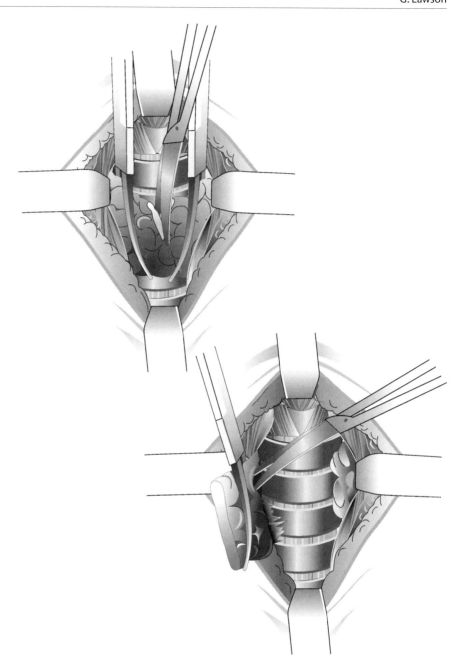

inferiorly based flap consisting of the anterior portion of a single tracheal ring is sutured to the inferior skin margin (Fig. 11.5).

During surgery, a special curved endotracheal tube (Montandon endotracheal tube) is introducing in the stoma and replaced by a tracheotomy tube at the end of the surgery. The placement begins with the tracheotomy tube at right angles to the trachea (Fig. 11.6); then as the tube is inserted, it is rotated so its axis is parallel to that of the trachea. The tracheotomy tube is sutured to the skin as an added precaution to prevent accidental dislodgement of the tube. To avoid subcutaneous emphysema, pneumothorax, and infection, a tracheotomy wound is never closed tightly around the tube.

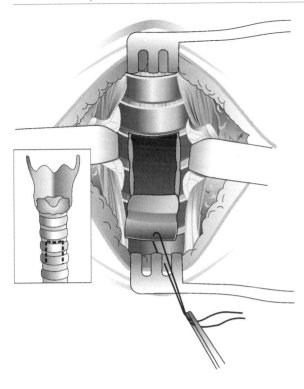

Fig. 11.5. Opening of the tracheal with an inferiorly based flap

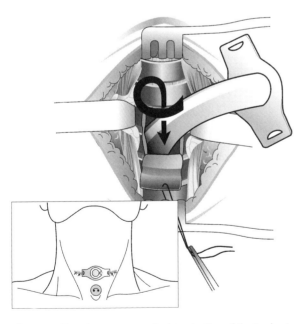

Fig. 11.6. Rotation movement for introduction of the tracheotomy tube

11.4.2 Percutaneous Dilatation Tracheotomy

Percutaneous dilatation tracheotomy (PDT) is a safe, simple, accepted alternative to conventional tracheotomy. Some studies [8–10] have demonstrated advantages of less cost, infection, bleeding, and operating time for PDT when compared to traditional open neck tracheotomy.

The procedure can be performed under local or general anesthesia. Nevertheless, there is no published proof in the literature to guarantee the safety of the technique in children, emergency situations, and patient with difficult airway management.

We strongly recommend this technique with good airway control by anesthetists or intensivists, ideally under direct vision with fiberscopy during the procedure. The surgery should be carried out by a skilled surgeon (or under his or her supervision), with the ability to perform a standard tracheotomy.

Anatomical suitability for PDT must be determined preoperatively with the patient's neck extended. A contraindication to the procedure is the inability to palpate the laryngeal landmark. The cricoid cartilage should be felt above the sternal notch. Similarly, the patient with a midline neck mass, a large thyroid gland, should be a candidate for conventional tracheotomy.

Patient received appropriate sedation, then positioned in supine position with the neck extended by using a shoulder roll. The patient's neck and upper chest are prepped and draped as for open neck tracheotomy.

Fiberoptic tracheobronchoscopy is carried out through the endotracheal tube. If needed, 2 ml of 4% lidocaine is injected into the trachea through the bronchoscope, and pulmonary toilet is performed. The distal extremity of the fiberscope is placed at the tip of the endotracheal tube, and the cuff is deflated.

Under fiberoptic vision, the endotracheal tube is slowly withdrawn from the trachea just below the level of the glottic opening and held securely to prevent accidental extubation. Laryngeal and tracheal landmarks are palpated. The light is visualized through the skin, and the tracheal rings are palpated to confirm the proper position of the tip of the tube.

A Teflon catheter introducer needle with a syringe attached is inserted between the first and second

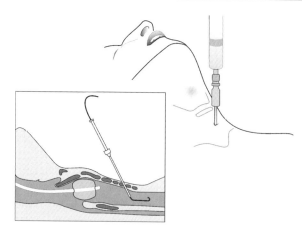

Fig. 11.7. Insertion of the needle

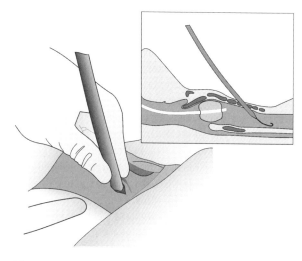

Fig. 11.8. Introduction of the Ciaglia dilatators

tracheal rings. Aspiration of air bubbles confirms entry into the trachea, and the location of the needle is verified endoscopically until a midline position is achieved inside of the trachea without puncturing the posterior tracheal wall (Fig. 11.7). The needle is removed and a J-tipped guidewire is threaded through the catheter into the trachea. The catheter is removed and replaced by the introducer dilator. A horizontal skin incision of 1.0–1.5 cm is then performed at the level of the puncture; a guiding catheter is placed over the guidewire after removal of the introducer dilator.

A hydrophilically coated Ciaglia Blue Rhino dilator is now introduced over the guiding catheter into the trachea until the 38F marking is identified endoscopically (Fig. 11.8). A tracheotomy tube with the

inner cannula replaced by a corresponding loading dilator from the Ciaglia' set is introduced over the guiding catheter into the trachea. The correct intratracheal position of the tracheotomy tube is confirmed endoscopically; the guidewire and guiding catheter are removed; and the inner cannula is put back. The respirator is disconnected from the endotracheal tube and is connected to the tracheostomy tube. The latter is fixed and adjusted, and the cuff is inflated. Final endoscopic control is performed through the tracheostomy tube; and if needed, excess secretions and/or blood are aspirated to prevent airway obstruction.

Postoperative chest radiography should be performed to ensure the absence of pneumothorax and pneumomediastinum.

The tracheotomy tube is first changed 7 days postoperatively.

11.4.3 Tracheotomy in the Pediatric Age Group

To prevent complications, preoperative planning is the first step to successful tracheotomy in a child. All patients should be examined and the airway secured before surgery. The surgical procedure is carried out in a manner similar to that in adults—in the operating room when possible.

More than in adults, care must be taken to avoid excessive dissection lateral to the trachea to prevent the possibility of recurrent nerve injury and dissection of air into the tissues. The thyroid isthmus is divided only if it cannot be retracted superiorly. The tracheal opening is a simple vertical incision made in the second and third tracheal rings. Nylon traction sutures are placed on either side of the incision line before the incision is performed and then after a second pair of traction sutures is placed along the cut edge of the trachea (Fig. 11.9). Those sutures will be helpful for the stoma opening and tracheostomy tube reinsertion. Excision of any anterior trachea wall during tracheotomy should be avoided in this age group.

Pediatric tracheostomy tubes generally have no cuff. The size of the tracheostomy tube is determined according to the age of the child with respect to the carina.

Fig. 11.9. Threads for traction are put in place for an easy opening

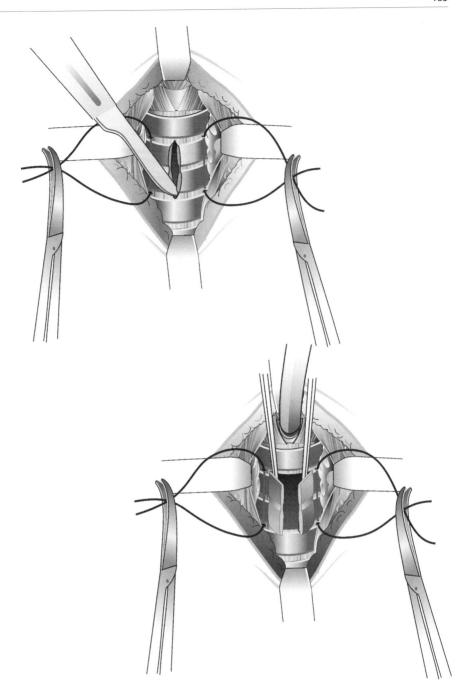

11.4.4 Bedside Open Tracheotomy

Intensive care unit patients are at higher risk for complications than other groups of patients because there frequently have multisystem diseases. When tracheotomy is required for these patients, they are taken to the operating room for conventional tracheotomy. Operating room time is expensive, in high demand, and often in short supply. On the other hand, moving critically ill patients is associated with a number of risks (e.g., accidental extubation, changes in the vital signs).

Open tracheotomy can also be performed at the bedside in the intensive care unit setting [11]. In such a situation, surgeons must ensure that proper lighting, some assistance, and proper equipment are available. Patients with unfavorable anatomy (morbid obesity, short and fat neck, cervical mass lesions, enlarged thyroid gland) should proceed to the operating room for a standard tracheotomy under ideal circumstances.

The surgical technique is the same as describe above for conventional open neck tracheotomy. The advantages of performing a tracheotomy at the bedside is that operating room coast are defrayed, the procedure is generally less expensive than a PDT, and the procedure can be performed as soon as the surgeons are available. As for main disadvantages, the procedure is more longer compare to PDT, it require transporting electrocautery, instrument trays and extra lighting from operating room to intensive care unit. Often there are no available trained operating room nurses and assistants.

11.4.5 Emergency Tracheotomy

11.4.5.1 Open Tracheotomy

It is widely accepted by head and neck surgeons that emergent tracheotomy is a procedure to be avoided. Nevertheless, in an acute airway emergency that cannot be handled by other option, tracheotomy should be considered.

Patients are positioned in supine position with the neck extended using a shoulder roll. The patient's neck and upper chest are prepared and draped as for open neck tracheotomy. A median vertical incision of 3–4 cm is performed starting at the level of the cricoid and extended to the sternal notch. The incision is continued through the skin, platysma, and subcutaneous tissues. The strap muscles are divided with retractors, and the thyroid isthmus is pushed inferiorly (or superiorly) with the index finger. The trachea is palpated and incised at about the second or third tracheal ring. The endotracheal tube or tracheostomy tube is introduced inside the trachea; sometimes a tracheal dilator is helpful during the introduction and so must be prepared as a part of the equipment for emergent tracheotomy.

The tracheostomy is securely fixed. As soon as the patient's situation allows, the tracheotomy is carefully assessed to control hemostasis, determine the exact location of the tracheal incision, and if needed perform appropriate revisions.

11.4.5.2 Cricothyroidotomy

Cricothyroidotomy is a rapid technique to create an opening in the cricothyroid membrane followed by placement of a stenting tube. The procedure is a good alternative to emergent tracheotomy. Its main advantage is that the cricothyroid membrane is near the skin surface and much less dissection is necessary. The major disadvantage is possible damage to the subglottis area, often because the cricothyrotomy tube is too large and/or is left in place for a long time.

The surgical technique is simple: The cricothyroid space is palpated, and a short, transverse incision is performed directly over the cricothyroid membrane. The knife is inserted into the cricothyroid membrane and twisted vertically to open it (Fig. 11.10). An endotracheal tube is inserted and secured.

When the patient's condition has stabilized, if respiratory support through the surgical airway is needed for more than 2–4 days the cricothyroidotomy should be converted to a conventional tracheotomy.

11.5 Complications of Tracheotomy

As for any surgical procedure, complications of tracheotomy may occur even with the use of optimal surgical techniques. Those complications can be generally divided into two categories: early and late.

1. Early complications (those occurring intraoperatively and early in the postoperative period)
   (a) Hemorrhage
   (b) Tracheoesophageal perforation
   (c) Recurrent nerve injury
   (d) Cricoid cartilage injury
   (e) Tracheostomy tube obstruction
   (f) Tracheostomy tube dislodgement
   (g) Pneumothorax
   (h) Pneumomediastinum
   (i) Subcutaneous emphysema
   (j) Wound infection

2. Late complications (those occurring in the late post-operative period)

(a) Infection

(b) Hemorrhage

(c) Granuloma

(d) Aspiration

(e) Laryngotracheal stenosis

(f) Subglottic stenosis

(g) Tracheoesophageal fistula

(h) Tracheomalacia

The best way to prevent complications during tracheotomy and in tracheotomized patients is a good knowledge of the following.

- Potential complications of tracheotomy
- Variety of strategies available for airway management
- Various surgical techniques for tracheotomy and their application
- Proper cannula selection based on the patient's anatomy and pathology
- Appropriate postoperative care for each specific situation

As soon as the complication is recognized, it must be managed efficiently to achieve the expected positive outcome.

11.6 Pearls and Tips

11.6.1 Pearls

- Tracheotomy stands out as one of the most helpful therapies in the management of compromised airway. In decision making for tracheotomy, appropriate solutions must be taken for each specific case, in order to avoid complications and life-threatening situations.
- The key features in preventing complications are good knowledge of:
  - The potential complications of tracheotomy.
  - The variety of strategies available for airway management.
  - The different surgical techniques for tracheotomy and their applications.

- The proper cannula selection according to the patient's anatomy and pathology.
- Appropriated routine and specific postoperative care.

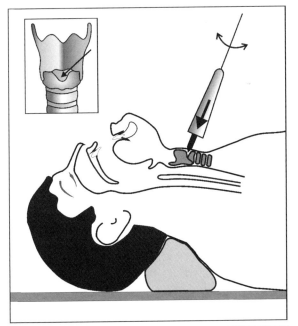

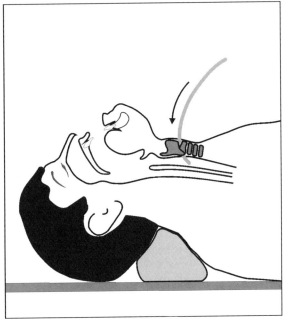

Fig. 11.10. Cricothyroidotomy

11.6.2 Practical Tips

- *Conventional or open neck tracheotomy*
  - Secure the airway first before performing the surgical procedure.
  - Be sure that efficient assistance and adequate equipment are available.
  - Dissecting in the midline to prevent
    - Bleeding from jugular vein, carotid artery, thyroid isthmus, or aberrant innominate arteries.
    - Injury to recurrent laryngeal nerves.
    - Pneumothorax or pneumomediastinum.
  - Secure the opening of the stoma, by suturing the anterior portion of a single tracheal ring to the inferior skin margin, and insert the tracheotomy tube into the trachea under direct vision to prevent false passage between the trachea and the sternum.
  - Prevent tracheotomy tube displacement by
    - Appropriate selection of the tube according to patient's anatomy.
    - Sewing the tracheotomy tube to the peristomal skin.
    - Setting the low-pressure cuff pressure under 25 mmHg.

- *Percutaneous dilatation tracheotomy (PDT)*
  - The principle contraindication to the PDT procedure is the inability to palpate the laryngeal landmarks.
  - Flexible bronchoscopy for endoscopic guidance is mandatory to
    - Visualize the trachea.
    - Confirm the proper position of the tip of the endotracheal tube.
    - Transilluminate for palpation of anatomic landmarks and visualize needle placement through the anterior tracheal wall.
    - Confirm the safe tracheal dilation and the proper tube placement.
  - Have a standard tracheotomy tray available.
  - Tracheotomy tube should be securely fixed to avoid accidental decannulation.
  - Never perform unnecessary change of the tracheotomy tube during the first post operative 3 days. If the tube replacement is inevitable, be prepared with:

- Endotracheal tube ready for patient re- intubation if need.
- A good preoxygenation of the patient.
- Tracheotomy dilatation forceps.
- Fiberscope ready for tracheal assessment.
  - When long-term tracheotomy is planed, it is preferable to perform conventional tracheotomy.

- *Emergency tracheotomy*
  - Depending on the severity and primary cause of the airway impairment.
    - Other airway management options should be considered.
  - All information related to the patient must be shared with the operating team and anaesthesiologist prior to the procedure.
  - Avoid
    - Percutaneous dilatation tracheotomy.
    - A high tracheotomy through or near the cricoid cartilage.
  - Cricothyroidotomy should be converted to conventional tracheotomy.

- *Tracheotomy in pediatric age group*
  - The tracheal opening must be a simple vertical incision.
  - Placed nylon traction sutures on either side of the incision line before tracheal opening.
  - Avoid any anterior trachea wall excision.
  - Tracheostomy tube size is determined according to the child's age.

References

1. Jackson C (1923) High tracheotomy and other errors: the chief causes of chronic laryngeal stenosis. Surg Gynecol Obstet 32:392
2. Jackson C, Jackson CL (1937) The larynx and its diseases. W.B. Saunders, Philadelphia, PA
3. Practice guidelines for management of the difficult airway (1993) A report by the American society of anaesthesiologists task force on management of the difficult airways. Anaesthesiology 78:597–602
4. Benjamin B (1993) Prolonged intubation injuries of the larynx: endoscopic diagnosis, classification, and treatment. Ann Otol Rhinol Laryngol 102(Suppl. 160):1–15
5. Stauffer JL, Olson DE, Petty TL (1981) Complications and consequences of endo-tracheal intubation and tracheostomy. Am J Med 70:65–75

6. Ciaglia P, Firsching R, Syniec C (1985) Elective percutaneous dilatation tracheostomy. A new simple bedside procedure: preliminary report. Chest 87:715–719

7. Holdgaard HO, Pedersen J, Jensen RH, Outzen KE, Midtgaard T, Johansen LV, Moller J, Paaske PB (1998) Percutaneous dilatational tracheostomy versus conventional surgical tracheostomy. Acta Anaesthesiol Scand 42:545–550

8. Ciaglia P, Graniero KD (1992) Percutaneous dilatation tracheostomy. Results and long term follow-up. Chest 101:464–467

9. Griggs WM, Myburgh JA, Worthley, LI (1991) A prospective comparison of a percutaneous tracheostomy technique with standard surgical tracheostomy. Int Care Med 17: 261–261

10. Hazard P, Jones C, Benitone J (1991) Comparative clinical trial of standard operative tracheostomy with percutneous tracheostomy. Crit Care Med 19:1018–1024

11. Wang SJ, Sercaz JA, Blackwell KE, et al (1999) Open bedside tracheotomy in intensive care unit. Laryngoscope 109: 891–893

Scarred Larynx

12a

Christoph Arens and Marc Remacle

Core Messages

> The vocal fold scar is an injury of variable severity sustained by the vibratory segment of the vocal cord.

> In many cases glottic scars are accompanied by glottic insufficiencies caused by vocal fold defects.

> A delay of 6 months is recommended before surgical treatment.

> Speech therapy is useful and can be sufficient in case of a minor scar.

> The main goal of surgery is to obtain a better closing and from there a better vocal fold vibration.

> Medialization may help achieve sufficient glottic closure but not a normal voice.

Treatment of laryngeal scars is one of the most challenging topics in laryngology. Vocal fold scars can result from voice abuse and misuse, acute, or chronic laryngitis especially in combination with reflux disease, acid ingestion, blunt or sharp trauma to the larynx [11, 14], and iatrogenic trauma during intubation [2]. It also may result as a sequel to vocal cord surgery for dysplasia or carcinoma in situ [16] (Fig. 12a.1).

Supraglottic scars predominantly affect respiration and deglutition, whereas glottic scars result in dysphonia and dyspnea. Symptoms associated with laryngeal scars are predominantly hoarseness, breathiness, voice effort, and voice fatigue [2]. In severe cases, aphonia and aspiration may be present sometimes in combination with a tracheotomy.

Glottic scars can be divided in four types.

Type I: mucosal, submucosal level—mild to moderate glottic insufficiency, reduced vibration

Type II: glottic insufficiency in a round anterior commissure region—anterior moderate defect; scars involving the vocalis muscle—no vibration, mild glottic insufficiency

Type III: glottic insufficiency—scar formation adherent to the inner perichondrium and the cartilage defect up to the supraglottic region, twisted arytenoids

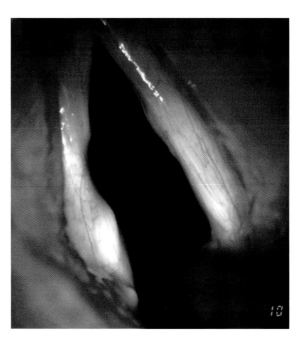

Fig. 12a.1. Scar of the left vocal cord after intubation

C. Arens (✉)
Universitätsklinikum Magdeburg A.ö.R.,
Universitätsklinik für Hals-, Nasen- und Ohrenheilkunde,
Klinikdirektor, Leipziger Str. 44, 39120 Magdeburg, Germany
e-mail: christoph.arens@med.ovgu.de

M. Remacle, H. E. Eckel (eds.), *Surgery of Larynx and Trachea,*
DOI: 10.1007/978-3-540-79136-2_12a, © Springer-Verlag Berlin Heidelberg 2010

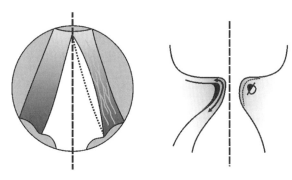

Fig. 12a.2. Type I. Scar of the vocal fold

Type IV: glottic insufficiency—anterior web formation, round anterior commissure, bilaterally reduced vibration

12a.1 Type I Scar of the Vocal Fold

The type 1 scar is an injury of variable severity sustained by the vibratory segment of the vocal cord [4, 6] (Fig. 12a.2). It affects Reinke's space and the vocal ligament. Vocal fold scars represent reparative disorganized tissue consisting mainly of fibrocytes producing collagen type I in the vibrating layer of the vocal fold, particularly the superficial layer of the lamina propria [22]. In contrast, the pliability of the vocal fold during phonation is guaranteed predominantly by fibers consisting of collagen type III as well as elastic fibers reaching into the basal layer of vocal fold mucosa. Depending on the severity of a scar, the vibration of the vocal fold can be completely impaired, leading to dysphonia. Scars can be localized in a single spot or can be present throughout the complete vocal fold. In many cases, glottic scars are accompanied by glottic insufficiencies caused by vocal fold defects.

Benninger et al. presented three rules: (1) The more mucosa excised, the more scar-forming activity of the lamina propria is stimulated. (2) Mucosal excision needs to be limited to precisely what is diseased or absolutely required. (3) Because fibroblast collagen is highest in the deeper layers of the lamina propria, the dissection must be kept superficial.

On stroboscopic examination, amplitude and mucosal waves show asymmetrical vibrations. The vocal cord defect may be visible. As with sulcus-vergeture, management is difficult [19].

A delay of 6 months is recommended before surgical treatment. Speech therapy is useful and can be sufficient in case of a minor scar [16, 20].

Scar surgery of the vocal folds should break up stiff scars to restore better elasticity and replace lost volume to gain complete glottic closure [3]. Laryngeal framework medialization, unilateral or bilateral, has been proposed [5, 9].

Microphonosurgery, similar to what is proposed for sulcus-vergeture can also be realized [18]. The epithelium, frequently atrophic must be freed from the deep part of the lamina propria. It is necessary to recreate a zone of detachment between the submucosal tissue and the epithelium. Hydrotomy or injection of saline solution, vasoconstrictors, or steroids can be helpful (Fig. 12a.3a, b)

In case of atrophy, injection of homologous collagen or fat is proposed to restore the shape and the volume of the vocal fold [15, 18]. Hyaluronic acid can also be injected to improve the pliability of the vocal fold [6, 10] (Fig. 12a.4a, b).

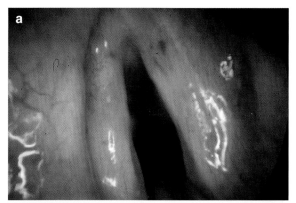

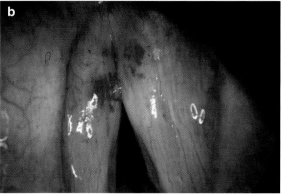

Fig. 12a.3. Bilateral superficial scar of the vocal cords. (**a**) Before. (**b**) After hyaluronic acid injection

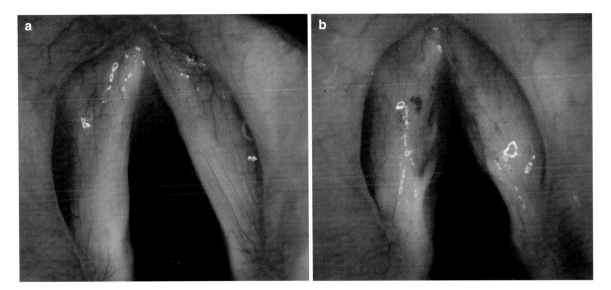

Fig. 12a.4. Bilateral scar of the vocal fold. (**a**) Before surgery. (**b**) After microsurgery: elevation of the epithelium, freeing of the subepithelial scar, and homologous collagen injection

These lesions are frequently bilateral and the two sides can be operated on at the same time. If the surgery has been difficult for one of the sides, it may be advisable to wait 6 months before approaching the other side.

Cordotomy is performed laterally. The scar formation is dissolved and the sliding flap prepared. Just by loosening the scars the mucosal flap drifts medially. In case of a volume deficit, we implant fat for an improved glottic closure leading to better vocal function (Fig. 12a.5).

The CO_2 laser technique thermal damage must be used with great caution to avoid thermal activation. This can be prevented by general avoidance of lasers in vocal fold surgery. Cold instruments are used to preserve as much mucosa as possible.

Other strategies that have recently shown advances include growth factor therapy [8] and cell therapy using stem cells or mature fibroblasts [12, 13]. The effects of these new treatments have not fully been confirmed clinically, but there seems to be great therapeutic potential in such regenerative medical strategies [7].

The management outcome, as in cases of sulcus-vergeture, may not be altogether satisfactory and the patient must be warned accordingly. The maximum benefit is not apparent until 4–5 months postoperatively [17]. The surgical treatment can be supported by antireflux agents.

Postoperative speech therapy is advisable to correct the excessive reactive supraglottic contraction. Bit by bit, as speech therapy progresses, the voice becomes stronger, more "comfortable," even if the timbre remains husky. Most of these patients feel improved because of the decreased voice fatigue, voice abuse, and dysthesia in the throat and the increased voice sound. Although complete restoration of the vocal cord may not be achieved, the surgery does improve glottic closure and the timbre [15, 17].

12a.2 Type II Scar (After Partial Cordectomy)

With type II cordectomy, the initial surgery leads to a mild to moderate loss of volume; it involves the vocalis muscle with the rigid scar formation not being able to be a sufficient counterpart to the normal vocal fold. This

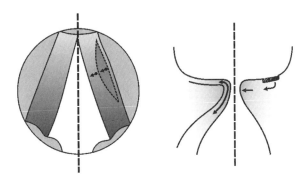

Fig. 12a.5. Lateral cordotomy and loosening of the scar

finding is often accompanied by a moderate anterior defect and a round anterior commissure (Fig. 12a.6). During videostroboscopy, reduced or absent amplitude of vibration with loss of the mucosal wave can be detected. Therefore, augmentation and medialization is needed to close the glottic gap. During microlaryngoscopy, a pouch is created and the scar formation dissected. During the second step, the vocal fold is augmented with septal cartilage or fatty/connective tissue. After implantation of the autologous tissue, the pouch is closed by several sutures (Fig. 12a.7). Medialization may help achieve sufficient glottic closure but not a normal voice.

Medialization thyroplasty, unilateral or bilateral, has been proposed [5, 9].

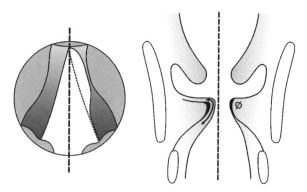

Fig. 12a.6. Type II glottic scar. Mild to moderate loss of volume involving the vocalis muscle with rigid scar formation

12a.3 Scar Type III (After Total or Enlarged Cordectomy)

With type III cordectomy, scar formation is adherent to the inner perichondrium and the cartilage (Fig. 12a.8). The huge defect also involves supraglottic structures. The arytenoid may be twisted. Glottic closure is impossible. These patients with huge defects can be aphonic and develop supraglottic phonation.

Therefore, a vocal pouch with its maximum at the glottic level has to be created. In these cases, it may be difficult to create a sufficient pouch without perforation at the subglottic level. Septal cartilage is placed in several layers in the pouch. Finally, the pouch is closed with 5–0 or 6–0 Vicryl sutures (Fig. 12a.9). Reconstruction of the anterior commissure and the volume in the posterior third of the glottis can be a problem. Sittel et al. [21] described a similar procedure transcervically that can be performed under local anesthesia. The cartilage is placed in a pocket that has been developed from the upper rim of the thyroid cartilage. The result is monitored endoscopically, and the patient can be asked to phonate. Finally, the cartilage is fixed in the pocked with sutures to the thyroid or with fibrin glue.

Benninger et al. [1] recommended medialization for glottic gaps of at least 1.5 mm. This procedure may be combined with lipoinjection in an attempt to reestablish the mucosal wave. In most cases of these huge defects, the created counterpart is stiff and immobile.

Laryngeal framework surgery is indicated only if it follows optimally managed voice therapy. The surgery

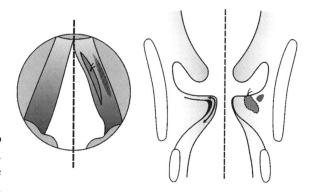

Fig. 12a.7. Type II glottic scar. A pouch is created, and the scar is dissected. In the second step, the vocal fold is augmented with septal cartilage or fatty/connective tissue

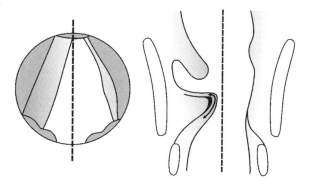

Fig. 12a.8. Type III glottic scar. Scar formation is adherent to the inner perichondrium and the cartilage

is advocated only when the posttherapy voice outcome does not meet the patient's requirements. Even when not entirely satisfied with their voice, patients often decline this complementary functional surgery.

After cordectomy, a minimum 6-month period is enforced before proceeding with framework surgery.

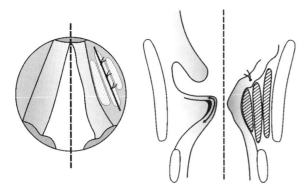

Fig. 12a.9. Type III glottic scar. A vocal pouch with maximum at the glottic level must be created. Septal cartilage is placed in several layers in the pouch

This surgery-free interval is respected to allow the scarring process to take place, to verify the absence of early recurrence, and to evaluate the voice rehabilitation achieved by voice therapy alone.

Laryngeal framework medialization is performed under general anesthesia. The patient is intubated with a no. 6 tube (8.2 mm outer diameter), the standard tube in microsurgery. The operation is performed under transnasal fiberscopic control. The landmarks used for establishing the thyroid cartilage window are standard.

The window is left intact to minimize the risk of tearing the fibrous tissue of the vocal cord bed during the dissection and positioning of the implant. The dissection, between the inner wall of the thyroid cartilage and the fibrous tissue that edges the window, requires meticulous care and must continue in close contact with the cartilage when the inner perichondrium is not identified. This undermining must cover a large enough area to ensure that the implant is put in place without fibrous tissue resistance and consequent tearing. This dissection is lengthier and more laborious than the dissection required for paralysis of the vocal cord.

The findings suggest that self-assessment scales are more significant for the indication of framework surgery than perceptual evaluation scales or acoustic and aerodynamic measures. The improvements produced by the latter seem limited, and the perceptual evaluation scales fail to cover a long enough listening period. In contrast, self-assessment allows the patients to examine their entire dynamic speech range. The patients in our experience notice improved resistance to vocal fatigue and report that phonation requires less effort.

Augmentation by collagen injection can be complementary.

12a.4 Scars Type IV (After Bilateral Resection Including the Anterior Commissure)

Lesions
   Glottic insufficiency
   Anterior web formation
   Round anterior commissure
   Bilaterally reduced vibration

Therapy
   Resection of anterior web formation or lesions
   Anterior mucosal flaps, stents

12a.4.1 Alternating Mucosal Flaps, Type IVa

A mucosal flap is at the surface of one vocal fold and is pedicled at the edge of the contralateral vocal fold (Fig. 12a.10a).

If necessary a second flap can be prepared (Fig. 12a.10b). Upside-down transposition of the flaps is achieved, and fixation is completed by suturing with 6.0 Vicryl (Fig. 12a.10c).

12a.4.2 Anterior Glottic Web Formation Type IVb

Endolaryngeal stent (according to Lichtenberger)

12a.5 Tips and Pearls

- Hyaluronic acid can be injected to improve the pliability of the vocal fold.
- Laryngeal framework medialization is performed under general anesthesia because the dissection, between the inner wall of the thyroid cartilage and the fibrous tissue that edges the window, requires meticulous care.
- The findings suggest that self-assessment scales are more significant for the indication of framework surgery than perceptual evaluation scales or acoustic and aerodynamic measures.

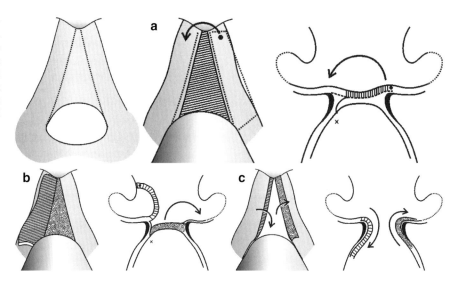

Fig. 12a.10. Anterior synechia, alternating mucosal flaps. (**a**) Mucosal flap at the surface of one vocal fold, pedicled at the edge of the contralateral vocal fold. (**b**) Preparation of a second flap. (**c**) Upside-down transposition of the flaps and fixation by suturing

References

1. Benninger MS, Alessi D, Archer S, Bastian R, Ford C, Koufman J, et al (1996) Vocal fold scarring: current concepts and management. Otolaryngol Head Neck Surg 115(5): 474–482
2. Berry DA, Reininger H, Alipour F, Bless DM, Ford CN (2005) Influence of vocal fold scarring on phonation: predictions from a finite element model. Ann Otol Rhinol Laryngol 114(11):847–852
3. Dailey SH, Ford CN (2006) Surgical management of sulcus vocalis and vocal fold scarring. Otolaryngol Clin North Am 39(1):23–42
4. Eller R, Heman-Ackah Y, Hawkshaw M, Sataloff RT (2007) Vocal fold scar/sulcus vocalis. Ear Nose Throat J 86(6):320
5. Friedrich G (1998) External vocal fold medialization:surgical experiences and modifications. Laryngorhinootologie 77(1): 7–17
6. Hansen JK, Thibeault SL (2006) Current understanding and review of the literature:vocal fold scarring. J Voice 20(1):110–120
7. Hirano S (2005) Current treatment of vocal fold scarring. Curr Opin Otolaryngol Head Neck Surg 13(3):143–147.
8. Hirano S, Bless DM, Nagai H, Rousseau B, Welham NV, Montequin DW, et al (2004) Growth factor therapy for vocal fold scarring in a canine model. Ann Otol Rhinol Laryngol 113(10):777–785
9. Isshiki N, Shoji K, Kojima H, Hirano S (1996) Vocal fold atrophy and its surgical treatment. Ann Otol Rhinol Laryngol 105(3):182–188
10. Jia X, Yeo Y, Clifton RJ, Jiao T, Kohane DS, Kobler JB et al (2006) Hyaluronic acid-based microgels and microgel networks for vocal fold regeneration. Biomacromolecules 7(12): 3336–3344
11. Kitahara S, Masuda Y, Kitagawa Y (2005) Vocal fold injury following endotracheal intubation. J Laryngol Otol 119(10): 825–827
12. Krishna P, Rosen CA, Branski RC, Wells A, Hebda PA (2006) Primed fibroblasts and exogenous decorin: potential treatments for subacute vocal fold scar. Otolaryngol Head Neck Surg 135(6):937–945
13. Lee BJ, Wang SG, Lee JC, Jung JS, Bae YC, Jeong HJ, et al (2006) The prevention of vocal fold scarring using autologous adipose tissue-derived stromal cells. Cell Tissue Organ 184(3–4):198–204
14. Lim X, Tateya I, Tateya T, Munoz-Del-Rio A, Bless DM (2006) Immediate inflammatory response and scar formation in wounded vocal folds. Ann Otol Rhinol Laryngol 115(12):921–929
15. Neuenschwander MC, Sataloff RT, Abaza MM, Hawkshaw MJ, Reiter D, Spiegel JR (2001) Management of vocal fold scar with autologous fat implantation:perceptual results. J Voice 15(2):295–304
16. Ramacle M, Lawson G, Hedayat A, Trussart T, Jamart J (2001) Medialization framework surgery for voice improvement after endoscopic cordectomy. Eur Arch Otorhinolaryngol 258(6):267–271
17. Remacle M, Lawson G (2007) Results with collagen injection into the vocal folds for medialization. Curr Opin Otolaryngol Head Neck Surg 15(3):148–152
18. Remacle M, Lawson G, Keghian J, Jamart J (1999) Use of injectable autologous collagen for correcting glottic gaps:initial results. J Voice 13(2):280–288
19. Rosen CA (2000) Vocal fold scar:evaluation and treatment. Otolaryngol Clin North Am 33(5):1081–1086
20. Rousseau B, Hirano S, Chan RW, Welham NV, Thibeault SL, Ford CN, et al (2004) Characterization of chronic vocal fold scarring in a rabbit model. J Voice 18(1):116–124
21. Sittel C, Friedrich G, Zorowka P, Eckel HE (2002) Surgical voice rehabilitation after laser surgery for glottic carcinoma. Ann Otol Rhinol Laryngol 111(6):493–499
22. Thibeault SL, Gray SD, Bless DM, Chan RW, Ford CN (2002) Histologic and rheologic characterization of vocal fold scarring. J Voice 16(1):96–104

Synechia of the Anterior Commissure

12b

György Lichtenberger[†]

Core Messages

> Thin, small webs mostly cause nothing or only mild dysphonia. If the web is big and thick, dysphonia and dyspnea may be present.

> The final diagnosis can be established by direct microlaryngoscopy combined with 0°–25°–45°–70° telescopes to determine the exact thickness of the membrane below the anterior commissure.

> Only very thin anterior commissure webs can be cured by simple endoscopic dissection of the membrane using laser or a microscalpel with a disposable sharp blade. In other cases, it is necessary, after dissection and division of the web, to fix a silicone sheet or keel between the deepithelialized parts of the dissected membrane.

> After dissecting the web, the wound surface is painted with mitomycin C to decrease fibroblast activity and the risk of recurrence.

> The keel is established using the endoextralaryngeal needle carrier of Lichtenberger. To achieve a good result, it is important that the keel appropriately covers the deepithelialized parts.

> After surgery the patient must be given broad-band antibiotics at least for 5 days. Administration of steroids during the first 3 days has proved advantageous. It is recommended that the position of the keel be checked after surgery.

> The keel is removed 3 weeks later by microlaryngoscopy after cutting the ends of the thread on the neck. The operation may be performed on small children.

12b.1 Diagnosis

Indirect laryngoscopy or magnifying indirect laryngoscopy are usually enough to establish the diagnosis in adults. Direct microlaryngoscopy may be necessary in children and newborns because of a lack of collaboration by other means. The final diagnosis can be established by direct microlaryngoscopy combined with 0°–25°–45°–70° telescopes to determine the exact thickness of the membrane below the anterior commissure.

12b.2 Preoperative Workup

The preoperative workup may include blood oxygen saturation monitoring and pulmonary function tests. In acquired cases, there may be an investigation for gastroesophageal reflux disease.

12b.3 Therapy

12b.3.1 Conservative Approach

In acute acquired cases, right after the damage is revealed, there is a chance to cover the rough deepithelialized surface with fibrin glue in an attempt to prevent adhesions. Mitomycin C may also be administered.

G. Lichtenberger
ORL-HNS, Szent Rokus Hospital & Institutions,
Gyulai P.u. 2, 1085 Budapest, Hungary

M. Remacle, H. E. Eckel (eds.), *Surgery of Larynx and Trachea*,
DOI: 10.1007/978-3-540-79136-2_12b, © Springer-Verlag Berlin Heidelberg 2010

12b.3.2 Surgical Approach

Only very thin anterior commissure webs can be cured by simple endoscopic dissection of the membrane using laser or a microscalpel with a disposable sharp blade. In other cases, it is necessary, after dissection and division of the web, to fix a silicone sheet, or keel, between the deepithelialized parts of the dissected membrane.

Surgical techniques with outer exposure of the larynx, mostly after preliminary tracheostomy, are seldom used nowadays. The most frequently used procedure with outer exposure was described by Montgomery and Gamble [3]. The procedure is done mostly after preliminary tracheostomy. The larynx is opened by means of thyreotomy. The cartilage incision is made exactly in the midline, and the web is dissected. Afterward, an umbrella-like T-shaped silicone keel is placed in the anterior commissure between the vocal cords (Fig. 12b.1). When the keel is in the appropriate place, the soft tissues and skin are closed above the larynx. Six weeks later the keel is removed after the wound surfaces are healed.

Endoscopic-microlaryngoscopic techniques with fixation of a keel or sheet in the anterior commissure by Nessel for 2–3 weeks without tracheostomy can be done using extraendolaryngeal sutures. The anterior commissure web is dissected by performing direct microlaryngoscopy. Two thick serum needles are pushed through the larynx from outside to inside. One needle is pushed through the cricothyroid and the other through the thyreohyoid membrane. Afterward, one thread is pushed through the first needle and then the other thread through the second needle. The ends of the threads are grasped with microforceps, which is not always easy owing to bleeding from the stitching canal making it difficult to find the ends of the threads. After grasping the ends of the

threads, they are pulled out and are tightened and knotted outside the laryngoscope. A silicone sheet is then fixed on the thread. The ends of the thread are pulled back, and the sheet is placed between the two parts of the dissected web in the anterior commissure. Having positioned the sheet in the appropriate place, the ends of the threads are tightened and knotted on a piece of silicone tube placed on the skin of the neck [4] (Fig. 12b.2).

Endoscopic-microlaryngoscopic technique with fixation of a keel or sheet in the anterior commissure for 2–3 weeks without tracheostomy using endoextralaryngeal sutures by Lichtenberger [1, 2] is also available. here, the anterior commissure web is dissected by performing direct microlaryngoscopy. The web may be dissected using laser or a microscalpel holder with a safety lock by Lichtenberger with disposable sharp blades (Fig. 12b.3).

Both dissection options have advantages and disadvantages. With laser there is less bleeding, but tissue loss and delayed wound healing are present. When performing the same intervention with a disposable sharp blade, there is more bleeding but there is no tissue loss and more rapid healing occurs. It seems that the laser technique is indicated if there is a thick web causing not only

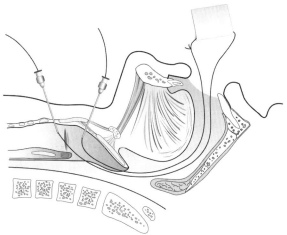

Fig. 12b.2. Endoscopic-microlaryngoscopic technique with fixation of a keel or sheet in the anterior commissure by Nessel

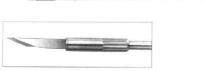

Fig. 12b.3. Microscalpel holder with safety lock and disposable blades by Lichtenberger

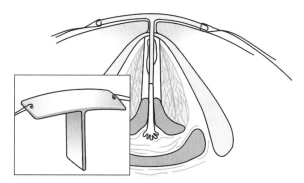

Fig. 12b.1. Surgical technique with outer exposure of the larynx according to Montgomery and Gamble. A T-shaped silicone keel is placed in the anterior commissure betwwen the vocal cords

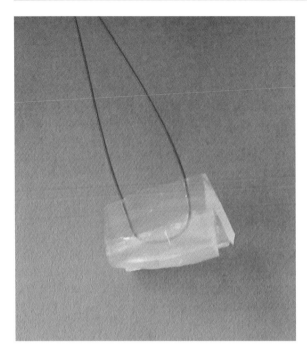

Fig. 12b.4. Silicone keel for endoscopic management of an anterior commissure web

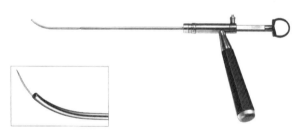

Fig. 12b.5. Needle carrier instrument by Lichtenberger

dysphonia but also dyspnea. In such cases, the most important factor is the patient's breathing, with the voice being of only secondary importance. In contrast, when there is a thin web that cannot be managed without interposition (keel or sheet) and the patient suffers only dysphonia, use of a sharp blade may be better because it does not cause tissue loss, which is important if the aim is to improve the voice of the patient.

After dissecting the web, the wound surface is painted with mitomycin C (0.2–0.6 mg/ml), a step that is repeated two more times. The introduction of mitomycin C after dissection of the web may further improve the results.

A homemade silicon keel is used (Fig. 12b.4). This keel is chosen from the series of keels made from a medical grade silicone block. Before fixing the keel on the thread, the chosen keel is placed in the anterior commissure without fixation. if the size and shape of the keel are appropriate, the thread is then placed through the keel.

Placing the thread through the keel is important for two reasons: The first is the safety factor—to prevent the thread cutting through the silicone keel. The other reason is that when the thread is placed appropriately it covers the deepithelialized areas in a craniocaudal direction. Afterward, the operation is continued with the endoextralaryngeal needle carrier (Fig. 12b.5).

One end of the fixing thread is led through a specially designed curved needle. Then the needle is placed in the distal, curved end of the device, and the needle carrier is pushed through the laryngoscope. (The use of the Weerda or Steiner laryngoscope can be recommended for this purpose.)

The distal bent, blunt end of the needle carrier is placed below the anterior commissure, and the special needle is pushed through the larynx with one end of the thread (Fig. 12b.6a). It is important that the thread

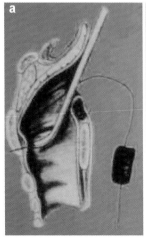
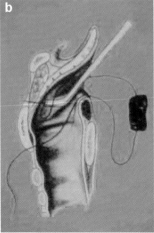
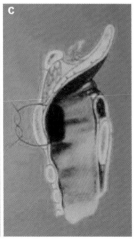

Fig. 12b.6. a–c
Endoextralaryngeal keel
fixation technique by
Lichtenberger

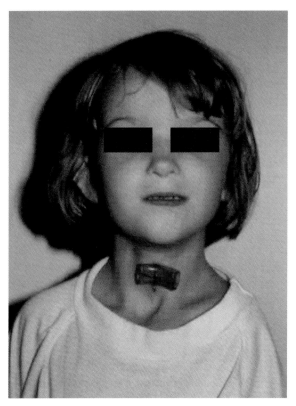

Fig. 12b.7. Small child after dissection of the web and fixing a keel with the endoextralaryngeal suture technique

goes through the thyroid cartilage, ensuring a stable position, not through the membranes (as in other techniques), to avoid an unstable position and dislocation of the keel with the consequence of re-scarring.

Then the silicone keel is fixed on the thread and the same procedure is repeated, but now the stitching occurs with the other end of the thread above the anterior commissure (Fig. 12b.6b). The ends of the thread are pulled after the keel is placed in the appropriate place; the thread ends are pulled and tightened on a bent silicone tube on the skin of the neck (Fig. 12b.6c). Three weeks later, the keel is removed by microlaryngoscopy after cutting the ends of the thread on the neck.

The operation may be performed on small children (Fig. 12b.7) and newborns. However, in infants < 1 year of age, it must be ensured that the anterior edge of the keel is not sharp. Otherwise, the keel may cut through the soft thyroid cartilage, as happened in one of our first cases.

To achieve a good result, it is important that the keel appropriately covers the deepithelialized parts of the larynx. This can be verified by endoscopy (Fig. 12b.8).

It is necessary to have a series of keels from which to choose the most suitable one. A silicone sheet can also be introduced in some adults. However, in these cases it must be taken into consideration that crustation may develop around the sheet, narrowing the lumen of the larynx temporary. The use of a thin sheet is not recommended in children because it cannot be fixed appropriately and it may move through the stitched canal, threatening the results of the surgery.

12b.4 Tips and Pearls

- The whole procedure should be done under totally sterile conditions.
- It means that not only the devices are sterile as with a simple microlaryngoscopy.
- The skin is disinfected, and the patient is covered with drapes before the operation.
- The keel of appropriate size is chosen from the series of homemade, medical grade silicone keels.
- An atraumatic, thin, specially curved needle is used.
- The keel should cover the deepithelialized areas in every direction.
- The silicone tube placed on the neck should have a bent shape to prevent decubitation of the skin at the two ends of the tube.
- The keel and the thread must be removed after 20–21 days in adults and after 14 days in children.

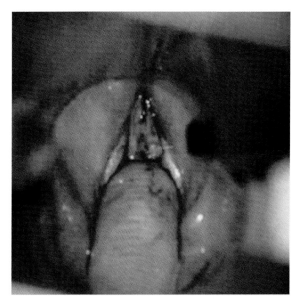

Fig. 12b.8. Endoscopic picture about the keel fixed in the anterior commissure

References

1. Lichtenberger G, Toohill RJ (1991) The endo-extralaryngeal needle carrier. Otolaryngol Head Neck Surg 105(5):755–756
2. Lichtenberger G, Toohill RJ (1994) New keel fixing technique for endoscopic repair of anterior commissure webs. Laryngoscope 104(6 Pt 1):771–774
3. Montgomery WW, Gamble JE (1970) Anterior glottic stenosis. Experimental and clinical management. Arch Otolaryngol 92(6):560–567
4. Nessel E (1968) A suggestion for a simplified management of the vocal fold synechia. HNO 16(9):284–287

Anastasios G. Hantzakos

Core Messages

> Accurate staging is of paramount importance for the decision-making process.

> Positron emission tomography has been used increasingly for staging and follow-up of patients with head and neck cancer

> Patient preference, physician expertise, and toxicity issues are important factors when determining clinical management for individuals.

> Surgical treatment remains superior to conservative treatment in reference to disease control, but the latter is superior in terms of organ preservation.

> External radiotherapy alone and/or brachytherapy may offer an excellent outcome in early-stage disease.

> Altered fractionation radiotherapy and concomitant chemoradiation have resulted in improved locoregional control of locally advanced disease.

> For locally advanced disease, concomitant chemoradiation appears to confer a reproducible survival benefit; the optimal time-dose regimen has not yet been defined for this approach.

> Altered fractionation radiotherapy and chemoradiation increase acute toxicity profile.

> Concomitant chemoradiotherapy should be the gold standard after resection in patients at high risk of failure or for patients not suitable for chemotherapy.

> Targeted chemoradiotherapy with monoclonal antibodies appears to be a promising approach, with a high therapeutic index

Although the human larynx and hypopharynx are considered distinct anatomical entities, this is not entirely the case. Their coexistence in the same wide anatomical area makes them share their anatomical borders to a great extent. Under this context, a hypopharyngeal malignancy can easily spread and invade the larynx and vice versa. Thus, laryngeal and hypopharyngeal cancer share common features and so are examined together in this chapter.

13a.1 Epidemiology of Laryngeal and Hypopharyngeal Cancer

Laryngeal cancer constitutes 1–2% of all malignancies diagnosed worldwide. The incidence of laryngeal cancer is estimated to be approximately 12,000 annually in the United States and approximately 2300 annually in the United Kingdom [52, 77]. Laryngeal cancer is seven times more common in men than in women [63]. Tables 13a.1 and 13a.2 show the estimates of the age-standardized incidence and mortality rates per 100,000 worldwide [62] and the age-adjusted incidence, mortality, and survival of patients with hypopharyngeal and laryngeal cancer in the United States [69].

A. G. Hantzakos
First Department of Otorhinolaryngology – Head & Neck Surgery of the University of Athens Medical School, Hippocrateion General Hospital, Athens, Greece
e-mail: ahantza@gmail.com

M. Remacle, H. E. Eckel (eds.), *Surgery of Larynx and Trachea,*
DOI: 10.1007/978-3-540-79136-2_13a, © Springer-Verlag Berlin Heidelberg 2010

Table 13a.1. Estimates of age-standardized incidence and mortality rates per 100,000 worldwide

Site	Incidence		Mortality	
	Male	Female	Male	Female
Hypopharynx	3.6	0.7	2.4	0.5
Larynx	5.7	0.7	3.1	0.4

Modified from Parkin et al. [62]

A recent epidemiological study from the National Cancer Institute's Surveillance Epidemiology and End Results (SEER) program in the United States [29] showed that there were drops in the incidence of hypopharyngeal and laryngeal cancer by 35% and 26%, respectively, from 1975 to 2001. From the same study, mortality trends for the period 1990–2001 are also encouraging: There were drops of 30% and 6% in hypopharyngeal and laryngeal cancer-related deaths, respectively. In the case of larynx, where mortality did not fall as much as the incidence, these trends suggest a decrease in the underlying initiation of the disease and either less successful treatment, changing risk factors, changing tumor biology, or a combination of the three. Another retrospective, longitudinal study of 158,426 cases of laryngeal squamous cell carcinoma diagnosed between the years 1985 and 2001, by review of the National Cancer Data Base (NCDB) in the United States, revealed that treatment patterns have changed with an increase in nonsurgical management with irradiation alone and with chemoradiation. Analysis of the NCDB identified a decrease in survival from the 1980s to the 1990s. Five-year relative survival for laryngeal squamous cell carcinoma recorded in the NCDB ranged from a high of 68.1% in 1985 to a low of 62.8% in 1993. Alarmingly, the increase in nonsurgical management parallels the increase in mortality across the years of study for which survival analysis was performed (1985–1996) [44]. These results have stimulated further discussion among the involved medical specialties

in reconsidering the treatment strategies in laryngeal cancer.

Geographic variation of laryngeal and hypopharyngeal cancer data may reflect the different habits of people of diverse cultures as well as environmental and occupational differences. For the male population, the incidence varies from 0.3 per 100,000 in Iceland to 17 per 100,000 in Bas-Rhin, France. Among women, the differences are less pronounced [19, 62]. A study analyzing whether there were any changes in incidence and prognosis of hypopharyngeal carcinoma diagnosed between 1960 and 1989 in Sweden [80] showed a significant decrease in the age-standardized incidence (ASI) for women, with an average decrease of 2% per year ($p < 0.001$), which was most evident in rural counties. The male patients, on the contrary, showed a significant increase of about 1.5% per year ($p < 0.001$). Overall, incidence rates appear to be higher among men in urban areas. Interestingly, a recent publication from Germany [13] showed a significant increase in the mortality rate of laryngeal cancer among females, whereas there is a significant decrease among males. The latter is being preceded or accompanied by a decrease of the corresponding incidence rates, suggesting a lower prevalence of the respective risk factors.

Tobacco and alcohol have long been recognized as the leading causes of head and neck cancer [85]. Although tobacco and alcohol are independent risk factors, it is often difficult to separate their contribution as they usually coexist and appear to act synergistically in multiplying the incidence of laryngeal and hypopharyngeal cancer. Accordingly, Tuyns et al. [79] found a 43-fold increased risk for cancer of the larynx for smokers of more than 26 cigarettes a day and heavy drinkers. Possible environmental carcinogens that have been implicated in head and neck carcinogenesis include polycyclic aromatic hydrocarbons, asbestos, wood dust,

Table 13a.2. Age-adjusted incidence, mortality, and survival of patients with hypopharyngeal and laryngeal cancer in the United States

Site	Annual incidence per 100,000	Percent of all head and neck sites	Incidence ratio in males/females	Mortality per 100,000	5-Year relative survival (1992–1997)
Hypopharynx	0.9	7	1.5/0.4 3.7	0.1	32%
Larynx	3.7	27	6.5/1.4 4.6	1.3	64.5%

Modified from Ries et al. [68]

welding fumes, industrial heat, formaldehyde, nickel, and chromium. Asbestos exposure has been reported to increase the risk of laryngeal cancer by 1.4- to 15.0-fold [27, 71]. Gustavvson and colleagues [40] reported an approximately twofold increased risk of pharyngeal and laryngeal cancer following a more than 8 years of exposure to welding fumes.

13a.2 Staging and Workup

Accurate staging is of paramount importance for the decision-making process because it allows a uniform description and diagnosis, which leads to treatment and outcome. Despite its imperfections, the basis remains the World Health Organization's (WHO) TNM classification system (Tables 13a.3 and 13a.4), which is determined by the size and extent of the tumor and the presence of nodal and distal metastases. For glottal cancer, the American Joint Committee on Cancer (AJCC) clinical staging system is also widely accepted in U.S. practice and literature.

Upon clinical suspicion of a lesion in the area of the larynx or hypopharynx, indirect laryngoscopy and careful fiberoptic endoscopic examination is of paramount importance for further investigation. Inspection of the problem initiates further workup. Direct laryngoscopy accompanied by pharyngoesophagoscopy under general anesthesia permits closer inspection of the lesion with its local spread and allows a biopsy. Direct laryngoscopy has been routinely applied since the emergence of endolaryngeal surgery reported by Kleinsasser [46], but newer tools have recently been added to the diagnostic armamentarium. Systematic use of rigid endoscopes of various angles (0°, 30°, 70°, 120°) can provide a more accurate view of the larynx and hypopharynx, and it complements topographical assessment of the lesion. Contact endoscopy, initiated and mastered by Andrea [3], claims to offer in vivo and in situ evaluation of the mucosal surface for detection of potential malignant pathology.

Another diagnostic tool, direct autofluorescence laryngoscopy, has been applied to the assessment of suspected precancerous and cancerous laryngeal lesions; it is claimed to have a sensitivity rate of 97.3% and a specificity of 83.8% [55]. The autofluorescence diagnosis is based on the ability of oxidized flavin mononucleotide (FMN) in normal cells to emit green fluorescence when exposed to blue light. Neoplastic cells have a significantly lower concentration of FMN and therefore do not fluoresce to the same degree [8]. More recently, fluorescence spectroscopy, a technique for evaluating the physical and chemical properties of a substance by analyzing the intensity and character of light emitted in the form of fluorescence, emerged as a promising refinement of autofluorescence endoscopy [6].

Additionally, optical coherence tomography (OCT), a high-resolution optical imaging technique that produces cross-sectional images of living tissues using light, is claimed to identify invasion of the basement membrane reliably in patients with laryngeal cancer [7]. Moreover, narrow band imaging (NBI) is a novel optical technique that enhances the diagnostic capability of endoscopes in characterizing tissues by using narrow band width filters in video endoscope system. This filter cuts all wavelengths in illumination except two narrow wavelengths. One of these wavelengths is of 415 nm which corresponds to the peak absorption spectrum of hemoglobin to emphasize the image of capillary vessels on surface mucosa. Superficial lesions are identified by changes in the color tone and irregularity of surface mucosa during endoscopic examinations. This method claims to have high sensitivity and specificity in the diagnosis of laryngeal superficial cancer on the basis of abnormal intraepithelial microvessel changes [81]. Although promising, these additional diagnostic tools do not yet have documentation with adequate number of cases to justify their use in the diagnostic workup today.

13a.3 Imaging

An increasing number of imaging modalities are available for more accurate assessment. However, they are largely dependent on the special interest of the radiologist. It is therefore important that the most specialized available neck radiologist be consulted prior to final staging. Computed tomography (CT) with intravenous contrast enhancement and magnetic resonance imaging (MRI) of the neck in axial and coronal sections allow more precise imaging of soft tissue involvement (i.e., dissemination of the tumor to the preepiglottic and paraglottic spaces) and enlarged neck lymph nodes. For better imaging of the endolarynx, CT during inspiration is preferred as laryngeal surface anomalies are more accurately visualized.

Table 13a.3. World Health Organization TNM classification of carcinomas of the larynx

T – Primary tumor	
TX	Primary tumor cannot be assessed
T0	No evidence of primary tumor
Tis	Carcinoma in situ

Supraglottis

T1	Tumor limited to one subsite of supraglottis with normal vocal cord mobility
T2	Tumor invades mucosa of more than one adjacent subsite of supraglottis or glottis or region outside the supraglottis (e.g., mucosa of base of tongue, vallecula, medial wall of piriform sinus) without fixation of the larynx
T3	Tumor limited to larynx with vocal cord fixation and/or invades any of the following: postcricoid area, preepiglottic tissues, paraglottic space, and/or with minor thyroid cartilage erosion (e.g., inner cortex)
T4a	Tumor invades through the thyroid cartilage and/or invades tissues beyond the larynx, e.g., trachea, soft tissues of neck including deep/extrinsic muscle of tongue (genioglossus, hyoglossus, palatoglossus, styloglossus), strap muscles, thyroid, esophagus
T4b	Tumor invades prevertebral space, mediastinal structures, or encases carotid artery

Glottis

T1	Tumor limited to vocal cord(s) (may involve anterior or posterior commissure) with normal mobility
T1a	Tumor limited to one vocal cord
T1b	Tumor involves both vocal cords
T2	Tumor extends to supraglottis and/or subglottis, and/or with impaired vocal cord mobility
T3	Tumor limited to larynx with vocal cord fixation and/or invades paraglottic space, and/or with minor thyroid cartilage erosion (e.g., inner cortex)
T4a	Tumor invades through the thyroid cartilage, or invades tissues beyond the larynx, e.g., trachea, soft tissues of neck including deep/extrinsic muscle of tongue (genioglossus, hyoglossus, palatoglossus, styloglossus), strap muscles, thyroid, esophagus
T4b	Tumor invades prevertebral space, mediastinal structures, or encases carotid artery

Subglottis

T1	Tumor limited to subglottis
T2	Tumor extends to vocal cord(s) with normal or impaired mobility
T3	Tumor limited to larynx with vocal cord fixation
T4a	Tumor invades through cricoid or thyroid cartilage and/or invades tissues beyond the larynx, e.g., trachea, soft tissues of neck including deep/extrinsic muscle of tongue (genioglossus, hyoglossus, palatoglossus, styloglossus), strap muscles, thyroid, esophagus
T4b	Tumor invades prevertebral space, mediastinal structures, or encases carotid artery

N – Regional lymph nodes

NX	Regional lymph nodes cannot be assessed
N0	No regional lymph node metastasis
N1	Metastasis in a single ipsilateral lymph node, 3 cm or less in greatest dimension
N2	Metastasis as specified in N2a, 2b, 2c, below
N2a	Metastasis in a single ipsilateral lymph node, more than 3 cm but not more than 6 cm in greatest dimension
N2b	Metastasis in multiple ipsilateral lymph nodes, none more than 6 cm in greatest dimension
N2c	Metastasis in bilateral or contralateral lymph nodes, none more than 6 cm in greatest dimension
N3	Metastasis in a lymph node more than 6 cm in greatest dimension
Note:	Midline nodes are considered ipsilateral nodes

M – Distant metastasis

MX	Distant metastasis cannot be assessed
M0	No distant metastasis
M1	Distant metastasis

Stage grouping

Stage 0	Tis	N0	M0
Stage I	T1	N0	M0
Stage II	T2	N0	M0
Stage III	T1 T2	N1	M0
	T3	N0 N1	
Stage IVa	T1 T2 T3	N2	M0
	T4a	N0 N1 N2	
Stage IVb	T4b	ANY N	M0
	ANY T	N3	
Stage IVc	ANY T	ANY N	M1

From Barnes et al. [84]

Table 13a.4. WHO TNM classification of carcinomas of the hypopharynx

T – Primary tumor	
TX	Primary tumor cannot be assessed
T0	No evidence of primary tumor
Tis	Carcinoma in situ
T1	Tumor limited to one subsite of hypopharynx and 2 cm or less in greatest dimension
T2	Tumor invades more than one subsite of hypopharynx or an adjacent site, or measures more than 2 cm but not more than 4 cm in greatest dimension, without fixation of hemilarynx
T3	Tumor more than 4 cm in greatest dimension, or with fixation of hemilarynx
T4a	Tumor invades any of the following: thyroid/cricoid cartilage, hyoid bone, thyroid gland, esophagus, central compartment soft tissue*
T4b	Tumor invades prevertebral fascia, encases carotid artery, or invades mediastinal structures.

* Central compartment soft tissue includes prelaryngeal strap muscles and subcutaneous fat.

N – Regional lymph nodes

NX	Regional lymph nodes cannot be assessed
N0	No regional lymph node metastasis
N1	Metastasis in a single ipsilateral lymph node, 3 cm or less in greatest dimension
N2	Metastasis as specified in N2a, 2b, 2c
N2a	Metastasis in a single ipsilateral lymph node, more than 3 cm but not more than 6 cm in greatest dimension
N2b	Metastasis in multiple ipsilateral lymph nodes, none more than 6 cm in greatest dimension
N2c	Metastasis in bilateral or contralateral lymph nodes, none more than 6 cm in greatest dimension
N3	Metastasis in a lymph node more than 6 cm in greatest dimension

Note: Midline nodes are considered ipsilateral nodes

M – Distant metastasis

MX	Distant metastasis cannot be assessed
M0	No distant metastasis
M1	Distant metastasis

Stage grouping

Stage 0	Tis	N0	M0
Stage I	T1	N0	M0
Stage II	T2	N0	M0
Stage III	T1 T2	N1	M0
	T3	N0 N1	
Stage IVa	T1 T2 T3	N2	M0
	T4a	N0 N1 N2	
Stage IVb	T4b	Any N	M0
	Any T	N3	
Stage IVc	Any T	Any N	M1

From Barnes et al. [84]

moreover, for bony or cartilaginous involvement, CT appears to be superior to MRI [32].

Recently, 2-[^{18}F]-fluoro-2-deoxy-D-glucose (FDG) positron emission tomography (PET) has been used increasingly for the staging and follow-up of patients with head and neck cancer [72, 84]. FDG-PET is a functional imaging modality that uses abnormal tissue metabolism to detect neoplasms. The radioactive glucose analogue FDG is metabolized in normal tissue and neoplastic tissues in proportion to the rate of tissue glucose metabolism. FDG is metabolically trapped in the intracellular space. This occurs more in tumors than in normal tissues and can be used to identify tumors based on accelerated glycolytic rates using PET. A recent study has shown that pretreatment tumor FDG uptake in PET represents an independent prognostic factor in patients with advanced resectable squamous cell carcinoma (SCC) of the larynx and hypopharynx [70]. Accordingly, high FDG uptake is associated with poor survival of patients with advanced laryngopharyngeal SCC. However, there is controversial evidence in the current literature for its value as a routine examination for initial staging [41, 57].

13a.4 Treatment Options

13a.4.1 Open Partial Surgery

Complete eradication of the disease and preservation of maximum function is the ultimate goal during treatment planning. For a patient with laryngeal and/or hypopharyngeal cancer, this would ideally be to preserve phonation, respiration, and deglutition as close to normal as possible, regardless of the disease stage.

Histological type, surgical expertise of the physician, and patient preference influence treatment planning in different ways; however, careful staging is far and away the most important factor. It provides the mainframe in which the physician seeks the best treatment options. For late-stage disease, multidisciplinary discussion is of paramount importance for optimal decisions based on the aforementioned parameters. For the past decades, clinical research has been focusing on organ preservation strategies along with disease eradication. The resulting evolution of conservative and refinement of surgical approaches has enriched our treatment strategies but has also made the decision process more challenging.

Since the first total laryngectomy was undertaken by Billroth in 1873, many surgeons have attempted less amputative techniques for less-advanced disease stages as otorhinolaryngology–head and neck surgery evolved as a surgical subspecialty. Most techniques for partial laryngopharyngectomy emerged during the late 1950s, starting with Alonso [1] and Ogura [58, 59] and were further established during the 1960s by Laccourreye, who described the procedure of supracricoid hemi-laryngopharyngectomy for selected cases of hypopharyngeal and lateral laryngeal wall tumors. The outcome of these procedures in carefully selected cases was quite promising; 95% local control in the initial series by Laccourreye brought up new ideas for treating selected invasive cancer cases without compromising laryngeal and pharyngeal function. The concept of conservation laryngopharyngectomy was further forwarded by Piquet during the 1970s, who conceived cricohyoidopexy and cricohyoidoepiglottopexy as viable alternatives for the treatment of supraglottic and glottic cancers. Based on this concept, Laccourreye named it supracricoid partial laryngectomy. Not only did this procedure achieve local control of 95% in selected T3 and T4 laryngeal cancer cases, [47, 48, 82, 83], it improved quality of life compared to that achieved with total laryngectomy [82].

As for hypopharyngeal carcinoma, historical aspects of the surgical treatment of piriform sinus cancer, the most common location of hypopharyngeal malignancy, include various techniques that have brought varying rates of success. I selectively mention the techniques of Ogura [59] and, more recently, Barton [9] for tumors localized solely in the piriform sinus. Alonso [1] suggested vertical hemi-laryngopharyngectomy for a tumor located in the outer wall of the piriform sinus. In a prospective study of seven patients, Iwai [45] proposed removing the affected half of the hypopharynx together with the affected vertical half of the adjacent supraglottic and glottic larynx and the superior two-thirds of the cricoid cartilage. Segas et al. [73] described a variation of Iwai's technique whereby the cricoid cartilage was preserved when not involved, thus reducing the possibility of postoperative aspiration. Additionally, Hirano [43] proposed partial laryngopharyngectomy

with preservation of the vocal process of the unilateral true vocal cord and reconstruction of the defect with a pectoralis major myocutaneous flap in four selected cases where the mass was confined to the ipsilateral piriform sinus, arytenoepiglottic fold, arytenoid eminence, and paraglottic space at the level of the false vocal cord. In a series of 34 patients operated on during a 2-year period and followed up for a median of 48 months, Barzan [10] suggested a more amputative method, consisting of complete removal of the affected half of the hypopharynx and larynx, starting from the level of the hyoid bone with resection of its unilateral half and ending with removal of the unilateral half of the first two tracheal rings. As a general comment, the limited number of patients in these studies and the specific indications for their application cannot justify any solid conclusions as to which technique is best.

13a.4.2 Endoscopic Partial Surgery

With the introduction of endolaryngeal surgery by Kleinsasser, its indications have progressed from solely glottic tumors to include all laryngeal and hypopharyngeal areas. Its indications and application are further discussed in the following section.

13a.4.3 Conservative Treatment

13a.4.3.1 Definitive Radiotherapy

The application of radiotherapy as a treatment modality for laryngeal cancer was conceived and first applied by Schepegrell in 1903. Since its widespread use, many questions have arisen as to its correct application and the indications for use of the various modalities and combinations that have been attempted from time to time. Aiming at improved local control, advances in cell biology and cell growth have led to increases in the total radiation dose but with lower per-dose fractions (hyperfractionation), reductions in overall treatment time (acceleration), and a combination of these two strategies for the purpose of counteracting tumor clonogenic cell repopulation, the latter being a cause of potential failure for patients treated with conventional radiotherapy.

For example, a split-course accelerated radiotherapy regimen implements a twice-daily course schedule for a reduced overall treatment time (OTT), whereas partly accelerated fractionation with a concomitant boost integrates a simultaneous radiation boost to small volumes, similarly aiming at reducing the OTT. The radiotherapy community has been addressed frequently on (1) whether radiotherapy is a treatment option only in patients with early disease or is still a treatment option for advanced disease, and (2) if altered fractionation radiotherapy (hyperfractionation/accelerated regimen) is better than conventional radiotherapy for advanced disease.

Clinical research has also focused on whether altered fractionation could offer better results than conventional radiotherapy and which altered fractionation schedule may have an acceptable therapeutic index. A recent evidence-based review on radiation oncology in head and neck squamous carcinoma [28] concluded that external radiotherapy and/or brachytherapy are crucial treatment options in patients with early-stage disease. However, advanced tumors and small tumors with enlarged neck nodes are commonly less well controlled by conventional radiotherapy. The main factors that contribute in locoregional failure in more than 30–50% of cases with an ultimate poor 30% five-year survival rate [50] are a high burden of clonogenic cells, accelerated repopulation during the irradiation course, hypoxic cells with surrounding neoangiogenesis, and overexpression of growth factor receptors [5, 11].

More than 20 randomized trials exploring altered fractionation schemes have been published so far with more than 17,000 patients included in controlled clinical studies. Two major studies have attempted a comparison between the various radiotherapy strategies. The four-group Radiation Therapy Oncology Group (RTOG) 90–03 trial [37] compared conventional radiotherapy with hyperfractionation radiation treatment, split-course accelerated radiotherapy, and partly accelerated fractionation with a concomitant boost. A significant benefit was recorded for local control in the hyperfractionated and concomitant-boost groups, but there was no significant improvement in overall survival. Moreover, more acute toxic effects were recorded but without more late toxic effects.

On the other hand, the CHART (Continuous Hyperfractionated Accelerated Radiation Treatment) trial [33] compared conventional radiotherapy with the continuous strategy giving a total dose of 54 Gy over 12 successive days. Early reactions in mucosa and skin were more severe and more recent in the group with continuous radiotherapy than in those who received conventional radiotherapy; but after 3 months the tissue reactions did not differ between the groups. Moreover, disease-free survival was similar in the two groups except for laryngeal tumors, in which significantly better 3-year local control was recorded with continuous treatment than with conventional treatment—but only for T3 tumors (70% vs. 47%) and T4 lesions (78% vs. 38%).

Finally, a meta-analysis [21, 22] that included data from 6515 patients randomized in 15 trials of altered fractionation, including various head and neck primary sites, showed that altered fractionation radiotherapy produced a significant 3% benefit in 5-year survival. This led to the conclusion [53] that altered fractionation radiotherapy is undisputedly the treatment of choice for laryngeal cancer, particularly hyperfractionated radiotherapy or accelerated radiotherapy with a concomitant boost.

It should also be mentioned that newer radiotherapy techniques, such as three-dimensional conformal radiation therapy (3D CRT) and intensity-modulated radiotherapy (IMT) are currently being investigated for their potential to increase the therapeutic gain. It is being done by escalating the dose to the tumor in all three dimensions and avoiding toxic exposure to radiation in the vital organs and structures surrounding the tumor, thus improving locoregional control.

13a.4.3.2 Chemotherapy

The role of chemotherapy as a sole definitive treatment of hypopharyngeal and laryngeal cancer has been questioned. However, at the 1982 American Society of Clinical Oncology (ASCO) annual meeting, Decker et al. [30, 31] described 34 previously untreated patients who received two to three cycles of cisplatin and fluorouracil; 93% showed a clinically objective response, and 63% had a complete response. The issue of radiosensitivity in chemosensitive tumors was also brought up by the same team [34]. This correlation led researchers to use induction chemotherapy as a strategy to differentiate tumors that needed total laryngectomy from those could be treated conservatively in three randomized trials. Patients with a good response to chemotherapy would receive radiotherapy, whereas those who did not respond well would undergo total laryngectomy [35].

The VALSG (Department of Veterans Affairs Laryngeal Cancer Study Group) trial [76], followed by the French group [68] and the EORTC (European Organization for Research and Treatment of Cancer) [54] were included in a specific meta-analysis by the MACH-NC (Meta-Analysis of Chemotherapy on Head and Neck Cancer) group [65]. The study revealed the superiority of surgery over chemotherapy in terms of the 5-year survival rate (6% higher in the surgery group) but proved the benefit of laryngeal preservation in 58% of the patients in the chemotherapy group. Similar results emanated from another study focused on resectable hypopharyngeal tumors comparing those randomly assigned to receive induction chemotherapy of cisplatin and fluorouracil followed by surgery and radiotherapy versus those of induction radiotherapy followed by radiotherapy but reserving surgery for salvage [12]. Comparison with the findings of the EORTC trial further supports the belief that tumor chemosensitivity is of utmost importance for choosing radiotherapy instead of surgery after induction chemotherapy [53].

A more recent German meta-analysis [26] on 32 trials with a total of 10,225 patients has proven that a large survival benefit of 12 months was observed in favor of concomitant chemoradiation, regardless of whether conventional, hyperfractionated, or accelerated radiotherapy was used. The enhanced activity of radiotherapy, when combined concurrently with platinum derivatives and 5-fluorouracil, is thought to occur because of inhibition of repair of lethal and sublethal damage induced by radiotherapy; radiosensitization of hypoxic cells; reduction of tumor burden leading to an improved blood supply, synchronization, and redistribution of tumor cells into the more sensitive G_2-M cell cycle phase; and finally induction of apoptosis [51].

Although quite effective, it should be stressed out that no larynx-preserving approach offers a survival advantage with respect to total laryngectomy and appropriate adjuvant therapy. In particular, concomitant chemoradiation may also be used for larynx preservation in selected patients with stage III cancer when total laryngectomy is the only surgical option or when the functional outcome with surgery is expected to be unsatisfactory [64]. Tumor penetration through cartilage into soft tissues, skin, and/or base of tongue involvements are clinical evidence of extensive disease; and therefore such patients are considered poor

candidates for laryngeal preservation. To achieve the best outcome, surgical treatment of the neck can be recommended for patients with nodal involvement treated with chemoradiation [64]. The RTOG guidelines advise surgeons to perform chemoradiation following by a neck dissection in N1 patients with incomplete resolution of neck disease and for all patients initially staged N2a or N2b (and N2c when the node is > 3 cm or persistent) or N3. Pfister et al. [64] stated that neck dissection should be performed within 15 weeks after completing chemoradiotherapy. With the popularization of FDG-PET in the posttreatment follow-up, some groups [2, 66] are investigating whether negative FDG-PET after chemoradiotherapy in patients with N2–N3 disease predicts for a high pathological complete response rate (> 80%) in the neck and a low overall nodal relapse rate (< 10%). Moreover, it is claimed that patients with high FDG uptake may be better treated by surgical resection followed by chemoradiotherapy [70].

In an effort to maximize the therapeutic result, researchers are investigating the effect of various substances compared to the traditional cisplatin-fluorouracil regimen. Induction chemotherapy with multiagents, including taxanes, might help select patients who may benefit from a definitive chemoradiation approach [67]. So far, however, the superiority of induction chemotherapy followed by concomitant therapies over concomitant chemoradiotherapy or targeted therapy combined with radiotherapy has not been adequately substantiated. Thus, induction chemotherapy including taxanes followed by concomitant chemoradiotherapy should remain an investigational approach [28].

The idea of adding radiosensitizers to traditional chemotherapy for the purpose of providing enhanced radiation-induced tumor cell killing with minimum toxicity has been discussed recently. A large Danish trial [61] has revealed improved locoregional control at 4 years (52% vs. 33%, $p = 0.006$) and longer disease-specific survival in patients with laryngeal and pharyngeal squamous cell carcinoma with the addition of *nimorazole*, a radiosensitizer with electron-affinity hypoxic action. It proved to be less toxic and clinically relevant. At the moment, nimorazole appears to be the only hypoxic cell sensitizer with evidence-based proven efficacy. *ARCON* (accelerated radiotherapy with carbogen and nicotinamide) and *tirapazamine* have also been tested, but their efficacy as radiosensitizers remains to be further investigated. The former causes vasodilation to reduce transient or acute hypoxia and allows breathing of carbogen to overcome chronic hypoxia [16]; the latter is a cytoxin-bioreductive compound that has shown a high hypoxic/toxicity ratio in preclinical studies [38].

Further developments in molecular biology and cancer genetics have drawn the researchers' attention in a different direction. The research for biological profiles that can predict chemosensitivity or radiosensitivity would result in predicting the likelihood of laryngeal preservation. The incidence of laryngeal preservation was significantly higher in patients whose tumors overexpressed P53, but this overexpression was not adequate to predict survival [24]. A few years later, the same group of researchers concluded that T stage, P53 overexpression, and an increased proliferating-cell nuclear-antigen index were independent predictors of successful organ preservation [25]. Furthermore, the same team, from the University of Michigan, investigated the expression of Bcl-2 family proteins in advanced laryngeal squamous cell carcinoma and concluded that five of seven tumors that overexpressed Bcl-2 had a complete response, whereas reduced expression of Bcl-2 L1 was associated with laryngeal preservation and decreased BAX expression with complete responses [78]. Moreover, angiogenesis seemed to be of interest as patients with vessel counts that were higher than the mean were three to five times more likely to need total laryngectomy than were those with counts below the mean [75]. A study from Memorial Sloan-Kettering Cancer Center confirmed the predictive value of P53 for an unfavorable outcome in laryngeal preservation [60].

The fact that epidermal growth factor receptor (EGFR) overexpression has been shown in preclinical models to be correlated with radiosensitivity has led to a new era of induction chemotherapy [11]. It has been shown in cellular and animal models that radiation therapy can upregulate EGFR expression and that EGFR activation enhances survival of cancer cells after radiotherapy. This biological effect may contribute to the repopulation effect that takes place during a conventional course of radiotherapy. Increased levels of EGFR expression have been correlated with a poor prognosis [39].

The introduction of monoclonal antibodies (cetuximab), which block epidermal growth factor (EGF) and tumor growth factor-α (TGFα), has added a new strategy to induction chemoradiation. Cetuximab is a mouse–human chimeric antibody of the immunoglobulin G1 (IgG1) subclass that binds to EGFR (HER-1, cERBB1). It acts by binding to EGFR and thereby effectively blocks phosphorylation and activation of EGFR tyrosine kinase. Cetuximab treatment alone demonstrates cytostatic effects on cell growth in most of the tumor cell lines that have been studied to date [28].

Preclinical and clinical data appear to support the hypothesis that EGFR inhibitors effectively radiosensitize cancer expressing high levels of EGFR [11, 49]. A large Phase III multiinstitutional study by Bonner et al. [20] compared radiotherapy alone with radiotherapy plus weekly cetuximab in patients with stage III–IV squamous cell carcinoma of the head and neck for the purpose of comparing locoregional control. There was an absolute improvement of 13% in overall 3-year survival for cetuximab-treated patients (44% vs. 57%, $p = 0.03$). Local toxicity was not increased to the point to alter the local therapeutic index. On the contrary, this approach offered a higher local therapeutic index than radiotherapy alone, as reflected by the higher therapeutic outcome with the same mucosal toxicity. Two large studies by the RTOG—RTOG 0522 (Phase III trial exploring cisplatin radiotherapy with and without cetuximab) and RTOG 0234 (Phase II trial looking for the outcome and feasibility of cetuximab added to weekly cisplatin with irradiation in high-risk resected patients) [28]—are currently ongoing, and their results are anxiously awaited by the therapeutic community.

Corvò [28] has reviewed the various treatment modalities and the probability of severe acute and late toxicity after altered fractionation radiotherapy and the association of irradiation with a radiosensitizer, chemotherapy, or targeted therapy. The results are shown in Table 13a.5. Whereas there was an increased probability of epidermitis with accelerated radiotherapy than with the remaining modalities, mucositis appeared with the highest probability after accelerated radiotherapy and concomitant chemoradiotherapy. The latter had also the highest probability for showing hematological toxicity and systemic side effects. Cetuximab targeted radiotherapy showed the highest probability of acneiform rash, followed by increased probability of systemic side effects and xerostomia with the conventional two-dimensional radiotherapy technique.

Table 13a.5. Probability of severe acute and late toxicity after altered fractionation radiotherapy; association of irradiation with radiosensitizer, chemotherapy, or targeted therapy

Severe toxicity	Accelerated RT	Hyperfractionated RT	Radiosensitizer RT*	Concomitant CT-RT	Targeted therapy - RT**
Epidermitis	++	+	+	+	+
Mucositis	+++	++	++	+++	+
Hematological toxicity	-	-	-	+++	+
Systemic side effects	-	-	+	+++	++
Acneiform rash	-	-	+	-	+++
Xerostomia with 2D technique	++	++	++	++	++
Xerostomia with 3D-IMRT technique	+	+	+	+	+
Late mucosal atrophy	+	+	+	++	+
Fibrosis	+	+	+	+	+

From Corvò [28]

RT, radiotherapy; CT, chemotherapy; IMRT, intensity-modulated radiotherapy; 2D, 3D, two- and three-dimensional, respectively
+, ++, +++: low, increased, and high probability of severe toxicity, respectively; incidence may vary according to radiotherapy technique, fractionation and total doses, primary site, chemotherapy regimen, and timing
*Nimorazole
** Cetuximab

13a.4.3.3 Photodynamic Therapy

Photodynamic therapy is the use of light-sensitive drugs to selectively identify and destroy diseased cells. When administered, these compounds accumulate and are retained to a greater degree in malignant tissues than in normal tissues. The drug remains inactive until it is activated by laser. The resulting photochemical reaction leads to the production of oxygen radicals, thereby destroying diseased cells without affecting surrounding normal tissues [18].

This treatment modality for cancer was first reported by Manyak et al. [56] in 1988. Several studies have shown photodynamic therapy to be effective in the treatment of T1 and T2 cancers of the larynx [17, 74]. In particular, these series demonstrated the efficacy of Photofrin-mediated photodynamic therapy as a curative treatment for T1 (85–91% of cases) and T2 (62% of cases) squamous cell carcinomas of the larynx. Further advantages of photodynamic therapy are no scarring, excellent voice preservation, repeatability, minimal side effects, and performance as an outpatient procedure.

13a.5 Criticisms and Conclusions

As ongoing research is focusing on accurately specifying the indications for conservative versus interventional treatment, many questions remain to be answered and form subjects of criticism among laryngeal and hypopharyngeal cancer therapists. More specifically, there are no clear indications that the combination of irradiation and multiagent chemotherapy is superior to irradiation plus high-dose cisplatin [16]. Additionally, more data about compliance and late toxicity are needed to support whether concomitant chemotherapy with altered fractionation can be used safely [16]. Although induction polychemotherapy followed by concomitant chemoradiotherapy has shown promising results, its superiority over concomitant chemoradiation alone is yet to be proven. For patients with intermediate-risk (T2–T3 N1) disease, further trials are required to answer whether chemoradiotherapy is indeed better than intensified radiotherapy alone [15]. Hope is also offered to patients with locally advanced carcinoma who are unfit for chemotherapy; for those patients, it would be reasonable to attempt altered fractionation radiotherapy or targeted therapy-radiotherapy [42]. As for patients older than 65 years, the current studies do not prove any important outcome benefit from modification by fractionation or chemoradiotherapy [21, 23].

Molecular biology has provided new data that may alter our approach to laryngeal and hypopharyngeal cancer. EGFR overexpression in tumors may predict a worse prognosis if the patient is treated with conventional radiotherapy [4]; such patients may be more likely to benefit from hyperfractionated accelerated radiotherapy [14] or moderately accelerated radiotherapy [36]. Finally, emerging data showing that the presence of a subset of Human Papilloma Virus (HPV) in patients with oropharyngeal cancers is related to a favorable prognosis [83], indicate that HPV infection could be an important prognostic factor for squamous cell carcinoma of the head and neck.

References

1. Alonso JM (1950) La Chirurgie Conservatrice pour le Cancer du Larynx at de l' Hypopharynx. Ann. Otolaryngol. (Paris) 67:567–575

2. Al-Sarraf M (2002) Treatment of locally advanced head and neck cancer: historical and critical review. Cancer Control 9:387–399

3. Andrea M (1995) Contact endoscopy during microlaryngeal surgery: a new technique for endoscopic examination of the larynx. Ann Otol Rhinol Laryngol 104(5):333–339

4. Ang KK, Berkey BA, Tu X, et al (2002) Impact of epidermal growth factor receptor overexpression on survival and pattern of relapse in patients with advanced head and neck carcinoma. Cancer Res 62:7350–7356

5. Antognoni P, Corvò R, Zerini D, Orecchia R (2005) Altered fractionation radiotherapy in head and neck cancer: clinical issues and pitfalls of "evidence-based medicine". Tumori 91:30–39

6. Arens C, Reussner D, Neubacher H, Woenckhaus J, Glanz H (2006) Spectrometric measurement in laryngeal cancer Eur Arch Otorhinolaryngol 263:1001–1007.

7. Armstrong W, Ridgway J (2006) Optical coherence tomography of laryngeal cancer. Laryngoscope 116(7):1107–1113

8. Baletic N, Petrovic Z, Pendjer I, Malicevic H (2004) Autofluorescent diagnostics in laryngeal pathology. Eur Arch Otorhinolaryngol 261:233–237

9. Barton RT (1973) Surgical treatment of carcinoma of the pyriform sinus. Arch Otolaryngol 97:337–339

10. Barzan L, Comoretto R (1993) Hemipharyngectomy and hemilaryngectomy for pyriform sinus cancer: reconstruction with remaining larynx and hypopharynx and with tracheostomy. Laryngoscope 103:82–86

11. Baumann M, Krause M (2004) Targeting the epidermal growth factor receptor in radiotherapy: radiobiological mechanisms, preclinical and clinical results. Radiother Oncol 72:257–266

12. Beauvillain C, Mahe M, Bourdin S, et al (1997) Final results of a randomized trial comparing chemotherapy plus radiotherapy with chemotherapy plus surgery plus radiotherapy in locally advanced resectable hypopharyngeal carcinomas. Laryngoscope 107:648–653

13. Becker N, Altenburg HP, Stegmaier C, Ziegler H (2007) Report on trends of incidence (1970–2002) of and mortality (1952–2002) from cancer in Germany. J Cancer Res Clin Oncol 133:23–35

14. Bentzen SM, Atasoy BM, Daley F, et al (2005) Epidermal growth factor receptor expression in pretreatment biopsies from head and neck squamous cell carcinoma as a predictive factor for a benefit from accelerated radiation therapy in a randomized controlled trial. J Clin Oncol 23:5560–5567

15. Bernier J (2004) Chemoradiation in locally advanced head and neck cancer: new evidence, new challenges. Expert Rev Anticancer Ther 4:335–339

16. Bernier J, Bentzen SM (2006) Radiotherapy for head and neck cancer: latest developments and future perspectives. Curr Opin Oncol 18:240–246

17. Biel MA (1994) Photodynamic therapy and the treatment of neoplastic diseases of the larynx. Laryngoscope 104: 399–403

18. Biel MA (20020 Photodynamic therapy in head and neck cancer. Curr Oncol Rep 4:87–96

19. Blot WJ, Devesa SS, McLaughlin JK, Fraumeni JR JF (1994) Oral and pharyngeal cancers. Cancer Surv 19/20:23–42

20. Bonner JA, Harari PM, Giralt J, et al (2006) Radiotherapy plus cetuximab for squamous-cell carcinoma of the head and neck. N Engl J Med 354:567–578

21. Bourhis J, Amand C, Pignon JP (2004) Update of MACH. NC (Meta-analysis of chemotherapy in Head & Neck Cancer) database focused on concomitant chemoradiotherapy. Proc Am Soc Clin Oncol 22–488

22. Bourhis J, Etessami A, Wilbault P, et al (2004) Altered fractionated radiotherapy in the management of head and neck carcinomas: advantages and limitations. Curr Opin Oncol 16:215–219

23. Bourhis J, Overgaard J, Audry H, et al (2006) Hyperfractionated or accelerated radiotherapy in head and neck cancer:a metaanalysis. Lancet 368:843–854

24. Bradford CR, Zhu S, Wolf GT, et al (1995) Overexpression of p53 predicts organ preservation using induction chemotherapy and radiation in patients with advanced laryngeal cancer. Otolaryngol Head Neck Surg 113:408–412

25. Bradford CR, Wolf GT, Carey TE, et al (1999) Predictive markers for response to chemotherapy, organ preservation, and survival in patients with advanced laryngeal carcinoma. Otolaryngol Head Neck Surg 121:534–538

26. Budach W, Her T, Budach V, Belka C, Dietz K (2006) A meta-analysis of hyperfractionated and accelerated radiotherapy and combined chemotherapy and radiotherapy regimens in unresected locally advanced squamous cell carcinoma of the head and neck. BMC Cancer 6:28

27. Burch JD, Howe GR, Miller AB, Semenciw R (1981) Tobacco, alcohol, asbestos, and nickel in the etiology of cancer of the larynx: a case-control study. J Natl Cancer Inst 67:1219–1224

28. Corvò R (2007) Evidence-based radiation oncology in head and neck squamous cell carcinoma. Radiother Oncol 85:156–170

29. Davies L, Welch G (2006) Epidemiology of head and neck cancer in the United States Otolaryngol Head Neck Surg 135:451–457

30. Decker D, Drelichman A, Jacobs J, et al (1982) Adjuvant chemotherapy with high dose bolus cis-diamminodichloroplatinum II (CDD) and 120 hour infusion 5-fluorouracil (5-FU) in stage III and IV squamous cell carcinoma of the head and neck. ASCO annual meeting, Saint Louis:abstr C-757

31. Decker DA, Drelichman A, Jacobs J, et al (1983) Adjuvant chemotherapy with cis-diamminodichloroplatinum II and 120-hour infusion 5-fluorouracil in stage III and IV squamous cell carcinoma of the head and neck. Cancer 51: 1353–1355

32. DeSanto LW (1982) Current concept in otolaryngology:the options in early laryngeal carcinoma. N Engl J Med 306: 910

33. Dische S, Saunders M, Barrett A, et al (1997) A randomised multicentre trial of CHART versus conventional radiotherapy in head and neck cancer. Radiother Oncol 44:123–136

34. Ensley J, Jacobs J, Weaver A, et al (1982) Initial cis-platinum combination predicting response to radiotherapy in patients with advanced epidermoid cancers of the head and neck. ASCO annual meeting, Saint Louis:abstr C-767

35. Ensley JF, Jacobs JR, Weaver A, et al (1984) Correlation between response to cisplatinum-combination chemotherapy and subsequent radiotherapy in previously untreated patients with advanced squamous cell cancers of the head and neck. Cancer 54:811–814

36. Eriksen JG, Steiniche T, Overgaard J (2005) The influence of epidermal growth factor receptor and tumor differentiation on the response to accelerated radiotherapy of squamous cell carcinomas of the head and neck in the randomized DAHANCA 6 and 7 study. Radiother Oncol 74:93–100

37. Fu KK, Pajak TF, Trotti A, et al (2000) A radiation therapy oncology Group (RTOG) phase III randomized study to compare hyperfractionation and two variants of accelerated fractionation to standard fractionation radiotherapy for head and neck squamous cell carcinomas:first report of RTOG 9003. Int J Radiat Oncol Biol Phys 48:7–16

38. Gandara DR, Lara PN, Golberg Z, et al (2002) Tirapazamine:the prototype for a novel class of therapeutic agent targeting tumor hypoxia. Semin Oncol 29:102–109

39. Gregoire V, Eisbruch A, Hamoir M, Levendag P (2006) Proposal for the delineation of the nodal CTV in the node-positive and post-operative neck. Radiother Oncol 79: 15–20

40. Gustavsson P, Jakobsson R, Johansson H, Lewin F, Norell S, Rutkvist LE. 1998 Occupational exposures and squamous cell carcinoma of the oral cavity, pharynx, larynx, and oesophagus: a case-control study in Sweden. Occup Environ Med 55:393–400

41. Hafidh MA, Lacy PD, Hughes JP, Duffy G, Timon CV. (2006) Evaluation of the impact of addition of PET to CT and MR scanning in the staging of patients with head and neck carcinomas Eur Arch Otorhinolaryngol 263: 853–859

42. Harari PM (2005) Promising new advances in head and neck radiotherapy. Ann Oncol 16:vi13–9

43. Hirano M, Kurita S, Yoshida T et al (1988) Partial laryngo-pharyngectomy for pyriform sinus carcinoma. Technique and preliminary results. Auris Nasus Larynx 15:129–136

44. Hoffman H, Porter K, Karnell L, et al (2006) Laryngeal cancer in the Unites States:changes in demographics, patterns of care, and survival. Laryngoscope 116(9 Pt. 2 Suppl. 111):1–13

45. Iwai H., Koike Y., Nagahara K (1975) Subtotal pharyngolaryngectomy conservation surgery for carcinoma of sinus pyriformis extending toward the larynx. Arch. Oto-Rhino-Laryng 209:271–276

46. Kleinsasser O (1962) Die Laryngomikroskopie (Lupen-laryngoskopie) und ihre Bedeutung für die Erkennung der Vorerkrankungen und Fröhformen des Stimmlippenkarzinoms. Arch Ohren Nasen Kehlkopfheilkd 180:724–727

47. Laccourreye H, Laccourreye O, Weinstein G, et al 1990 Supracricoid laryngectomy with cricohyoidopexy: a partial laryngeal procedure for selected supraglottic and transglottic carcinomas. Laryngoscope 100:735–741

48. Laccourreye H, Laccourreye O, Weinstein G, et al (1990) Supracricoid laryngectomy with cricohyoidoepiglottopexy: a partial laryngeal procedure for glottic carcinoma. Ann Otol Rhinol Laryngol 99:421–426

49. Lammering G (2005) Molecular predictor and promising target:will EGFR now become a star in radiotherapy? Radiother Oncol 74:89–91

50. Laskar SG, Agarwal JP, Srinivas C, Dinshaw KA (2006) Radiotherapeutic management of locally advanced head and neck cancer. Expert Rev Anticancer Ther 6:405–417

51. Lawrence TS, Blackstock WA, McGinn C (2003) The mechanism of action of adiosensitization of conventional chemotherapeutic agents. Semin Radiat Oncol 13:13–21

52. Lee DJ (2002) Definitive radiotherapy for squamous carcinoma of the larynx. Otolaryngol Clin North Am 32:1013–1033

53. Lefebvre JL (2006) Laryngeal preservation in head and neck cancer:multidisciplinary approach. Lancet Oncol 7: 747–755

54. Lefebvre JL, Chevalier D, Luboinski B, et al (1996) Larynx preservation in pyriform sinus cancer: preliminary results of a European Organization for Research and Treatment of Cancer phase III trial. J Natl Cancer Inst 88:890–899

55. Malzahn K, Dreyer T, Glanz H, Arens C (2002) Autofluorescence endoscopy in the diagnosis of early laryngeal cancer and its precursor lesions. Laryngoscope 112:488–493

56. Manyak MJ, Russo A, Smith PD, Glatscin E (1988) Photodynamic therapy. J Clin Oncol 6:380–391

57. Muylle K, Castaigne C, Flamen P (2005) 18F-fluoro-2-deoxy-D-glucose positron emission tomographic imaging: recent developments in head and neck cancer. Curr Opin Oncol 17(3):249–253

58. Ogura JH, Jurema AA, Watson RK (1960) Partial laryngo-pharyngectomy and neck dissection for pyriform sinus cancer. Conservation surgery with immediate reconstruction. Laryngoscope 22:737–747

59. Ogura JH, Mallen RW (1965) Partial laryngopharyngectomy for supraglottic and pharyngeal carcinoma. Tr Am Acad Ophthalmol Oto-Laryngol 69:832–845

60. Osman I, Sherman E, Singh B, et al (2002) Alteration of p53 pathway in squamous cell carcinoma of the head and neck:impact on treatment outcome in patients treated with larynx preservation intent. J Clin Oncol 20:2980–2987

61. Overgaard J, Hansen HS, Overgaard M, et al (1998) A randomized double-blind phase III study of nimorazole as

hypoxic radiosensitizer of primary radiotherapy in supra glottic larynx and pharynx carcinoma. Results from the Danish Head and Neck Cancer Study (DAHANCA). Protocol 5–85. Radiother Oncol 46:135–146

62. Parkin DM, Muir CS, Whelan SL, Gao Y-T, Ferlay J, Powell J (1992) Cancer incidence in five continents, vol VI. IARC Scientific Publications, Lyon

63. Parkin DM, Pisani P, Ferlay J (1999) Global cancer statistics. CA Cancer J Clin 49:33–64

64. Pfister D, Laurie SA, Weinstein GS, et al (2006) American Society of Clinical Oncology Practice Guidelines for the use of larynx preservation strategies in the treatment of laryngeal cancer. J Clin Oncol 24:3604–3693

65. Pignon JP, Bourhis J, Domenge C, Designe L (2000) Chemotherapy added to locoregional treatment for head and neck squamous-cell carcinoma:three meta-analyses of updated individual data. Lancet 355:949–955

66. Porceddu SV, Jarmolowski E, Hicks RJ, et al (2005) Utility of positron emission tomography for the detection of disease in residual neck nodes after chemo-radiotherapy in head and neck cancer. Head Neck 27:175–181

67. Posner MR (2005) Paradigm shift in the treatment of head and neck cancer: the role of neoadjuvant chemotherapy. Oncologist 10:11–19

68. Richard JM, Sancho-Garnier H, Pessey JJ, et al (1998) Randomized trial of induction chemotherapy in larynx carcinoma. Oral Oncol 34:224–228

69. Ries LAG, Eisner MP, Kosary CL, et al (1973–1998) SEER Cancer Statistics Review. National Cancer Institute. Bethesda, MD

70. Roh JL, Pae KH et al (2007) 2-[18F]-Fluoro-2-deoxy-D-glucose positron emission tomography as guidance for primary treatment in patients with advanced-stage resectable squamous cell carcinoma of the larynx and hypopharynx Eur J Surg Oncol 33(6):790–795

71. Rothman KJ, Cann CI, Flanders D, Fried MP (1980) Epidemiology of laryngeal cancer. Epidemiol Rev 2:195–209

72. Ryan WR, Fee Jr WE, Le QT, Pinto HA (2005) Positron-emission tomography for surveillance of head and neck cancer. Laryngoscope 115:645–650

73. Segas JV, Hantzakos AG, Tzagaroulakis AM, Adamapoulos GK (2001) A novel technique in the operative treatment of pyriform sinus carcinoma. Acta Otolaryngol 121(4): 529–533

74. Schweitzer VG (2001) PHOTOFRIN-mediated photodynamic therapy for treatment of early stage oral cavity and laryngeal malignancies. Lasers Surg Med 29:305–313

75. Teknos TN, Cox C, Barrios MA, et al (2002) Tumor angiogenesis as a predictive marker for organ preservation in patients with advanced laryngeal carcinoma. Laryngoscope 112:844–851

76. The Department of Veterans Affairs Laryngeal Cancer Study Group (1991) Induction chemotherapy plus radiation compared with surgery plus radiation in patients with advanced laryngeal cancer. N Engl J Med 324:1685–1690

77. The Royal College of Surgeons of England, London (2000) Effective head & neck cancer management: Second consensus document. British Association of Otorhinolaryngologists, Head and Neck Surgeons, London

78. Trask DK, Wolf GT, Bradford CR, et al (2002) Expression of Bcl-2 family proteins in advanced laryngeal squamous cell carcinoma: correlation with response to chemotherapy and organ preservation. Laryngoscope 112:638–644

79. Tuyns AJ, Esteve J, Raymond L, et al (1988) Cancer of the larynx/hypopharynx, tobacco and alcohol: IARC international case-control study in Turin and Varese (Italy), Zaragoza and Navarra (Spain), Geneva (Switzerland) and Calvados (France). Int J Cancer 41:483–491

80. Wahlberg P, Andersson H, Biörklund A, Möller A (1998) Carcinoma of the hypopharynx: analysis of incidence and survival in Sweden over a 30-year period. Head Neck 20(8):714–719

81. Watanabe A, Taniguchi M, Tsujie H et al. (2009). The value of narrow band imaging for early detection of laryngeal cancer. Eur Arch Otorhinolaryngol 266(7):1017–1023

82. Weinstein GS, El-Sawy MM, Ruiz C, et al (2001) Laryngeal preservation with supracricoid partial laryngectomy results in improved quality of life when compared with total laryngectomy. Laryngoscope 111:191–199

83. Wenberger PM, Yu Z, Haffty BG, et al (2006) Molecular classification identifies a subset of human Papillomavirus-associated oropharyngeal cancers with favorable prognosis. J Clin Oncol 24:736–747

84. Wong RJ, Lin DT, Schoder H, et al (2002) Diagnostic and prognostic value of [(18)F]fluorodeoxyglucose positron emission tomography for recurrent head and neck squamous cell carcinoma. J Clin Oncol 20:4199–4208

85. Wynder EL, Bross IJ, Feldman RM (1957) A study of etiological factors in cancer of the mouth. Cancer 10: 1300–1323

86. Barnes L, Eveson JW, Reichart P, Sidransky D (eds.) (2005) World Health Organization Classification of Tumours. Pathology and genetics of head and neck tumours. IARC Press, Lyon

Endoscopic Approach

13b

Hans Edmund Eckel, Giorgio Perretti, Marc Remacle, and Jochen Werner

Core Messages

> Transoral laser surgery is suited for the curative treatment of most T1–T2 carcinomas of the glottic and supraglottic larynx.

> The main advantage of this minimal access approach is reduced perioperative morbidity and hospital stay. Tracheotomy is usually not required, but postoperative monitoring in an intensive or intermediate care unit may be needed following more extensive procedures.

> Shielding the endotracheal tube is essential to avoid serious airway complications (ignition of oxygen)

> Postoperative aspiration (following surgery for supraglottic tumors or following arytenoid cartilage resection), secondary bleeding, dental injuries, and mucosal tears are the most common complications and sequelae.

> Exhaustive technical equipment, including contemporary CO_2 laser systems and focusing devices, operating laryngoscopes, multiple suction devices, and specially designed instruments are required for successful endoscopic tumor surgery.

> Comprehensive training in head and neck surgery and specialized instruction in the use of medical lasers is mandatory for laryngologists performing these procedures.

H. E. Eckel (✉)
Department of Oto-Rhino-Laryngology,
A.ö. Landeskrankenhaus Klagenfurt, HNO, St. Veiter Str. 47,
A-9020 Klagenfurt, Austria
e-mail: hans.eckel@kabeg.at

Two novel approaches to the treatment of laryngeal and hypopharyngeal carcinoma have contributed to the spectrum of therapeutic options during the past two decades: transoral laser surgery, mostly used for early-stage carcinoma and sequential or concomitant chemotherapy and radiotherapy for organ preservation in advanced stages.

Although transoral approaches to head and neck carcinoma are certainly not new, they have long been given up for open surgical approaches that seemed more promising with regard to surgical radicality and oncological outcome. Transoral approaches were thought to be inadequate for oncological interventions because of what was believed to be limited visualization of the surgical field, bleeding, difficult manipulation, and inability to reconstruct soft tissue defects.

With technical advances in endoscopic surgery during the 1960s achieved by Kleinsasser [1] and his microlaryngoscopic technique of endolaryngeal microsurgery and the implementation of medical laser systems by Strong and Jako in the 1970s [2], things gradually changed beginning in the early 1980s. Clinical pioneers such as Grossenbacher, Motta, Rudert and Steiner in Europe and Vaughn, Davis, and Shapshay in North America were able to demonstrate that highly selected malignant lesions of the upper aerodigestive tract could now be operated on endoscopically with promising oncological and functional results.

These authors were able to show that transoral laser surgery provides advantages relating to its hemostatic effects and precision of tissue ablation. They reported that laser surgery causes minimal morbidity, offers good functional results, and provides a cost-effective alternative to open surgical procedures and to radiotherapy.

Therefore, transoral laser surgery is now a widely used surgical approach to small glottic and supraglottic carcinomas [3–6]. Moreover, successful treatment of

M. Remacle, H. E. Eckel (eds.), *Surgery of Larynx and Trachea*,
DOI: 10.1007/978-3-540-79136-2_13b, © Springer-Verlag Berlin Heidelberg 2010

stage II to IV lesions of the vocal folds, supraglottic larynx, oropharynx, and hypopharynx have repeatedly been reported in the literature [5–8]. The data presented in these studies indicated that transoral laser surgery leads to oncological results that are comparable to those attained with more conventional treatment modalities in selected groups of patients, and the surgical trauma- and treatment-related co-morbidites are reduced.

13b.1 Preoperative Diagnostic Procedures

The endoscopic management of laryngeal and hypopharyngeal tumors requires a meticulous preoperative evaluation of the patient (in terms of adequate exposure of the surgical field under microlaryngoscopy) and of the lesion itself. All available technical tools (including both endoscopy and imaging) should be employed to define the superficial and deep extension of the tumor precisely. Moreover, regional lymph nodes should be assessed before planning the most appropriate treatment with a simultaneous or delayed procedure on the neck.

Endoscopy represents the first-line diagnostic procedure to be considered as the gold standard for clinical tumor staging of the larynx and hypopharynx. Flexible and rigid fiberoptic endoscopes coupled to videolaryngoscopy allow us to obtain clear, magnified images of the superficial extension of the lesion, with the unique opportunity to assess laryngeal mobility and sensation. With glottic tumors, special consideration should be paid to evaluate uni- or bilateral vocal cord involvement, anterior commissure extension, and supra- or subglottic spread. With supraglottic and hypopharyngeal tumors, the precise evaluation of neoplastic extension to critical anatomical areas—e.g., the glottic plane, ventricle, aryepiglottic folds, piriform sinus, valleculae, base of the tongue—is of paramount importance to modulate the endoscopic surgical resection. In this light, the possibility of tailoring the resection intraoperatively based on microlaryngoscopic evaluation of the tumor allows the surgeon an additional degree of freedom not conceivable with the conservative open-neck approaches. In fact, resection of supraglottic tumors (e.g., involving the anterior commissure) are best performed by an endoscopic route. Currently, vocal cord and arytenoid mobility cannot be evaluated by objective measurements, and their function can only be expressed by generic terms ranging from impaired vocal cord mobility (due to a tumor mass or limited vocal muscle invasion) to fixation (for deep muscle infiltration or paraglottic space, cricoarytenoid joint, or recurrent nerve involvement).

Even though associated with a high degree of intra- and interjudge variability because of its subjectivity and the possibility of false-positive findings for adjacent inflammatory changes, preoperative videolaryngostroboscopy (VLS) by 70° or 90° rigid endoscopes allows macroscopic evaluation of glottic lesions and patterns of mucosal wave correlated with the degree of vocal ligament involvement. In fact, maintenance of the mucosal wave is an indirect sign of an intraepithelial lesion (up to carcinoma in situ), whereas a reduced or absent mucosal wave is suspicious for neoplasms transgressing the basal membrane into the lamina propria (ranging from microinvasive to frankly invasive carcinomas).

From a clinical point of view, rigid endoscopy under local anesthesia for supraglottic and hypopharyngeal tumors is not fully reliable owing to the difficulty of properly evaluating bulky tumors obscuring the anterior commissure and vocal cords, the ventricle, and the piriform sinus. In such a scenario, a flexible fiberscope is by far the most useful tool to evaluate vocal cord and/or arytenoid mobility as well as piriform sinus symmetrical expansion during phonation and swallowing.

Subsequently, a more detailed multiperspective endoscopic view of the larynx can be obtained by 0° and angled (30°, 70°, 120°) rigid telescopes during microlaryngoscopy. In this way, zones of the larynx and hypopharynx (anterior and posterior commissures, bottom and roof of the ventricle, subglottis, apex of the piriform sinus, and postcricoid area) traditionally considered "dark" can be adequately visualized (Fig. 13b.1). Adjunctive information can be obtained by combining the use of angled telescopes with special probes or microinstrumentation to evert and palpate the free edge of the true vocal cords, lift the false vocal folds to inspect the ventricle, and divaricate the arytenoids. Additionally, accurate palpation of the base of tongue and medial wall of the piriform sinus, arytenoid mobilization, displacement of the epiglottis to evaluate anterior commissure involvement, and exploration of the piriform sinus apex and postcricoid region can also be performed in the same setting of the intraoperative diagnostic workup. Moreover, adjunctive staging information can be derived from surgical maneuvers performed at the beginning of the endoscopic resection, such as infrapetiolar exploration to evaluate minimal

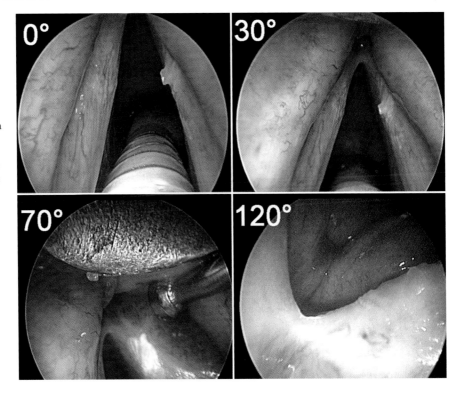

Fig. 13b.1. Intraoperative rigid endoscopy by 0° and angled (30°, 70°, 120°) telescopes of a leukoplastic lesion of the middle third of the right vocal cord clearly defines its superficial extension. Lifting the right false vocal fold by means of a curved suction tip coupled to a 70° rigid telescope allows exclusion of lateral extension to the floor and bottom of the ventricle

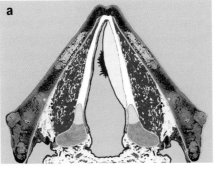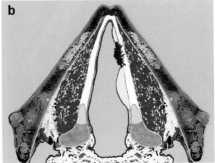

Fig. 13b.2. Two similar lesions of the middle third of the right vocal fold. (**a**) Complete mucoligamentous hydrodissection after intraoperative saline infusion (SI) into Reinke's space; the lesion is therefore limited to the overlying mucosal epithelium. (**b**) Incomplete ballooning of the epithelial layer due to initial involvement of the lamina propria

inner thyroid lamina involvement and transtumoral resection (e.g., at the level of the mid-suprahyoid epiglottis) to exclude preepiglottic space invasion [5].

In cases of glottic cancer limited to the true vocal cord, subepithelial saline infusion (SI) by means of an appropriately angled needle allows further confirmation of preoperative VLS findings regarding involvement of the lamina propria by the neoplastic growth. Complete hydrodissection of the mucoligamentous plane, with consequent ballooning and lifting of the lesion from the underlying intermediate layer of the lamina propria suggests purely intraepithelial confinement of the neoplastic nests. Moreover, the mechanical expansion of Reinke's space after SI facilitates subsequent removal of the lesion itself, serving as a heat sink to protect the vocal ligament from thermal damage in the case of a laser procedure. An incomplete or absent mucoligamentous hydrodissection after SI has the same implications as a reduced or absent mucosal wave as detected on the VLS, and it is associated with transgression of the basal membrane by neoplastic cells through the vocal ligament (Fig. 13b.2). Even SI in

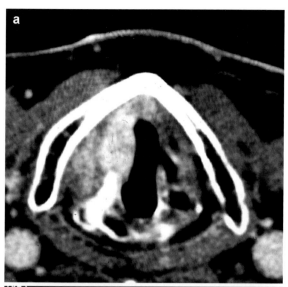

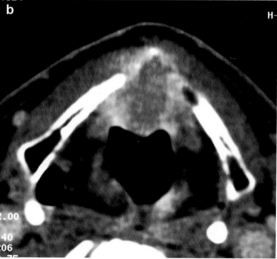

Fig. 13b.3. Preoperative axial computed tomography (CT) scans after contrast medium administration. (**a**) Right paraglottic space involvement of a tumor extending from the anterior commissure (with increased thickness) to the arytenoid cartilage (sclerosed and without the normal fat tissue posterolateral to its body). (**b**) Anterior transcommissural lesion involving the preepiglottic space and massively eroding the thyroid cartilage at the level of its notch, beyond the external perichondrium, with possible initial infiltration of the deep layer of the strap muscles

Reinke's space is associated with possible drawbacks, mainly concerning false-negative cases in the event of limited lamina propria involvement by a few nests of neoplastic cells. For this reason, the results of intraoperative SI should always be integrated with those of preoperative VLS. If the two tests give conflicting results, the cordectomy should be tailored according to

the more pessimistic scenario (i.e., as if they were both positive for vocal ligament involvement). Applying such a simple diagnostic algorithm in the University of Brescia, Italy, the combination of VLS and SI obtained specificity, sensitivity, positive predictive values (PPV), negative predictive values (NPV), and accuracy of 89%, 100%, 88%, 100%, and 94%, respectively [9].

Integration of endoscopic findings with those from radiological imaging is nowadays an essential prerequisite for correct staging and treatment of any neoplastic lesion of the larynx and hypopharynx. As a matter of fact, relying on the endoscopic information alone can lead to clinical underdiagnosis in 40–55% of cases [10] with consequent inappropriate therapeutic planning and less effective locoregional oncological control. Recently, computed tomography (CT) (with particular emphasis on the multislice technique) and magnetic resonance imaging (MRI) are playing a definite role in imaging for preoperative assessment of laryngeal and hypopharyngeal cancer. CT scanning presents some unique advantages, making this diagnostic tool the gold standard in the modern radiological assessment of these tumors. Its reduced examination time with minimal patient compliance needed and wide availability make it a sound diagnostic tool. Only a few elements of uncertainty arise, such as in the presence of minimal thyroid cartilage erosion and paraglottic space involvement. In such selected cases, subsequent MRI scans can increase diagnostic accuracy, even though roughly 20% of them display movement artifacts, thereby reducing the imaging quality (Fig. 13b.3).

The radiological checklist for the endoscopic surgeon should therefore always include an assessment of invasion of the visceral spaces (with particular reference to submucosal supracommissural and/or subcommissural extension, posterolateral paraglottic space invasion, and preepiglottic space involvement), laryngeal framework infiltration, and tumor extension beyond laryngeal sites (e.g., base of the tongue, soft tissues and major vessels of the neck, prevertebral fascia) (Fig. 13b.4).

The N category plays a definitive role in terms of prognosis of these tumors, particularly when dealing with supraglottic and hypopharyngeal bulky lesions. Combining clinically evident and occult lymph nodes metastases from intermediate (T2–T3) supraglottic and hypopharyngeal tumors, more than 30% can be expected to present regional disease at the time of diagnosis. In this respect, the gold standard imaging technique is ultrasonography examination of the neck

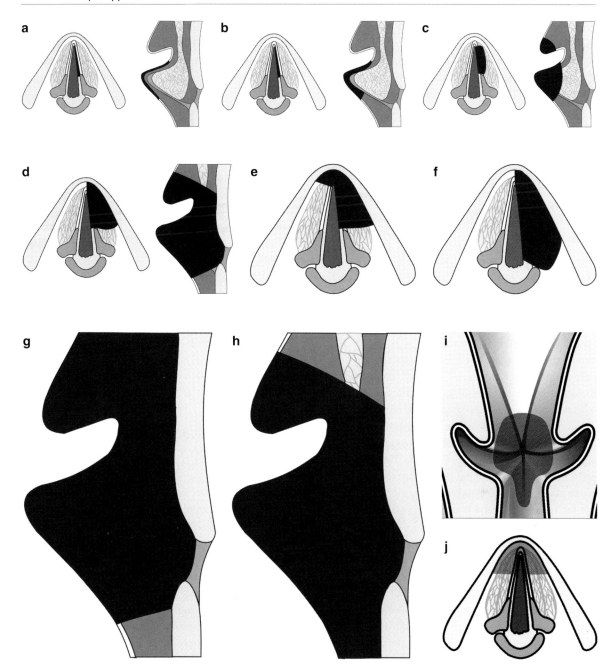

Fig. 13b.4. Endoscopic cordectomy. Proposal for a classification by the Working Committee, European Laryngological Society that is a synthesis of the year 2000 classification and the 2007 modification. (**a**) Subepithelial cordectomy (type I). (**b**) Subligamental cordectomy (type II). (**c**) Transmuscular cordectomy (type III). (**d**) Total or complete cordectomy (type IV). (**e**) Extended cordectomy encompassing the contralateral vocal fold (type Va). (**f**) Extended cordectomy encompassing the arytenoid (type Vb). (**g**) Extended cordectomy encompassing the ventricular fold (type Vc). (**h**) Extended cordectomy encompassing the subglottis (type Vd). (**i, j**) Cordectomy for cancers arising from the anterior commissure (type VI). (Reprinted with permission (From Remacle et al. [12, 13], with permission)

combined with fine-needle aspiration cytology of suspicious lymph nodes. Such a technique surpasses the diagnostic accuracy of CT and MRI, allowing detection of occult metastatic foci in nodes < 5 mm in greatest diameter. Precise preoperative assessment of the neck status can play a decisive role in choosing between an endoscopic procedure alone or an endoscopic procedure combined with simultaneous or delayed, unilateral or bilateral neck dissection.

13b.1.1 Surgical Technique

The CO_2 surgical laser is clearly the preferred laser system for oncological surgery of the larynx. It is coupled to an operating microscope and is generally set at an output power of 2–6 W in a super pulse or continuous mode at a spot size of approximately 0.8 mm^2. Patients are intubated transorally (using a laser-shielded tube) for surgery except for those who have a preexisting tracheotomy. Various laryngoscopes, including bivalved adjustable laryngoscopes, are used to expose the larynx. Repeated readjustment and repositioning of the laryngoscope is frequently required to achieve optimal exposition of the surgical field. Two suction devices should be available throughout the operation: One is mounted on the operating laryngoscope, and the other is handled by the surgeon throughout the intervention and is used to evacuate the plume and manipulate the tissue.

Specimens are resected in one piece whenever possible. In every case, the tumor must be resected with sufficient safety margins—which is equally important during laser surgery and open approaches—and R0 resection must be confirmed histologically. The development of modern laser systems permits laser application with lower power settings so that charring and necrosis of specimen margins could be reduced in comparison to older laser systems. Thus, the pathologists can accurately evaluate the resection margins.

Dissection of a tumor in two or more portions (a concept introduced by W. Steiner, Göttingen, Germany) allows the surgeon to scrutinize the cutting surfaces under the microscope and make a more confident assessment of the depth of tumor invasion. Up to now, no definitive arguments could be found against piecemeal laser resection even if a higher risk of increased metastasis seems possible based on an animal experimental study [11].

However, those examinations were performed in a highly aggressive tumor model on lymphogenic metastatic spread, so further studies are required. Although the question is not yet settled, cutting through malignant tumors during surgery does not comply with the generally accepted basic concepts of oncological surgery. If large tumors are to be resected transorally, the surgeon has to weigh the advantages of transecting the tumor for easier handling of the specimen against the potential dangers of manipulation-related tumor spread.

Specimens should be oriented anatomically after removal to facilitate histopathological examination of the margins. The value of frozen sections remains unclear to date, and not all experienced laser surgeons use them routinely.

Patients should receive 250 mg of methylprednisolone intravenously during the intervention and 80 mg orally during the first 2–5 days after surgery depending on the extent of the surgery. Extubation is usually performed some 30 minutes after the end of the intervention, and patients must be closely observed after extubation for airway control.

13b.1.2 Classification of Procedures for Glottic Carcinoma

In the year 2000, the European Laryngological Society (ELS) Working Committee on Nomenclature proposed a classification of endolaryngeal procedures for the treatment of glottic dysplasia and carcinoma. They did so with the aim of reaching better agreement and uniformity concerning the extent and depth of resection of cordectomy procedures (guidelines) by offering reproducibility to laryngologists to allow relevant comparisons with the literature when presenting/publishing the results of cordectomy [12]. The classification was meant to be a synthesis of the categorizations available in the literature and the classifications that had been previously and separately presented by some authors. The aim was not to define or restrict therapeutic indications. Rather, by means of this common classification, the authors hoped to permit comparison of postoperative results achieved by different centers and to improve instruction and training of younger surgeons.

The classification described eight types of cordectomy: subepithelial cordectomy (type I); subligamental cordectomy (type II); transmuscular cordectomy (type III); total cordectomy (type IV); extended cordectomy including the contralateral vocal fold and the anterior commissure (type Va); one arytenoid cartilage (type Vb); subglottic structures (type Vc); or the ventricle and paraglottic space (type Vd). This classification was subsequently used by many surgeons to describe their endoscopic interventions. However, the classification did not propose any specific management for lesions originating in the anterior commissure, which have been included so far among the indications for type Va cordectomy. This situation was a source of discussion and possible confusion when comparing results from different studies.

To resolve this problem, a new cordectomy category, encompassing the anterior commissure and the anterior part of both vocal folds—type VI cordectomy—was proposed by the ELS Working Committee on Nomenclature in 2007 [13]. The members of the working committee thought that tumors with invasion of the thyroid or cricoid cartilages or arytenoid cartilage fixation were not suitable candidates for transoral laser surgery. Therefore, the classification does not include resection types for these advanced (T3 and T4) glottic carcinoma. A synthesis of the year 2000 classifications and the 2007 modification is given here (Fig. 13b.4 a–i).

13b.1.2.1 Subepithelial Cordectomy (Type I)

Subepithelial cordectomy is resection of the vocal fold epithelium, passing through the superficial layer of the lamina propria. This surgical procedure spares the deeper layers and thus the vocal ligament. Subepithelial cordectomy is performed for cases of vocal fold lesions suspected of premalignant or malignant transformation. As the entire epithelium is generally affected in various degrees of severity, it is usually necessary to resect it completely to avoid leaving in place a dysplastic or even carcinomatous area. In rarer cases where epithelial modifications are restricted to a segment of the vocal fold, the clinically normal epithelium may be preserved. Because subepithelial cordectomy ensures histopathological examination of the entire epithelium of the vocal fold, the main role of this surgical procedure is diagnostic. It can also be therapeutic if histological results confirm hyperplasia, dysplasia, or carcinoma in situ without signs of microinvasion. Indeed, by definition, these lesions are limited to the

epithelium. If, on the other hand, there are signs of invasive tumor spread, a further procedure is required.

13b.1.2.2 Subligamental Cordectomy (Type II)

Subligamental cordectomy is resection of the epithelium, Reinke's space, and the vocal ligament. It is performed by cutting between the vocal ligament and the vocal muscle. The vocal muscle is preserved as much as possible. The resection may extend from the vocal process to the anterior commissure. At a diagnostic level, this procedure is indicated for cases of severe leukoplakia when a lesion shows clinical signs of neoplastic transformation and stroboscopic examination indicates deep infiltration, or "vibratory silence." When palpated, this infiltration feels thickened and the mucosa cannot freely be moved over the underlying structures. At a therapeutic level, subligamental cordectomy is indicated for cases of microinvasive carcinoma or severe carcinoma in situ with possible microinvasion.

13b.1.2.3 Transmuscular Cordectomy (Type III)

Transmuscular cordectomy is performed by cutting through the vocalis muscle. The resection encompasses the epithelium, lamina propria, and part of the vocalis muscle. The resection may extend from the vocal process to the anterior commissure. Partial resection of the ventricular fold may be necessary to expose the entire vocal fold. Transmuscular cordectomy is indicated for small superficial cancers of the mobile vocal fold that reach the vocalis muscle without deeply infiltrating it.

13b.1.2.4 Total or Complete Cordectomy (Type IV)

Complete cordectomy extends from the vocal process to the anterior commissure. The depth of the surgical margins reaches the internal perichondrium of the thyroid ala. Sometimes the perichondrium is included with the resection. Anteriorly, the incision is made in the anterior commissure. It is important that the attachment of the vocal ligament to the thyroid cartilage is cut. Complete cordectomy is indicated for T1a cancer infiltrating the vocalis muscle. Extension of a neoplasm may spread as far as the anterior commissure without involving it.

13b.1.2.5 Extended Cordectomy Encompassing the Contralateral Vocal Fold (Type Va)

Extended cordectomy was meant to include the anterior commissure and, depending on the extent of the tumor, either a segment or the entire contralateral vocal fold. This approach is somewhat controversial because resection around the anterior commissure is technically difficult and leads to poor phonatory results. This resection type is now commonly replaced by type VI cordectomy.

13b.1.2.6 Extended Cordectomy Encompassing the Arytenoid (Type Vb)

Extended cordectomy encompassing the arytenoid is indicated for vocal fold carcinoma involving the vocal process or the arytenoid cartilage posteriorly. The arytenoid cartilage should be mobile. The cartilage is partially or totally resected. The posterior arytenoid mucosa may be preserved if this decision seems oncologically sound.

13b.1.2.7 Extended Cordectomy Encompassing the Ventricular Fold (Type Vc)

According to certain schools, total cordectomy can be extended to the mucosa of Morgagni's ventricle, the paraglottic tissues, and the ventricular fold. This procedure (type Vc) is indicated for ventricular cancers or for transglottic cancers that spread from the vocal fold to the ventricle. The specimen encompasses the ventricular fold and Morgani's ventricle.

13b.1.2.8 Extended Cordectomy Encompassing the Subglottis (Type Vd)

If necessary, cord resection can be continued underneath the glottis to expose the cricoid cartilage (Fig. 13b.8). In selected cases, this extended cordectomy (type Vd) is suitable for T2 carcinoma with limited subglottic extension without cartilage invasion.

13b.1.2.9 Cordectomy for Cancers Arising from the Anterior Commissure (Type VI)

Type VI cordectomy is indicated for cancer originating in the anterior commissure, extended (or not) to one or both vocal folds, without infiltration of the thyroid cartilage. The surgery comprises anterior commissurectomy with bilateral anterior cordectomy. If the tumor is in close contact with the cartilage, resection can encompass the anterior angle of the thyroid cartilage. To remove Broyle's ligament, the incision must be started above the insertion plane of the vocal folds, at the base of the epiglottic insertion, and is extended through Broyle's ligament. To achieve this resection, it may be necessary to resect the petiole of the epiglottis and the anterior parts of the ventricular folds to ensure sufficient visualization. Resection of the anterior commissure may include the subglottic mucosa and cricothyroid membrane because cancers of the anterior commissure tend to spread toward the lymphatic vessels of the subglottic area.

13b.1.3 Supraglottic Carcinomas

Among the indications for laser surgery in patients with laryngeal cancer, surgical treatment of supraglottic carcinoma plays a prominent role. This is mainly due to the often better functional results than those achieved with open partial resection [14, 15]. Of course, there remain indications for open surgery, which is, again, a reason why head and neck surgeons should be trained in the complete field of laryngeal surgery and not focus uniquely on one treatment method [6, 16, 17]. In the following, however—and this is the objective of this chapter—laser surgery of supraglottic carcinoma is described with its main aspects.

The main advantage of transoral laser microsurgery is that the resection can be tailored to the extent of the tumor [5, 18, 19]. Instead of using an open technique, the surgeon can proceed according to the often clear delineation between healthy and affected tissue provided by the operating microscope.

Endoscopic laser surgery is most appropriate for resecting carcinomas on the free edge of the epiglottis, central suprahyoid carcinomas, and carcinomas located on the lingual surface of the epiglottis, on the margins of the ventricular fold, or on the aryepiglottic folds.

En bloc resection is mainly possible for small, circumscribed carcinomas of the supraglottis; the technique is comparable to resection of early glottic cancer. Laser microsurgery can be recommended because carcinomas in this area can be resected with more sufficient safety margins compared to glottic carcinomas. The postoperative functional results are highly satisfactory.

Tumor infiltration of carcinomas of the infrahyoid epiglottis is rather difficult to determine preoperatively, particularly in the area of the petiole. Thus, it is often also difficult to stage T1 and T3 carcinomas preoperatively. However, clinical experience shows that infiltration of the preepiglottic space must be considered with all carcinomas of the infrahyoid region. In cases of infiltration, laser surgery is not contraindicated; but this surgery requires complete exposure of the tumor after division of the preepiglottic fat pad. This goal may best be achieved by cutting through the vallecula with the laser. Bleeding of the vessels is controlled with conventional electrocautery or by means of titanium clips, which have proved to be appropriate. The medial glossoepiglottic fold is divided, requiring splitting the suprahyoid epiglottis in the sagittal plane. Parasagittal incision must also be considered occasionally if it facilitates exposure of lateral supraglottic structures (e.g., the aryepiglottic fold). After exposure of the preepiglottic fat and the laryngeal aspect of the tumor-bearing infrahyoid epiglottis, the tumor is divided in the sagittal direction, and the incision is performed vertically. Sometimes the advanced-stage tumor requires transverse incision of the lesion. If tumor infiltration into the thyroid cartilage or one of the arytenoid cartilages is found, these areas can be included in the resection. Depending on the extent of resection, unilateral arytenoid resection causes more or less significant postoperative swallowing difficulties. Resection of both arytenoid cartilages must be avoided to prevent persistent severe postoperative dysphagia with aspiration. The surgeon must always be aware when resecting extensive lesions that the resection margins may extend from inside the larynx into the subcutaneous tissue of the neck.

In contrast to open surgery, nasogastric tube feeding can usually be limited to only a few days, and temporary tracheostomy can generally be avoided. Thus, the endoscopic technique can be considered mostly superior to conventional open surgery with regard to quality of life, especially during the first postoperative weeks. Furthermore, there is no age limit compared to open supraglottic partial laryngectomy. Transoral CO_2 laser surgery can be called the method of choice for tumor resection of lesions in the above-mentioned sites and

stages as the functional results and the obviously better oncological results are superior to those attained with primary radiochemotherapy.

Of course, this does not mean that supraglottic partial laryngectomy performed with CO_2 laser is a risk-free method. The author has seen cases in which there was significant postoperative bleeding or persistent functional deficits such as swallowing difficulties with aspiration. However, this is no criticism of laser surgery in itself but should emphasize the risks and make surgeons more aware to the importance of careful postoperative follow-up. Regarding the risk of postoperative bleeding, it must be ensured that patients are under continuous supervision during the postoperative phase so they can be adequately treated in case of an emergency, including provision of rapid intubation if required.

At this point, the limitations and complications of transoral laser surgery of laryngeal carcinomas must be mentioned. Several publications have reported on this topic since 1971, and a series of possible complications has been identified: local infection, emphysema, fistulation, bleeding, respiratory distress due to stenosis or edema, swallowing difficulties, and aspiration pneumonia [20, 21]. The complication rate is determined mainly by the experience of the surgeon. Furthermore, it became obvious that the complications are less frequent after laser surgery of early laryngeal cancer than after laser treatment of advanced carcinoma.

Large supraglottic tumors can also be resected transorally when the tumor can be clearly exposed and the intervention is performed by an experienced surgeon. In these cases, laser surgery is much less limited by the technical possibilities than by the functional outcome. The patient may, for example, experience postoperative swallowing difficulties depending on the extent of the resection in the arytenoid region. It was mentioned previously that the resection of both arytenoid cartilages should be avoided because it would cause significant postoperative dysphagia with inevitable aspiration. Similar problems may occur when unilateral resection of the arytenoid cartilage is performed together with resection of the corresponding base of the tongue.

Even the laryngeal skeleton may be affected by postoperative complications. Most frequently it is observed in patients who have received pre- or postoperative radiochemotherapy. Protracted chondritis is sometimes seen, including formation of cartilaginous or bony sequestra that can often but not always be removed by a transoral access. Laser surgical treatment of advanced laryngeal carcinomas requires a particularly high degree of experience and technical training of the surgeon. It is easy to see that it is difficult to resect advanced supraglottic carcinomas through a narrow tube—far more difficult than tumor resection by an open approach. If piecemeal resection is applied, it requires a high degree of concentration by the surgeon and close cooperation with the pathologist to assess the adequacy of the resection margins accurately. Hence, we can understand the need for intensive training programs in transoral laser microsurgery to achieve excellent results. Clinical training should start with laser surgery of circumscribed supraglottic lesions. After gaining more experience, the treatment spectrum can be enlarged to more extended supraglottic carcinomas.

Established oncological principles should always determine the most suitable treatment concepts of supraglottic cancer. This is especially true for advanced supraglottic tumors, although carcinomas in their initial stages must also be taken seriously. There are still controversial discussions between the surgery and radiooncology departments. This problem should be resolved in the future so a substantial interdisciplinary discussion in the sense of tumor conferences may be established. This objective can be achieved by recognizing the personal and method-specific limitations of the various treatment options. Categorical rejection of one form of treatment is as wrong as radical advocacy of others. This is also true for transoral laser microsurgery of the supraglottic larynx. There are definite indications for laser surgery, but there are also considerable anatomical and functional limitations.

When discussing the optimal treatment option for supraglottic carcinomas, it must be considered that the primary tumor can be successfully treated by surgery and/or radiotherapy in most cases. The frequently poor prognosis of the patients suffering from laryngeal squamous cell cancer is generally based on the lymphogenic metastatic spread of this tumor and on the occurrence of distant metastases that may be observed in the further course of the disease.

To define individual treatment strategies, interdisciplinary discussions relating to those issues must be pursued from various aspects so a consensus can be found. Only by understanding that treatment of oncology patients is a specialized discipline and accepting that these patients must be treated in specialized centers can we finally be able to offer patients an optimized, individual treatment concept that is supported by an internationally established consensus.

13b.2 Recurrences: Follow-Up, Diagnosis, and Management

The essential prerequisite for endoscopic management of laryngeal and hypopharyngeal tumors is ensuring adequate patient compliance to a compulsive postoperative follow-up. Tailored endoscopic resections often are performed within millimetric safe margins and such an ultraconservative approach is potentially dangerous if the patient escapes regular controls by the same surgeon who performed the procedure. Particularly when dealing with tumors at high risk of recurrence—T2 glottic cancer with anterior transcommissural extension, T3 glottic or supraglottic tumors with lateral extension to the bottom of the ventricle and paraglottic space, every hypopharyngeal tumor—an even more strict clinical and radiological follow-up is strongly recommended (Figs. 13b.5 and 13b.6).

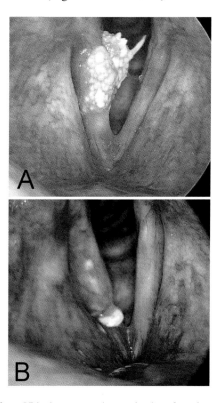

Fig. 13b.5. Videolaryngoscopic examination of a patient affected by a verrucous lesion of the middle third of the right vocal cord. The patient subsequently submitted to subligamental cordectomy (type II) (**a**). Videolaryngoscopic examinations of the same patient 9 months after surgery. A superficial leukoplasic lesion, suspicious for recurrence, was detected at the level of the anterior third of the residual vocal fold, requiring a second microlaryngoscopic procedure (**b**)

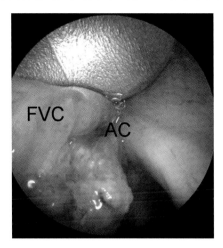

Fig. 13b.6. Intraoperative rigid endoscopy with a 70° telescope. Erythroplasic lesion involves the entire left vocal fold with massive extension to the floor, bottom, and roof of the ventricle. *AC*, anterior commissure; *FVC*, false vocal cord

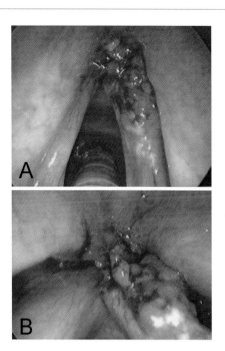

Fig. 13b.7. Superficial recurrence of mucosal dysplasia

In the University of Brescia experience, endoscopy under local anesthesia should be carried out at least every 2 months for the first 2 years after surgery and with decreasing frequency in the subsequent years. VLS can be added to the evaluation of patients treated for early glottic cancer, and the gold standard for all the other lesions remains VLS by rigid and/or flexible endoscopes. Video-recording and storage of serial postoperative controls can further assist in comparisons among clinical pictures possibly related to the healing process (granulomas, synechiae) or to suspicious recurrences and second tumors.

As previously described for the preoperative setting, strict cooperation between the endoscopic surgeon and an experienced radiologist is mandatory during follow-up. Our policy encompasses periodic CT scans (usually once a year during the first 2 years after surgery even in the absence of endoscopic abnormalities) in patients with T2–T3 glottic and supraglottic tumors. For hypopharyngeal lesions, we usually prefer MRI with the same time schedule. Any endoscopic abnormalities deemed not related to normal postoperative sequelae and with a possible deep pattern of disease progression should be immediately evaluated by the appropriate imaging examination. Neck monitoring should be performed with a closer attitude (ultrasonography every 4 months during the first 2 years) in patients with T3 glottic and T2–T3 supraglottic tumors submitted to a "wait and see" policy, and it can be used with longer intervals (once a year) in patients treated by neck dissection. In the case of suspicious ultrasonographic findings, fine-needle aspiration cytology is always recommended. The institutional strategy for postoperative oncological surveillance can vary widely depending on the site and stage of the primary lesion, local facilities, and population variables; but it should at least include evaluation of the chest once a year. Moreover, the recent introduction of positron emission tomography (PET)–CT scanning represents a potential tool for more effective and compulsive whole-body oncological follow-up.

Recurrences after endoscopic surgery can follow completely different patterns of progression. Aside from superficial persistence/recurrence of mucosal dysplasia with possible progression to invasive cancer (easily detected by endoscopic evaluation) (Fig. 13b.7), the main concerns of follow-up examination should always be directed to the early diagnosis of deep submucosal neoplastic progression to the visceral spaces, laryngeal framework, and soft tissues of the neck (Fig. 13b.8). Symptoms such as worsening dysphonia and progressive dysphagia with associated otalgia should always be taken into account, with a prompt, careful search for submucosal laryngohypopharyngeal bulging, impaired vocal cord and/or arytenoid mobility, and recurrent palsy. The presence of any of these clinical features should also prompt liberal use of CT or MRI of the neck and possibly the chest.

Fig. 13b.8. Video-laryngoscopic examination of a patient affected by erythroleukoplasic lesions involving both vocal cords (**a**). The patient submitted to an extended cordectomy (type Va) encompassing both false and true vocal folds. The patient was reevaluated 6 months later by flexible endoscope with detection of a suspicious area limited to the petiolar region. He was therefore submitted to CT scanning with detection of massive thyroid cartilage disruption (**b**). The patient underwent total laryngectomy (**c**). Cutting the specimen through a sagittal plane revealed massive infiltration of the preepiglottic space and cartilaginous framework (**d**)

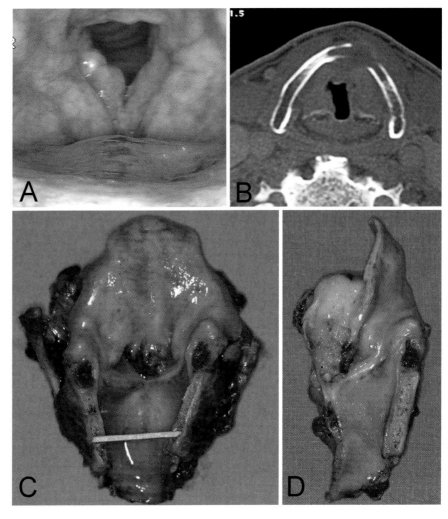

If there is a local recurrence, more re-treatment options are available after initial laser surgery than after initial radiotherapy or open surgery because wound complications as a result of previous irradiation are not encountered and the laryngeal framework is still intact, preventing early extralaryngeal spread of local failures [22]. Therefore, such recurrences allow further organ-sparing procedures if they are discovered in a timely way. In such situations, all treatment options are still available, such as further endolaryngeal surgery, conventional partial laryngectomy, radiotherapy, or total laryngectomy. Superficial persistence/recurrence either in subsites adjacent to the primary tumor or with a multifocal pattern resembling field cancerization usually has a favorable outcome when treated by further endoscopic resection. Complementary radiotherapy has a beneficial role in the presence of multiple local

recurrences after more than one surgical attempt and whenever the vocal outcome becomes a major issue while counseling the patient [23]. Oncological outcomes are usually not worsened in such a salvage scenario, being comparable to those observed in the primary therapeutic setting. By contrast, the situation of submucosal progression of residual neoplastic cells toward the deep visceral space is certainly much more difficult. Previous endoscopic removal of the natural barriers to tumor spread (Broyle's ligament, conus elasticus, vocal ligament, quadrangular membrane, epiglottis), though less important than with open-neck partial laryngectomy, makes the subsequent patterns of tumor diffusion unpredictable. However, preservation of the cartilaginous laryngeal framework during initial laser sugery prevent recurrences from spreading beyond the larynx.

For this reason, the use of endoscopic laser resection usually has been discouraged for infiltrating anterior commissure carcinoma because of inadequate exposure and the close proximity of underlying cartilage. Supracricoid open partial procedures may be more appropriate for these lesions as consistent data in the literature demonstrate that local control rates can be achieved with this technique that are clearly superior to those reported here [22].

13b.3 Sequelae and Functional Outcomes

One of the favorite arguments supporting radiotherapy for early glottic cancer has always been better vocal function when compared to cordectomy through thyrotomy and vertical partial laryngectomies [24]. Perhaps the most striking change that has emerged from the endoscopic approach is the possibility to precisely modulate the deep extent of resections in such a way that the term "cordectomy" alone is no longer appropriate to describe this procedure. In this light, the ELS classification allows one to define and clearly distinguish the extent of excision, which facilitates making meaningful comparisons between vocal outcomes after different types of cordectomy. Another consequence of such a classification is the possibility of comparing vocal outcome after endoscopic surgery with those achieved after radiotherapy.

Even though a truly complete voice evaluation has not yet been achieved, a comprehensive vocal analysis according to the ELS Working Committee [25] should include subjective evaluation using a questionnaire such as the Voice Handicap Index (VHI) [26], perceptual voice evaluation by a panel of Speech Pathologists and Otolaryngologists according to the GRBAS scale [27], and objective analysis by computerized systems including a number of parameters such as Fundamental Frequency, Jitter, Shimmer, and Noise to Harmonic Ratio. Following these guidelines, the University of Brescia retrospectively analyzed the functional outcomes after different types of cordectomy performed for early glottic cancer [28–31]. In those patients, we observed no statistically significant differences in the voice after types I and II cordectomy compared to a group of normal subjects. However, significant dysphonia has been documented only after type III, IV,

and V resections, mainly due to two key factors: anterior commissure synechiae (particularly after type Va cordectomy) and substantial glottic gap after removal of a significant amount of vocal muscle (more than one-third of its depth), necessitating a further phonosurgical procedure. Staged phonosurgery may be indicated in patients with severe dysphonia [32].

Fascinating future developments in the area of tissue engineering (e.g., replacement of the lamina propria by stem cells of autologous fibroblasts) will hopefully allow re-creation of the normal pliability of the vocal cord "cover" resected by endoscopic procedures. Nonetheless, the present state of the art of phonosurgery is limited to obtaining partial recovery of vocal function by purely acting on the medialization of the scarred vocal fold to close the glottic incompetence. In our experience, no adjunctive phonosurgical treatment was needed after types I and II cordectomy owing to the optimal postoperative conversational voice obtained after a standard voice therapy protocol and vocal hygiene, including voice rest for at least 2 weeks after surgery and smoking cessation. On the other hand, the glottic incompetence arising from wider resections could be corrected in different ways.

Our (Brescia) treatment policy is to restore good glottic closure immediately after type III cordectomy by a primary intracordal autologous fat injection (PIAFI) performed at the end of the endoscopic resection. Abdominal fat tissue is processed, avoiding any contact with air, and injected into the residual vocal muscle lateral to the vocal process (Fig. 13b.9). The increase in the neocord mass likely to be achieved is fine-tuned by precise modulation of the injection controlled by 30° rigid endoscopy. In this way, a near-normal conversational voice is obtained from the day after surgery owing to good glottic closure, which reduces vocal fatigue and social handicap. In particular, a comparison of vocal outcomes between patients treated by type III cordectomy alone with those submitted to this procedure followed by PIAFI showed a positive trend for the latter patients in terms of VHI and objective voice evaluations. Furthermore, a statistically significant improvement was reached in terms of the GRBAS scale. No complications or significant prolongation of the overall surgical time were observed as a result of PIAFI. A potential shortcoming of this technique is the variable resorption rate of the injected fat. However, this has not been observed to date during our short-term follow-up [33].

Fig. 13b.9. Primary intracordal autologous fat injection (PIAFI) after transmuscular cordectomy (type III). Note the glottic gap due to endoscopic resection (a) and its immediate correction after fat injection into the residual vocal muscle and paraglottic space (b)

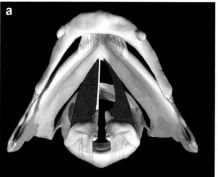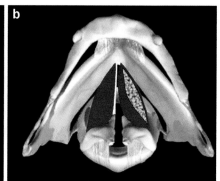

Other authors prefer to perform phonosurgical voice rehabilitation only following a disease-free interval of at least 6 months to 1 year. After this time, they may use standardized thyroplasty or vocal cord injection techniques [34–37].

After types IV and V cordectomy, a wider glottic gap usually reduces the possibility of good glottic closure, and the fibrotic nature of the neocord prevents any mucosal wave. After a mandatory lapse of at least 1 year, patients who are strongly motivated to improve vocal performance can be treated by personally tailored phonosurgical procedures, including medialization thyroplasty and/or anterior commissure laryngoplasty [37–39].

The first procedure is aimed at medializing the scarred neocord when a linear glottic gap is interposed between the operated side and the contralateral normal vocal fold in cases of type IV excision. In such a scenario, the use of autologous cartilage, titanium, or Gore-Tex implants allows us to modulate the amount of medialization precisely and gradually without any risk of mucosal penetration or overcorrection.

On the other hand, the anterior commissure laryngoplasty procedure is suggested in cases of "keyhole"-shaped anterior incompetence secondary to type Va cordectomy. Such a defect can be successfully corrected only by posteromedial displacement of the contralateral thyroid lamina under that of the more affected side. In this case, the normal vocal cord loses tension and is shortened with subsequent filling of the anterior "keyhole" gap. The reshaping of the thyroid cartilage is then stabilized by means of a rigid microplate (Fig. 13b.10).

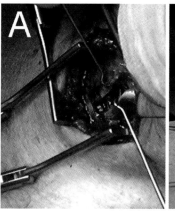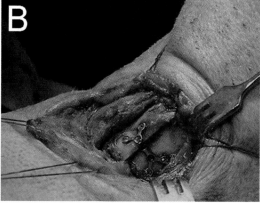

Fig. 13b.10. Intraoperative views during anterior commissure laryngoplasty according to Zeitels for correction of an anterior "'keyhole' gap after right type Va cordectomy. Thyrotomy is performed paramedially on the side of the less involved vocal cord (*left*) (**a**) to displace posteromedially the uninvolved thyroid lamina underneath the contralateral one (*right*). In such a way, detension of the left vocal fold combined with reshaping the anterior commissure closes the "keyhole" gap. This position is then maintained in place by a molded titanium microplate (**b**)

Our preliminary results after such phonosurgical approaches to the scarred vocal cord after types IV and V cordectomy showed improved glottic closure in 74% of patients when comparing the preoperative laryngoscopic examination with the postoperative one.

Swallowing is usually not impaired after standard types I–V cordectomy as defined by the ELS Classification. However, impairment may arise when the surgeon embraces more extended procedures to treat bulky T2 and T3 glottic tumors with significant subglottic and/or supraglottic extension, encompassing removal of both vocal cords, one or both the false vocal folds, the ventricle, and the petiole of the epiglottis (procedures that we usually define as endoscopic partial laryngectomy, or EPL, largely corresponding to the newly defined type VI cordectomy of the ELS classification) (Fig. 13b.11). A retrospective analysis of such patients treated at our institution revealed that they rarely needed postoperative nasogastric feeding tube (< 10% of cases and for a maximum 5 days), never required tracheostomy, and stayed in the hospital for a

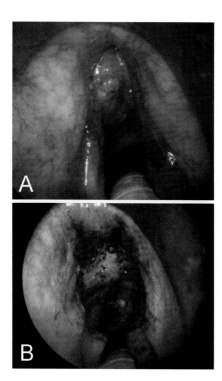

Fig. 13b.11. Intraoperative endoscopy of a T2 lesion with anterior transcommissural extension using a 0° rigid telescope (**a**). Laryngeal framework infiltration was ruled out by CT scans. Endoscopic partial laryngectomy was performed with exposure of the thyroid cartilage, cricothyroid membrane, and cricoid arch (**b**)

mean of 3 days. The postoperative voice after EPL turned out to be slightly better than that after supracricoid partial laryngectomy (SCPL) in patients matched for T category. However, the most important advantage of the endoscopic treatment when compared to the open-neck partial laryngectomy approach was in regard to the swallowing function. As a matter of fact, when we studied deglutition of patients treated by EPL, we found some kind of neovestibule and/or subglottic bolus aspiration in 20% of them by videoendoscopic examination of the swallow and in 27% by videofluoroscopy. These rates grew, respectively, to 57% and 71% when these diagnostic tools were applied to evaluating the swallow of patients treated by SCPL.

One of the most important advantages of endoscopic resection of supraglottic cancer compared to both radiotherapy and open-neck horizontal supraglottic laryngectomy is the possibility of excising the tumor within millimetric free margins while sparing adjacent uninvolved supraglottic subsites and structures such as hyoid bone, base of tongue musculature, prelaryngeal muscles, cartilaginous framework, and the external branch of the superior neurovascular pedicle (Fig. 13b.12). Such a cautious approach to laryngeal structures has a significantly better functional outcome in terms of perioperative morbidity and faster postoperative recovery of swallowing than that achieved with open-neck surgery.

A retrospective study was performed at our institution that compared two groups of patients affected by supraglottic tumors matched for T category and treated with horizontal supraglottic laryngectomy or endoscopic resections. A number of advantages become evident after endoscopic surgery [31]. All patients undergoing open-neck surgery needed both a tracheotomy and a nasogastric feeding tube compared to only 14% and 21%, respectively, of those who underwent endoscopic procedures. Moreover, when needed, the mean duration of tracheotomy and nasogastric feeding tube dependence were 35 and 19 days, respectively, for the open-neck group versus 4 and 5 days, respectively, for the endoscopic group. The mean hospitalization time was also significantly shorter after endoscopic procedures (10 vs. 26 days). A comprehensive evaluation of swallowing was performed by a subjective questionnaire employing the M.D. Anderson Dysphagia Inventory [40], videofluoroscopy, and videoendoscopic examination during deglutition of a colored gel. Even though subjective measurements by the M.D. Anderson

Fig. 13b.12. Modulation of endoscopic supraglottic resections from simple ventriculectomy (**a**, **b**), to partial (**c**, **d**), and complete (**e**, **f**) supraglottic laryngectomy

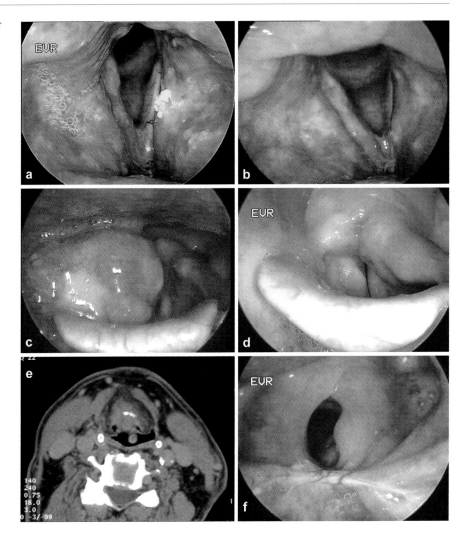

Dysphagia Inventory questionnaire showed similar results, there was a statistically significant difference when comparing the results obtained by the swallowing tests. Patients treated by open-neck surgery showed 36% and 80% rates of subglottic aspiration as detected by videoendoscopic evaluation of deglutition and videofluoroscopy, respectively, compared to 8% and 21% after endoscopic treatment, respectively. Therefore, in the case of supraglottic tumors, impaired swallowing fundamentally affects patients' quality of life, whereas voice function usually does not represent a major concern. This assumption was confirmed by our comprehensive evaluation of the voice by VHI, GRBAS, and objective analysis, which showed no statistically significant differences between the two groups and a matched control population.

Early hypopharyngeal tumors certainly play a minor role among the indications for endoscopic surgery. For their nature (submucosal spread and early lymph node metastases) and late diagnosis (related to the silent areas where these tumors grow and the peculiar socioeconomic status of the patients usually affected by these lesions), hypopharyngeal malignancies are often diagnosed in an advanced stage. However, there is a relative paucity of open-neck conservative approaches that can be applied to these lesions. Thus, endoscopic management can certainly play a definitive role as an alternative to the costly, highly morbid organ preservation protocols in strictly selected early tumors of the hypopharynx.

As in the case of supraglottic lesions, the main sequels of endoscopic procedures for hypopharyngeal lesions are usually related to swallowing, which can be significantly hampered for a prolonged time. A nasogastric feeding tube or, more frequently, percutaneous endoscopic gastrostomy (PEG) may be needed during the long-lasting rehabilitative training protocol of swallowing. In Steiner's experience [5], 27% of 129 patients regained oral feeding on the first postoperative day without the need for a nasogastric feeding tube. In the remaining patients, a feeding tube was positioned and held in place for a mean of 9 days after surgery (range 1–25 days). A definitive gastrostomy tube was left in only two patients with severe aspiration but who refused total laryngectomy. Tracheotomy is usually not an issue so long as resection does not involve extensive adjacent supraglottic areas. Voice is generally not affected at all except in case of tumors involving the posterior half of the medial wall of the piriform sinus. When treating these lesions, in fact, the endoscopic surgeon can be forced to cause temporary or persistent damage to the recurrent nerve at its point of entry in the posterior paraglottic space.

13b.4 Tips and Pearls

- Tumors with complete fixation of one arytenoid cartilage are usually not suited for transoral laser surgery.
- Tumors arising from the anterior commissure are particularly difficult to expose and resect. Perform preoperative imaging (CT or MRI) prior to surgery and consider open (supracricoid) partial laryngectomy as a surgical alternative to laser surgery.
- With rare exceptions, subglottic carcinomas are not suited for transoral surgery.
- Perform adequate imaging of the larynx in the presence of supraglottic lesions to assess the true extent of the tumor before planning endoscopic surgery.
- Use laser-shielded tubes when performing CO_2 laser surgery for laryngeal tumors.
- Use two suction devices—one to evacuate the smoke and one to suction blood and manipulate the tissue during surgery.
- Administer perioperative antibiotic prophylaxis in all cases that require exposure of laryngeal cartilages.
- Insert a feeding tube at the end of the procedure in patients with supraglottic tumors or with resection of one arytenoid cartilage.

- Use dental protection to avoid dental trauma.
- Inspect the pharynx and oral cavity at the end of the operation to identify mucosal tears and bleeding.

References

1. Kleinsasser O (1962) [laryngomicroscopy (lens laryngoscopy) and its importance in the diagnosis of premorbid diseases and early forms of carcinoma of the labium vocale.]. Arch Ohren Nasen Kehlkopfheilkd 180:724–727
2. Strong MS, Jako GJ (1972) Laser surgery in the larynx. Early clinical experience with continuous CO_2 laser. Ann Otol Rhinol Laryngol 81:791
3. Ambrosch P (2007) The role of laser microsurgery in the treatment of laryngeal cancer. Curr Opin Otolaryngol Head Neck Surg 15:82–88
4. Eckel HE, Thumfart W, Jungehulsing M, Sittel C, Stennert E (2000) Transoral laser surgery for early glottic carcinoma. Eur Arch Otorhinolaryngol 257:221–226
5. Steiner W, Ambrosch P, Hess CF, Kron M (2001) Organ preservation by transoral laser microsurgery in piriform sinus carcinoma. Otolaryngol Head Neck Surg 124:58–67
6. Werner JA, Dunne AA, Folz BJ, Lippert BM (2002) Transoral laser microsurgery in carcinomas of the oral cavity, pharynx, and larynx. Cancer Control 9:379–386
7. Eckel HE, Staar S, Volling P, Sittel C, Damm M, Jungehuelsing M (2001) Surgical treatment for hypopharynx carcinoma: Feasibility, mortality, and results. Otolaryngol Head Neck Surg 124:561–569
8. Steiner W, Fierek O, Ambrosch P, Hommerich CP, Kron M (2003) Transoral laser microsurgery for squamous cell carcinoma of the base of the tongue. Arch Otolaryngol Head Neck Surg 129:36–43
9. Peretti G, Piazza C, Berlucchi M, Cappiello J, Giudice M, Nicolai P (2003) Pre- and intraoperative assessment of midcord erythroleukoplakias: A prospective study on 52 patients. Eur Arch Otorhinolaryngol 260:525–528
10. Nakayama M, Brandenburg JH (1993) Clinical underestimation of laryngeal cancer. Predictive indicators. Arch Otolaryngol Head Neck Surg 119:950–957
11. Sapundzhiev NR, Dunne AA, Ramaswamy A, Sitter H, Davis RK, Werner JA (2005) Lymph node metastasis in an animal model: Effect of piecemeal laser surgical resection. Lasers Surg Med 36:371–376
12. Remacle M, Eckel HE, Antonelli A, Brasnu D, Chevalier D, Friedrich G, Olofsson J, Rudert HH, Thumfart W, de Vincentiis M, Wustrow TP (2000) Endoscopic cordectomy. A proposal for a classification by the working committee, european laryngological society. Eur Arch Otorhinolaryngol 257: 227–231
13. Remacle M, Van Haverbeke C, Eckel H, Bradley P, Chevalier D, Djukic V, de Vicentiis M, Friedrich G, Olofsson J, Peretti G, Quer M, Werner J (2007) Proposal for revision of the european laryngological society classification of endoscopic cordectomies. Eur Arch Otorhinolaryngol 264:499–504
14. Rudert HH, Hoft S (2003) Transoral carbon-dioxide laser resection of hypopharyngeal carcinoma. Eur Arch Otorhinolaryngol 260:198–206

15. Rudert HH, Werner JA, Hoft S (1999) Transoral carbon dioxide laser resection of supraglottic carcinoma. Ann Otol Rhinol Laryngol 108:819–827

16. Dunne AA, Davis RK, Dalchow CV, Sesterhenn AM, Werner JA (2006) Early supraglottic cancer: How extensive must surgical resection be, if used alone? J Laryngol Otol 120:764–769

17. Dunne AA, Folz BJ, Kuropkat C, Werner JA (2004) Extent of surgical intervention in case of n0 neck in head and neck cancer patients:An analysis of data collection of 39 hospitals. Eur Arch Otorhinolaryngol 261:295–303

18. Rudert H (1988) [laser surgery in ent surgery] laser-chirurgie in der hno-heilkunde. Laryngol. Rhinol. Otol.(Stuttg) 67:261

19. Steiner W, Vogt P, Ambrosch P, Kron M (2004) Transoral carbon dioxide laser microsurgery for recurrent glottic carcinoma after radiotherapy. Head Neck 26:477–484

20. Klussmann JP, Knoedgen R, Wittekind C, Damm M, Eckel HE (2002) Complications of suspension laryngoscopy. Ann Otol Rhinol Laryngol 111 (11):972–976

21. Sesterhenn AM, Dunne AA, Werner JA (2006) Complications after co(2) laser surgery of laryngeal cancer in the elderly. Acta Otolaryngol 126:530–535

22. Eckel HE (2001) Local recurrences following transoral laser surgery for early glottic carcinoma: Frequency, management, and outcome. Ann Otol Rhinol Laryngol 110:7–15

23. Peretti G, Piazza C, Bolzoni A, Mensi MC, Rossini M, Parrinello G, Shapshay SM, Antonelli AR (2004) Analysis of recurrences in 322 tis, t1, or t2 glottic carcinomas treated by carbon dioxide laser. Ann Otol Rhinol Laryngol 113:853–858

24. Bron LP, Soldati D, Zouhair A, Ozsahin M, Brossard E, Monnier P, Pasche P (2001) Treatment of early stage squamous-cell carcinoma of the glottic larynx: Endoscopic surgery or cricohyoidoepiglottopexy versus radiotherapy. Head Neck 23:823–829

25. Dejonckere PH, Bradley P, Clemente P, Cornut G, Crevier-Buchman L, Friedrich G, Van De Heyning P, Remacle M, Woisard V (2001) A basic protocol for functional assessment of voice pathology, especially for investigating the efficacy of (phonosurgical) treatments and evaluating new assessment techniques. Guideline elaborated by the committee on phoniatrics of the european laryngological society (els). Eur Arch Otorhinolaryngol 258:77–82

26. Benninger MS, Ahuja AS, Gardner G, Grywalski C (1998) Assessing outcomes for dysphonic patients. J Voice 12:540–550

27. Piccirillo JF, Painter C, Fuller D, Haiduk A, Fredrickson JM (1998) Assessment of two objective voice function indices. Ann Otol Rhinol Laryngol 107:396–400

28. Manfredi C, Peretti G (2006) A new insight into postsurgical objective voice quality evaluation: Application to thyroplastic medialization. IEEE Trans Biomed Eng 53:442–451

29. Peretti G, Piazza C, Balzanelli C, Cantarella G, Nicolai P (2003) Vocal outcome after endoscopic cordectomies for tis and t1 glottic carcinomas. Ann Otol Rhinol Laryngol 112:174–179

30. Peretti G, Piazza C, Balzanelli C, Mensi MC, Rossini M, Antonelli AR (2003) Preoperative and postoperative voice in tis-t1 glottic cancer treated by endoscopic cordectomy: An additional issue for patient counseling. Ann Otol Rhinol Laryngol 112:759–763

31. Peretti G, Piazza C, Cattaneo A, De Benedetto L, Martin E, Nicolai P (2006) Comparison of functional outcomes after endoscopic versus open-neck supraglottic laryngectomies. Ann Otol Rhinol Laryngol 115:827–832

32. Sittel C, Eckel HE, Eschenburg C (1998) Phonatory results after laser surgery for glottic carcinoma. Otolaryngol Head Neck Surg 119:418–424

33. Bolzoni Villaret A, Piazza C, Redaelli De Zinis LO, Cattaneo A, Cocco D, Peretti G (2007) Phonosurgery after endoscopic cordectomies: I. Primary intracordal autologous fat injection after transmuscular resection:Preliminary results. Eur Arch Otorhinolaryngol 264(10):1179–1184

34. Friedrich G, de Jong FI, Mahieu HF, Benninger MS, Isshiki N (2001) Laryngeal framework surgery: A proposal for classification and nomenclature by the phonosurgery committee of the european laryngological society. Eur Arch Otorhinolaryngol 258:389

35. Friedrich G, Remacle M, Birchall M, Marie JP, Arens C (2007) Defining phonosurgery:A proposal for classification and nomenclature by the phonosurgery committee of the European laryngological society (els). Eur Arch Otorhinolaryngol 264(3):251–256

36. Sittel C (2004) Polydimethylsiloxane particles are not experimental in the human larynx. J Biomed Mater Res B Appl Biomater 69:251

37. Sittel C, Friedrich G, Zorowka P, Eckel HE (2002) Surgical voice rehabilitation after laser surgery for glottic carcinoma. Ann Otol Rhinol Laryngol 111:493–499

38. Zeitels SM (2004) Optimizing voice after endoscopic partial laryngectomy. Otolaryngol Clin North Am 37:627–636

39. Zeitels SM, Hillman RE, Franco RA, Bunting GW (2002) Voice and treatment outcome from phonosurgical management of early glottic cancer. Ann Otol Rhinol Laryngol Suppl 190:3–20

40. Chen AY, Frankowski R, Bishop-Leone J, Hebert T, Leyk S, Lewin J, Goepfert H (2001) The development and validation of a dysphagia-specific quality-of-life questionnaire for patients with head and neck cancer:The m. D. Anderson dysphagia inventory. Arch Otolaryngol Head Neck Surg 127:870–876

Open Partial Resection for Malignant Glottic Tumors

13c

Christoph Arens

Core Messages

> The quality of primary treatment is crucial for the results of laryngeal tumor therapy and the patient's life.

> Endoscopic resection was not able to replace open partial resection totally.

> Patient selection is based on the tumor's extent, the surgeon's expertise, and patient's expectations and/or demands.

> The main indication for open partial resection are glottic cancers with involvement of supraglottic or subglottic structures, one-sided slightly impaired mobility, or extension into the anterior commissure to the other vocal fold.

> Contraindications for oncological reasons include invasion of the thyroid cartilage, arytenoid fixation, interarytenoid invasion, subglottic extension with involvement of the cricoid cartilage, lesions that extend outside the larynx, and preepiglottic space invasion.

13c.1 Introduction

Several surgical options for treating laryngeal carcinoma can be used that allow resecting the tumor with oncologically safe margins and preservation of laryngeal function. The quality of the primary treatment is crucial for the results of laryngeal tumor therapy and the patient's life. Treatment includes addressing regional lymphatic drainage. The treatment strategy is based on the primary site of the tumor, its extension into the laryngeal structures, and the existence of regional and distant metastases.

Transcervical open partial resection for glottic cancer found its earliest application in the treatment of glottic malignant tumors. As these tumors produce early symptoms, the patients often present with localized disease. The first transcervical cordectomy for a vocal fold carcinoma was carried out by Brauers in 1834 [1]. Around the turn of the 19th century, cordectomy was the most frequently practiced procedure, and it produced rather good results for certain indications [2].

Despite some trials on laryngeal preservation as an alternative to total laryngectomy, the era of partial resection started in the 50th of the last century. Among the pioneers of function-preserving laryngeal surgery was Leroux-Robert, who advocated frontolateral partial resection [3]. Several modifications of open partial resection were described over the following years by Lore, Conley, Ogura, Silver, Mayer, and Piquet. It was predominantly Italian and French head and neck surgeons who developed and advocated open partial resections as extensive as subtotal laryngectomy for more advanced glottic cancer.

C. Arens
Universitätsklinikum Magdeburg A.ö.R.,
Universitätsklinik für Hals-, Nasen- und Ohrenheilkunde,
Klinikdirektor,
Leipziger Str. 44, 39120 Magdeburg, Germany
e-mail: christoph.arens@med.ovgu.de

M. Remacle, H. E. Eckel (eds.), *Surgery of Larynx and Trachea,*
DOI: 10.1007/978-3-540-79136-2_13c, © Springer-Verlag Berlin Heidelberg 2010

Conditions for the development of partial resection were the knowledge of tumor spread and laryngeal function as well as improved endoscopic diagnosis. This led to an exact pretherapeutic classification of tumor spread and reliable posttherapy follow-up. In 1962, Kleinsasser introduced the microscope into direct laryngoscopy and laryngeal surgery [4, 5].

During the last two decades, open partial resection was at least partially replaced by transoral endoscopic resection via microlaryngoscopy. After a phase that saw endoscopic resection of T3–T4 cancers, endoscopic resection became a helpful additional method of surgical therapy for laryngeal cancer, but it did not push open partial resection completely out of the picture. Conservation surgery for glottic cancer still includes transcervical open partial resection as well as transoral endoscopic resection.

13c.2 Selection of Patients for Open Partial Laryngeal Resection

Patient selection is based on the tumor's extent, the surgeon's expertise, and the patient's expectations and/or demands. In 1988, Kleinsasser presented three arguments for performing open partial resection [6]: (1) excellent access to the tumor; (2) adaptation of extending the resection to the tumor size; (3) the possibility of immediate reconstruction

With a T1 vocal fold cancer, the tumor is limited to the vocal cord, with normal clinical mobility. In case of sufficient tumor exposition through the operating microscope, these carcinomas can normally be resected by a transoral endoscopic approach. Dysplastic lesions, carcinoma in situ, and T1a vocal fold carcinoma are the most appropriate lesions for microlaryngoscopic transoral resection. Superficial involvement of the anterior commissure (bilateral Tis and T1b) is not a contraindication for an endoscopic approach. However, with deeper invasion of Broyle's tendon secondary to the large anterior defect, the oncological and functional results may be unsatisfactory. Therefore, in most cases of T1, a vocal fold carcinoma with deep involvement of the anterior commissure, and with T1b tumors, we prefer an open transcervical approach. We also perform open partial resection for small glottic cancers in case of inadequate exposure.

Indications for open partial resection are glottic cancers with involvement of supraglottic or subglottic structures or one-sided, slightly impaired mobility, extension into the anterior commissure to the other vocal fold or in tumors after resection leading to glottic insufficiency and thus to an impaired voice and a decreased quality of life.

T2 glottic cancers are an inhomogeneous group of lesions. Due to large tissue defects after endoscopic removal of large T1 and T2 tumors transoral resection should not be the treatment of choice for functional reasons. T2 carcinomas that extend to the ventricle or the paraglottic space or that present with fixation of the vocal fold posteriorly with highly differentiated squamous cell carcinoma and expanding borders are suitable for a vertical partial resection in carefully selected cases. The craniocaudal diameter should not extend more than 2 cm. Open partial resection of T2 tumors with involvement of the anterior commissure should be performed cautiously because of possible cartilage infiltration and invasion or even penetration of the cricothyroid ligament. Depending on the tumor site and grading, neck dissection has to be performed.

Similar to large T2 vocal fold carcinomas, T3 tumors may require open partial resection in selected cases. Arytenoid infiltration and tumor grading are especially important to the decision making about whether to perform an open partial resection. With T3 glottic carcinoma, a neck dissection should be performed simultaneously.

With T4 glottic carcinomas, vertical partial resection is not a therapeutic option. Surgery with total removal of the thyroid cartilage, such as cricohyoidopexy (CHP) or cricohyoidoepiglottopexy (CHEP), may be indicated. These surgical techniques can be used as an alternative to laryngectomy. There are many advantages of vertical partial resection in comparison to cricohyoidopexy. By using vertical partial resection, the patient is able to phonate naturally at the glottic level postoperatively. Phonation at the supraglottic level remains an exception after transcervical resection leading to unfavorable functional results. Additionally, aspiration is prevented by a reconstructed, functioning glottic sphincter. The indication for open partial resection with glottic reconstruction also depends on the patient's request for an immediately sonorous voice with sufficient volume to maintain quality of life.

13c.3 Contraindications

Contraindications for oncological reasons include invasion of the thyroid cartilage, arytenoid fixation, interarytenoid invasion, subglottic extension with involvement of the cricoid cartilage, lesions that extend outside the larynx, and preepiglottic space invasion. As all of the patients have to be tracheotomized for several days, the surgery is contraindicated in elderly patients and patients with severe cardiopulmonary disease.

13c.4 Surgical Techniques

The authors prefer a midline incision from the superior thyroid incision down to the trachea in order to perform a tracheotomy as the first step. Alternatively, two horizontal incisions may be possible but do not provide the same good overview of the larynx. The medial cervical fascia is carefully prepared and the infrahyoid muscles pulled aside. The isthmus of the thyroid gland with the entire pretracheal and prelaryngeal tissue is resected including the prelaryngeal Delphian node. The technique of thyreotomy is nearly the same as it was during the early 20th century [7–9, 13, 14].

The perichondrium is paramedially incised vertically to ensure good protection of the medial thyrofissure afterward. The cartilage is divided in the midline or paramedian with a circular or oscillating saw, ensuring that the underlying tissue is not damaged. Then, the spot where the anterior laryngeal artery penetrates the cricothyroid ligament is found, indicating the exact midline. After medial incision of the cricothyroid membrane, the soft tissues of the larynx are incised with a blunt curved knife (Herrmann) up to the petiolus.

The endolaryngeal surface is now totally exposed for examination and resection under the operating microscope. Depending on the site and size of the lesion in the glottis, a cartilage window can be resected with the tumor in a small frame at the upper and lower border of the thyroid.

Generally, the vocal fold is not completely resected. The tumor resection is adapted to the extent of the lesion. If possible, the tumor is resected in one bloc. Additionally, we perform circular lateral as well as deep resections for free margins. This helps the pathologist determine the resection margins more exactly. For immediate control, frozen sections can be carried out. In any case of positive margins, the patient must undergo revision surgery.

According to its volume and extent, the defect is reconstructed by a false cord flap including parts of the epiglottis if necessary [7, 9–12]. This flap, pedicled cranioposteriorly, is fixed as far forward as possible into the anterior commissure with respect to the exact insertion of Broyle's tendon. Sometimes the glottic level of the flap has to be filled up with fat or cartilage. The main idea of this type of resection is that there is least one straight vertical margin to establish a new anterior commissure by a flap covered by healthy, well vascularized mucosa on at least at one side. For bilateral lesions with superficial tumor growth on the contralateral side, cordectomy type I, and if necessary type II, can be applied. Exact reconstruction of the anterior commissure is important for achieving a good functional result. It should be reconstructed in the typical V-shape for good glottic closure, especially with advanced resection. The functional result of the operation is predominantly influenced by the remaining volume of the vocalis muscle and the flap. The thyrofissure is closed with 2–0 Vicryl sutures via three pairs of drill holes performed before the split of the thyroid.

Before closure we create a so-called Miculicz stent (latex glove filled with cotton gauze), which is inserted in the laryngeal lumen to prevent bleeding and swelling. The external perichondrium is then closed with 3–0 Vicryl suture. The stent can be taken out 1 day after surgery. The distal end of the stent is led out through the cricothyroid ligament and fixed to the cuffed tracheal cannula. Only in patients with large flaps involving the laryngeal ventricle is a feeding tube recommended.

13c.5 Reconstructive Surgery for Glottic Defects

Resection and reconstruction vary depending on the site, size, and growth of the tumor. According to the site and size of the tumor, there are different thyroid cartilage resections. These resections respect the reconstruction of the anterior commissure, in contrast to most of the previously published modifications of laryngeal

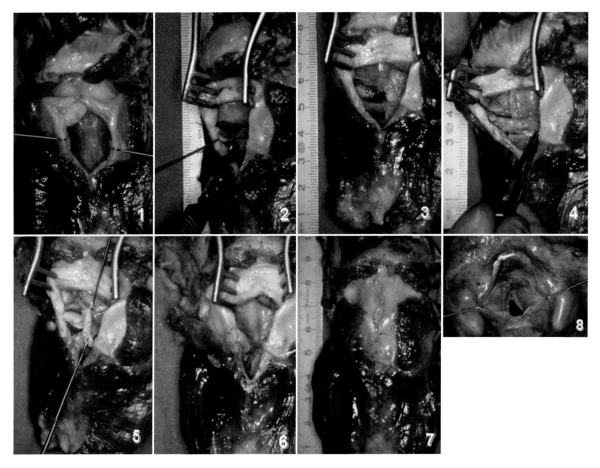

Fig. 13c.1. 1–8 Figures present a open partial resection of the right vocal fold with cordectomy in a cadaver larynx. A false cord flap is transposed to the glottis level for immediate reconstruction

partial resections, especially the frontolateral resection from Leroux-Robert, which results in a round anterior commissure with mostly a bad functional outcome. Several examples are shown in Figures 13c.1–13c.4.

13c.6 Postoperative Care

The Miculicz stent has to be fixed thoroughly and removed on the first postoperative day. The patient must be watched closely because the stent may cause acute respiratory distress if it is acutely displaced. In most cases, the tracheal cannula can be removed within 24 hours after surgery. With advanced resections, the tracheal cannula can stay in place up to 1 week, and a feeding tube

may be necessary. Temporary swallowing dysfunction after extended cordectomy is rare. When present, it is mostly caused by edema in the arytenoid region.

Regular follow-up care is required for all patients with head and neck cancer, preferably at least every 6–12 weeks during the first postoperative year. Additionally, postoperative voice therapy may significantly improve the functional outcome. In some patients the flap becomes atrophic, leading to glottic insufficiency and development of supraglottic phonation. In these cases, medialization of the flap with septal cartilage or fat injection can be carried out after 2 years of tumor-free survival. Secondary to the pull-down of the ventricular fold, cystic lesions may develop that may mimic a recurrence underneath the flap. In these cases, diagnostic microlaryngoscopy with adjustment procedures to the flap is mandatory.

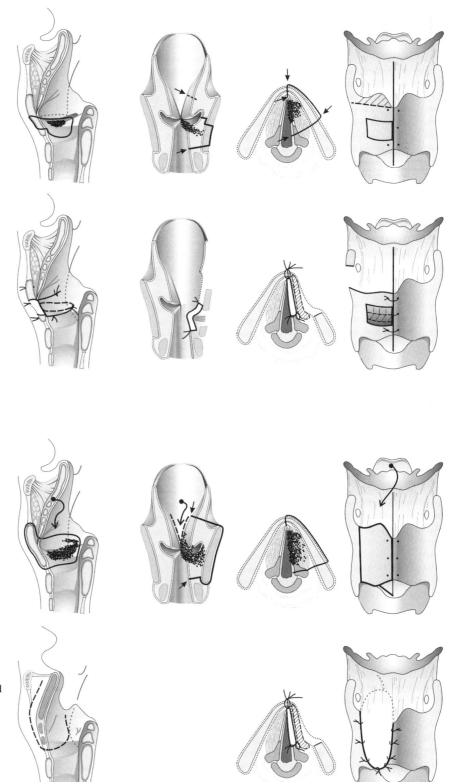

Fig. 13c.2. T2 vocal fold carcinoma. Primary glottic reconstruction can be performed immediately after tumor resection during the same procedure by reconstructing the vocal fold or creating a counterpart for the intact contralateral vocal fold. Depending on the defect, a ventricular fold flap or an enlarged ventricular fold flap with parts of the epiglottis is transpositioned to the glottic level and fixed by sutures to create a sufficient glottic closure. In this case, the carcinoma was excised with a cartilage window. To create more volume for the new vocal fold, parts of the upper rim of the ipsilateral thyroid are placed underneath the flap

Fig. 13c.3. T2–T3 vocal fold carcinoma with involvement of the ventricular fold, resulting in a large defect including major parts of the thyroid cartilage. In these cases, an epiglottis sliding flap can be performed [9–11, 15, 16]

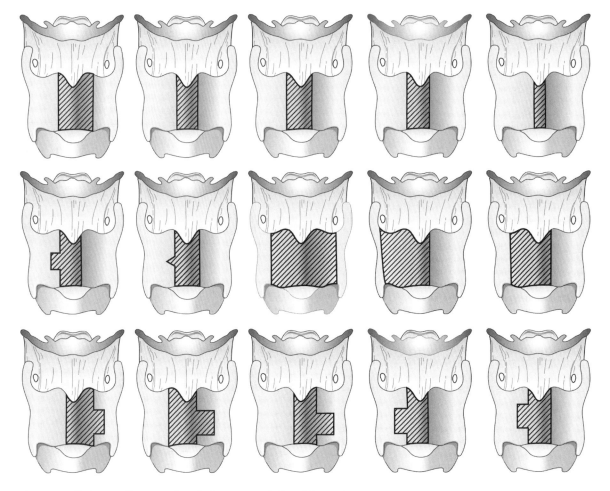

Fig. 13c.4. Various cartilage resections during open vertical partial resections

References

1. Brauers (1834) zit. bei Kahler, O.: Die bösartigen Neuerungen des Kehlkopfs. In: Denker A, Kahler O (eds) Handbuch der Hals-Nasen-Ohrenheilkunde, Bd. V. Springer, Berlin, 1929 (S.441)
2. Bruns V (1978) Die Laryngektomie zur Entfernung intralaryngealer Neubildungen. Berlin 1887, zit. bei Kahler, O.: Die bösartigen Neuerungen des Kehlkopfs. In: Denker A, Kahler O (eds) Handbuch der Hals-Nasen-Ohrenheilkunde. Bd. V. Springer, Berlin 1929 (S.441)
3. Leroux-Robert J (1975) A statistical study of 620 laryngeal carcinomas of the glottic region personally operated upon more than five years ago. Laryngoscope 85:1440–1452
4. Kleinsasser O (1962) Die Laryngomikroskopie (Lupenlaryngoskopie) und ihre Bedeutung für die Erkennung der Vorerkrankungen und Frühformen des Stimmlippenkarzinoms. Arch Ohrenheilkd 180:724–727
5. Kleinsasser O (1965) Weitere technische Entwicklung und erste Ergebnisse der "endolaryngealen Mikrochirurgie". Laryngol Rhinol Otol 44:711–727
6. Kleinsasser O (1988) Tumors of the larynx and hypopharynx. Thieme-Verlag, Stuttgart/New York

7. Neel HB, Devine KD, DeSanto LW (1980) Laryngofissure and cordectomy for early cordal carcinoma: outcome in 182 patients. Otolaryngol Head Neck Surg 88:79–84
8. Daly JF, Kwok FM (1975) Laryngofissure and cordectomy. Laryngoscope 85:1290–1297
9. Friedman M, Toriuni DM (1987) Glottic reconstruction following hemilaryngectomy:false cord advancement flap. Laryngoscope 97:882–884
10. Tucker HM, Wood BG, Levine H, Katz R (1979) Glottic reconstruction after near total laryngectomy. Laryngoscope 89:609–618
11. Sedlacek K (1965) Predni a lateralni rekonstrukcni laryngektomie se stazenim epiglottis. Ceskoslovenska Otolaryngol 14:328–334
12. Kambic V, Radsel Z, Smid L (1976) Laryngeal reconstruction with epiglottis after vertical hemilaryngectomy. J Laryngol Otol 90:467–473
13. LeJeune FE, Lynch MG (1955) The value of laryngofissure. Ann Otol Rhinol Laryngol 64:256–262
14. McGavran MH, Spjut H, Ogura J (1959) Laryngofissure in the treament of laryngeal carcinoma: a critical analysis of success and failure. Laryngoscope 69:44–53
15. Kleinsasser O (1987) Chirurgische Behandlung der Larynx- und Hypopharynxkarzinome. In: Kleinsasser O (ed.) Tumoren des larynx und des hypopharynx. Thieme Verlag, Stuttgart

Surgery for Laryngeal and Hypopharyngeal Cancer

13d

Open Neck Approach—Partial and Reconstructive Laryngectomy

Dominique Chevalier

13d.1 Introduction

The larynx and pharynx are both important for swallowing, voice, and breath. Any surgery at this level may have a negative impact. Many of these operations require a temporary tracheotomy and a nasogastric tube. Decision making is based on evaluation of the patient, the tumor, the local resources and expertise, and the possibility of functional salvage, if any [15].

13d.2 Specific Assessment

13d.2.1 Direct Pharyngolaryngoscopy

Direct endoscopic examination of the pharynx, larynx, and esophagus is performed under general anesthesia. It is conducted with rigid endoscopes and 30° and 70° rigid telescopes to improve the quality of the mucosal assessment, particularly in the case of a small cancer [8]. This examination is an indispensable diagnostic tool and has several goals.

- It allows multiple mucosal biopsies for histological examination.
- It provides an accurate evaluation of superficial tumor spread.
- Systematic examination of the entire upper aerodigestive tract and the esophagus allows detection of synchronous cancers.

During this step, careful palpation of the true vocal cord and the tumor is important for evaluating the depth of the lesion. In addition, drawings, pictures, and/or video recording of the tumor are helpful to the clinician for decision making at the time of the multidisciplinary meeting.

13d.2.2 Diagnostic Imaging

Imaging techniques are becoming more precise and are routinely used to complement the clinical and endoscopic assessments of patients with laryngeal and hypopharyngal carcinomas.

D. Chevalier
Service ORL Hospital Huriez, Centre Hospitalier et Universitairee de Lille, Rue Michel Polonovski, 59037 Lille Cedex, France
e-mail: d-chevalier@chru-lille.fr

M. Remacle, H. E. Eckel (eds.), *Surgery of Larynx and Trachea*,
DOI: 10.1007/978-3-540-79136-2_13d, © Springer-Verlag Berlin Heidelberg 2010

Computed tomography (CT) is currently the most useful imaging modality [22]. The goal of CT is accurate assessment of the location and size of the primary cancer and detection of any extension to the neck either directly or through lymphatic metastasis. CT examination must be performed from the nasopharynx to the upper mediastinum with and without intravenous contrast enhancement. In case of a small laryngeal tumor, CT is preferably performed before endoscopy and biopsy to avoid inflammation, which may result in overestimating cancer infiltration. CT also allows the use of dynamic maneuvers such as the Valsalva and phonation.

Knowing the natural course of the tumor, it is important to assess carefully the anatomical areas of the larynx and hypopharynx. A cancer of the vocal cord or the ventricle may extend into the paraglottic space, and a supraglottic cancer can extend into the preepiglottic space. Preepiglottic extension is easily detected after image reconstruction in the sagittal plane. Laterally, laryngeal cancer may extend to the thyroid cartilage, which acts as a temporary barrier against extension into the neck. The CT scan allows one to explore, in the same session, the upper aerodigestive tract and the lung.

Metastatic lymph nodes are frequently encountered with carcinoma of the supraglottis. The probability of metastatic involvement of a lymph node is associated with the following criteria seen on imaging.

- Size > 10 mm (12 mm in the subdigastric area)
- Central necrosis with heterogeneity and peripheral enhancement
- Circular shape

For evaluating carcinoma of the subglottis, CT scans yield important information regarding superior mediastinal and retropharyngeal lymph nodes where clinical examination is not feasible.

Magnetic resonance imaging (MRI) is performed with the use of an anterior neck coil and application or use of a protocol that consists of axial, T2-weighted fast spin echo and T1-weighted spin echo images. Then, following intravenous administration of gadolinium, axial, sagittal, and coronal T1-weighted spin echo images are obtained. MRI is more sensitive for detecting minimal neoplastic invasion to the cartilage than CT [4], whereas CT is more specific. MRI has superior resolution for demonstrating soft tissue details. Nevertheless, because of its susceptibility to motion-induced artifact, MRI is not routinely performed when staging of cancer of the larynx.

Ultrasonography is helpful for assessing cervical lymph nodes. It is a simple, noninvasive, rapid, highly sensitivity technique for detecting subclinical lymph node metastasis, but its reliability is operator-dependent. It is a useful method for follow-up and can be combined with fine-needle aspiration to confirm histological invasion.

13d.3 Partial Surgery for Laryngeal Cancer

The larynx is divided into three parts.

- Supraglottis, which includes the lingual and laryngeal surface of the epiglottis, aryepiglottic folds, arytenoid cartilages, false vocal folds, ventricle
- Glottis, which includes the true vocal cords and the anterior and posterior commissures
- Subglottis, which is the area of the larynx inferior to the glottis

Many partial procedures have been described, providing a wide choice of conservative treatments with the goal to cure while preserving laryngeal functions. We select here the most used frequently used and published procedures.

13d.3.1 Cordectomy

Most of the patients who undergo cordectomy are treated through an endoscopic approach, which is considered safe. When an endoscopic procedure is not feasible owing to anatomical or technical considerations, the external approach is still possible. The main indication is T1 glottic cancer involving the true vocal cord without extension to the anterior commissure.

The surgical technique is as follows: After a horizontal incision, the thyroid cartilage is exposed and a midline thyrotomy is performed. The larynx is opened after section of the cricothyroid membrane and the anterior commissure. The inner perichondrium is elevated on the tumor side, and the true vocal cord is removed under direct vision. The anterior commissure is reconstructed by anchoring the remaining vocal cord to the thyroid cartilage, which is sutured on the midline. The strap muscles and the external perichondrium are closed [10].

We recommend that the area be carefully assessed for local extension. This step is not indicated in cases of deep extension into the vocal muscle due to the high risk of local recurrence. Patients can swallow easily the day after the procedure and be discharged from the hospital quickly as no tracheotomy is needed.

Few publications have become available since the development of endoscopic procedure. Lefebvre [14] reported a 5-year local control rate of 94% and a 5-year survival rate of 87%.

The following guidelines can help avoid complications.

- The most important point is to confirm the indication(s). It is important to be sure that the tumor does not involve the vocal muscle because in that case there is a high risk of local recurrence.
- As no tracheotomy is performed, a small drain is necessary to avoid subcutaneous emphysema.

13d.3.2   Frontolateral Vertical Laryngectomy

Frontolateral vertical laryngectomy, described by Leroux-Robert, consists in a vertical laryngectomy with removal of the anterior commissure. It is performed less frequently than cordectomy. It is considered an alternative in cases of exposition failure due to anatomical considerations. This procedure is indicated for surgical treatment of T1b glottic cancer with extension close to the anterior commisure but without deep invasion to it.

After a horizontal incision, the thyroid cartilage is exposed and a lateral thyrotomy is performed on both sides close to the midline The larynx is opened after section of the cricothyroid membrane on the tumor-free side. The inner perichondrium is elevated on the tumor side, and the true vocal cord with the anterior commissure attached to the thyroid cartilage is removed under direct vision of the tumor. The remaining vocal cord is sutured anteriorly to the thyroid cartilage, which is then sutured at the level of the midline. The strap muscle and the external perichondrium are closed. It is important to suture the petiole of the epiglottis to the thyroid cartilage anteriorly to avoid postoperative stenosis.

In our experience, the results are good: The 5-year survival rate was 83%, and the local control rate was 96%. In a recent review, Brumund [3] reported the results of a series of 270 patients at the ENT and Head and Neck Surgery Department of the Georges Pompidou European Hospital and confirmed excellent results. The 5-year actuarial survival rate was 83.1% for T1 lesions and 67.2% for T2 lesions. He found that the actuarial local control ranged from 96.2% (T1) to 68.2% (T2).

This surgical technique is safe and can be performed without tracheotomy. Therefore, careful hemostasis must be done at time of closure to avoid complications.

13d.3.3   Frontal Anterior Laryngectomy with Epiglottoplasty

Bouche [2] and Sedlacek in 1965 and Kambic in 1977 expressed interest in using the epiglottis to reconstruct the larynx. In 1979, Tucker [23] published a series of patients who underwent "near-total laryngectomy," which was in fact frontal anterior resection of the larynx using the epiglottis to close the larynx anteriorly. This procedure allowed resection of both false and true vocal cords with the anterior part of the thyroid cartilage. The reconstruction is done anteriorly to close the remaining larynx with the epiglottis. Functional results are usually good, and the procedure can be performed in the elderly.

Frontal anterior laryngectomy with epiglottoplasty is indicated to treat glottic cancer classified as T1b or T2. It is still indicated in cases of superficial anterior commissure extension.

To begin this operation, a tracheotomy is necessary. The thyroid cartilage is exposed, and two lateral thyrotomies are performed at least 1.5 cm from the midline. The larynx is opened superiorly through the petiole of the epiglottis. Inferiorly, the cricothyroid membrane is transected at the level of the superior border of the cricoid cartilage. The inner perichondrium is elevated on both sides, and then both false and true vocal cords with the anterior commissure attached to the thyroid cartilage are removed. The epiglottis is pulled downward, and its anterior face is dissected close to the cartilage; the hyoepiglottic ligament is transected. The epiglottis is sutured laterally to the remaining thyroid cartilage and inferiorly to the cricoid cartilage. The strap muscle and the external perichondrium are closed. Note that the hyoepiglottic ligament must be transected to allow suture of the petiole with the cricoid cartilage mucosa without tension and both ventricles must be removed with the specimen.

During follow-up, the tracheostomy tube is capped if the airway is sufficient. Usually it can be done at day 4, but sometimes edema occurs after this time and it is wise to keep the tracheotomy tube (smallest size as possible) in place until the patients begins swallowing. The nasogastric tube is removed when the patient is able to swallow liquids, which means at least between days 12 and 18.

Local control and survival rates for this operation are excellent. Giovanni [9] reported a 5-year survival and local control rates of 86% and 92%, respectively. Mallet [17] confirmed those results in a series of 65 patients with 5-year survival and local control rates, respectively, of 82% and 94%. As with other partial laryngectomies, all patients had hoarseness and weakness of the voice. Aspiration can occur during the postoperative course, and speech therapy is mandatory.

To avoid complications, it is necessary to suture the epiglottis to the thyroid cartilage laterally. If not there is a possible risk of stenosis.

13d.3.4 Supracricoid Partial Laryngectomy with Cricohyoidoepiglottopexy

After the publications of Majer [16] and Labayle, Piquet [19, 20] published the first report of a series of patients with glottic cancer who were treated with supracricoid partial laryngectomy with cricohyoidoepiglottopexy. The aim was to perform a large or subtotal resection of the larynx to decrease the local recurrence rate of glottic cancer that had been initially treated with transcartilaginous techniques. This technique was frequently used in France and Italy and then gained popularity in Europe and other countries. The main problem with it consists in the postoperative course and the higher risk of aspiration in comparison with other partial laryngectomies.

There are some major points of which to take note.

- This technique allows removal of a large part of the larynx.
- Use of the epiglottis can improve functional results.
- At least one functional cricoarytenoid joint must be preserved.
- Subglottic extension is associated with a higher risk of recurrence.

Cricohyoidoepiglottopexy (CHEP) is indicated to treat glottic carcinomas with deep invasion into the vocal muscle and that are close to the thyroid cartilage but without extension through it. CHEP is indicated in cases of impaired motion of the true vocal cord, but the arytenoid cartilage must be still mobile. The subglottic extension must also be carefully assessed; when the extension goes farther than the superior border of the cricoid cartilage, CHEP is contraindicated. CHEP is indicated for bilateral glottic cancer with or without anterior commissure invasion but without extension to the petiole of the epiglottis. Using the UICC classification, CHEP is indicated for T2 and selected T3 glottic cancers.

The surgical technique starts with elevating the anterior flap, after which the midline raphe of the strap muscles is divided. Sternohyoid and thyrohyoid muscles are transected close to the hyoid bone. The superior border of the thyroid cartilage is dissected, and the inferior constrictor muscles are transected at the posterior border of both thyroid cartilage ala. To avoid injuring the inferior laryngeal nerve, the inferior cornu of the thyroid cartilage is transected and left in place on the side(s) of remaining arytenoids(s) cartilage(s). With the same intent concerning the superior laryngeal nerves, both superior cornu are preserved. The superior border of the cricoid cartilage is dissected, and on the tumor side the mucosa and inner perichondrium can be elevated to enlarge the margins during the resection. The larynx is opened by transecting the inferior part of the epiglottis and that of the preepiglottic space. The incision is performed anterior to the arytenoid cartilage, and both true and false vocal cords are removed. When necessary (T3 lesions), arytenoid cartilage can be removed. It is important to spare the posterior mucosa, which is then sutured anteriorly and can be useful for improving the vocal result. Inferiorly, the cricothyroid membrane is transected, and the specimen is removed.

Closure is performed by impaction of the cricoid cartilage to the hyoid bone using three or four sutures (Vicryl no. 2). The needle passes under the cricoid cartilage, through the inferior part of the epiglottis, and around the hyoid bone with part of the base of the tongue. Care must be taken superiorly to avoid injury of both hypoglossal nerves. The needle is grasped close to the midline of the hyoid bone. The strap muscles are then sutured, the skin flap is closed over a drain, and a tracheotomy tube is inserted.

Note that it is important to save at least one mobile cricoarytenoid unit. Furthermore, the inferior and superior laryngeal nerves must be protected and spared. Another important point is that during the resection both ventricles must be totally removed to avoid a cyst, which can create laryngeal stenosis.

During follow-up, the tracheotomy tube is capped if the airway is sufficient. Usually it can be done at day 4, but sometimes edema occurs after this time; thus, it is safer to keep a tracheotomy tube (smallest size possible) until the beginning of swallowing. Some authors advocate early removal, but care must be done to avoid severe dyspnea and we think it is better to do it when the risk of edema disappears. The nasogastric tube is removed when the patient is able to swallow liquids, which means between days 12 and 18 at the earliest.

Aspiration frequently occurs and decreases progressively. Speech therapy is always mandatory and should continue after the patient is discharged from the hospital.

As the goal is to decrease the risk of local recurrence, it is clear that wide resection of the larynx provides excellent oncological results. In our experience, the results are good, with a 5-year survival rate of 78% and a local control rate of 94.3%. These results have been confirmed by other teams, with a local control rate that ranges between 90% and 96% [7, 11, 21].

There are certain measures that can help avoid complications: (1) At time of closure, superior stitches should encircle the base of the tongue and the hyoid bone. These stitches must be close to the midline to avoid injury of the hypoglossal nerves and lingual artery. (2) During closure, the petiole of the epiglottis must be encircled by the needle to avoid stenosis.

13d.3.5 Supracricoid Partial Laryngectomy with Cricohyoidopexy

Following the work of Majer and Rieder, supracricoid partial laryngectomy with cricohoidopexy was described by Labayle. It is similar to the CHEP technique but allows total removal of the supraglottis. To date, among the partial laryngectomy techniques, it allows the widest resection of the larynx. Because of the risk of aspiration, patient selection is important, and attention must be paid to the general status of their health [18].

The three major points to remember about this surgery are (1) The cricohyoidopexy (CHP) technique is similar to the CHEP. (2) The preepiglottic space and epiglottis are removed. (3) Functional results are less good than with other techniques.

The CHP technique is indicated for the following conditions.

- Supraglottic cancer without extension to the upper part of the preepiglottic space.
- Glottic cancer that has invaded the supraglottis, particularly when the site of origin is the anterior commissure. In that case, there is a high risk of extension to the inferior part of the prepiglottic space, and removal of the tumor is mandatory.
- Transglottic and supraglottic cancer with vocal cord fixation but without arytenoids cartilage fixation.

The surgical technique is similar to the CHEP technique, previously described. A neck dissection is routinely performed prior laryngeal surgery. The main difference is removal of the epiglottis with the prepiglottic space. That means that at time of dissection the inferior border of the fat of the prepiglottic space is divided from the hyoid bone and is totally removed with the specimen. If possible, at least one arytenoid cartilage is preserved. For reconstruction, there are no differences between the two operations, and the pexy is performed with four stiches crossing under the cricoid cartilage and the hyoid bone with the base of the tongue.

As the resection is large, aspiration occurs frequently. If possible, it is better to spare both arytenoid cartilages. Speech therapy must be initiated and continued after hospital discharge. The goal are swallowing (first) and optimizing voice result (second). Inferior and superior laryngeal nerves must be protected and spared.

As indicated for supraglottic cancer, the oncological results are good. Survival at 5 years ranges between 68% and 84%, and the local recurrence rate is low, between 0% and 16% [5, 12].

The follow-up for this operation are similar to those for the CHEP technique. The tracheostomy tube is capped if the airway is sufficient. Usually, it can be done at day 4, but sometimes edema occurs after this time, and it is safer to keep a tracheotomy tube (smallest size as possible) in place until the beginning of swallowing.

To avoid complications, one must remember that the larynx is very large, and the impaction of the cricoid cartilage and hyoid bone must be done at the same level. If the cricoid cartilage is located backward, the risk of aspiration is higher.

13d.3.6 Supraglottic Laryngectomy

Supraglottic laryngectomy was described by Alonso [1]. It consists in resecting the whole supraglottic portion of the larynx, including both ventricular folds and the epiglottis. Extensions of this procedure have been described (e.g., in the case of superior tumor extension with partial resection of the base of the tongue). It should be noted that supraglottic partial laryngectomy is the most classic technique and is widely performed. It allows resection of supraglottic cancer without deep extension into the prepiglottic space. Finally, the oncological and functional results are good when it is properly indicated and performed.

The main indications are a tumor of the epiglottis and the anterior part of the ventricular folds. Contraindications are invasion of the glottis and/or the ventricle, thyroid cartilage extension, impaired motion of the vocal cord, and tongue base extension.

The surgical procedure starts with incising and elevating the skin, after which bilateral neck dissection is performed. The infrahyoid muscles are transected at the level of the hyoid bone and reflected inferiorly to expose the superior part of the thyroid cartilage. The superior cornu is transected. The external perichondrium of the thyroid cartilage is elevated and reflected inferiorly at the level of the true vocal cords. Then the thyroid cartilage is transected horizontally on both sides. The larynx is entered superiorly in the valleculae after elevating the mucosa from the inferior edge of the hyoid bone. The surgeon moves close to the midline to have a large view of the operating field, after which the incision is enlarged laterally and inferiorly to expose the larynx. Both aryepiglottic folds are transected, and the incision is continued into the ventricles and anteriorly above the anterior commissure and true vocal cords. Closure is performed by impaction of the remaining thyroid cartilage to the base of the tongue and, if spared, the hyoid bone using three or four sutures (Vicryl no. 2). At the end, the perichondrium is sutured to the hyoid bone, and infrahyoid muscles are sutured superiorly and cover the surgical field.

Note that it is important to save both true vocal cords and to avoid injuring them during resection of the tumor. Inferior and superior laryngeal nerves must be protected and spared as well.

The oncological results are good, with a low recurrence rate of 5–15% for T1 and T2 supraglottic carcinomas. Survival is excellent as well. One of the main causes of failure is a second primary lesion.

During follow-up, the tracheostomy tube is capped if the airway is sufficient. Usually it can be done at day 4. The nasogastric tube is removed when the patient is able to swallow liquids, which means between days 10 and 16 at the earliest. Aspiration can occur but is less frequent than after supracricoid partial laryngectomy.

To avoid complications, during removal of the specimen it is important to keep in mind the exact level of the glottis. If it is injured, the functional result could be worse.

13d.4 Partial Surgery for Hypopharyngeal Cancer

Compared to laryngeal surgery, fewer partial pharyngectomy procedures are available for the surgical treatment of hypopharyngeal cancers with preservation of laryngeal and pharyngeal function. Because occult cervical metastasis is frequent, neck dissection should be performed systematically. Only a few patients are amenable to partial pharyngectomy. These procedures are associated with good local control of disease, but the patients have a poor prognosis owing to the high incidence of second primary tumors, co-morbidities, and metastasis.

13d.4.1 Posterior Partial Pharyngectomy

Important points to remember about posterior partial pharyngectomy include the following.

- The diagnosis is made late in the disease, as there are few indications it is present.
- Small, superficial tumors can be treated with endoscopic resection.

This procedure is indicated for tumors that are limited to the posterior and lower wall of the pharynx without extension to the piriform sinus or the larynx. Such tumors are routinely treated by radiotherapy.

During the workup, it is essential to assess the exact local extension because if the defect of the posterior wall is large it is necessary to perform an immediate reconstruction.

For the surgery, the pharynx can be opened anteriorly through a transhyoid approach. It is necessary to detach the suprahyoid muscles from the hyoid bone. The mucosa of the vallecula is then incised to open the surgical field and provide direct access to the tumor. After excising the tumor, the surgical defect is left open and the mucosal edges are sutured to the prevertebral fascia using resorbable sutures. The pharynx can be opened laterally when the tumor is large and reconstruction is needed. In this situation, bilateral neck dissection is performed first. The posterior wall of the hypopharynx is exposed, and the larynx and the base of the tongue are elevated to open the surgical field. The posterior wall mucosa is dissected from the prevertebral fascia. After opening the pharynx, the tumor is removed under direct vision in a monobloc specimen. Reconstruction is then performed using either a radial forearm free flap or a pectoralis major myocutaneous flap, which is less often employed because of its size [24].

13d.4.2 Partial Lateral Pharyngectomy (Trotter)

Using a lateral approach, the posterior two-thirds of the thyroid cartilage and the greater cornu of the hyoid bone are resected. Then the lateral wall of the piriform sinus is resected as along with the deep fascia and the thyrohyoid muscle. Primary closure is usually possible, but reconstruction with a local muscular flap is sometimes necessary. This procedure is indicated for cancer limited to the lateral wall of the piriform sinus.

13d.4.3 Supracricoid Hemipharyngolaryngectomy

Supracricoid hemipharyngolaryngectomy allows surgical treatment of large tumors of the upper part of the piriform sinus. The oncologic results are good when this surgery is properly indicated. The procedure is indicated for tumors of the medial wall of the piriform sinus without impaired mobility of the larynx and

located above the level of the superior border of the cricoid cartilage.

The surgery starts with ipsilateral neck dissection. Using a lateral approach, the ispsilateral thyroid ala and half of the hyoid bone are resected. Infrahyoid muscle are reflected inferiorly and the larynx is entered trough the vallecula. The preepiglottic space and the epiglottis are vertically transected. Resection is continued inferiorly above the superior border of the cricoid cartilage, the vocal cord is removed with the ventricle. At this point the lateral margin and the pyriform sinus are visualized and the vertical posterior resection is performed under direct vision. The defect is covered by apposition of the edges, after mobilization of the prevertebral muscles insertions that are sutured to the posterior border of the infrahyoid muscles.

Superiorly the pharynx is closed by suturing the remaining mucosa of the pharyngeal wall to the vallecula Then the edges of the previously spared infrahyoid muscles are sutured externally to the constrictor muscles. The entire pyriform sinus and the ispsilateral hemilarynx above the cricoid cartilage are removed with the tumor.

The postoperative course is often marked by slow recovery of swallowing ability and a risk of aspiration and bronchopulmonary infections. Patients may begin oral feeding, with caution, by the 10th postoperative day.

Laccourreye [13], in a series of 34 patients with cancer of the piriform sinus staged as T2, confirmed the reliability of this technique with 5-year actuarial local and 5-year actuarial regional control rates of 96.6% and 93.7%, respectively.

To avoid complications, closure of the pharynx with stitches must be accomplished without tension to avoid dysfunction of the cricopharyngeal muscle and aspiration.

13d.4.4 Supraglottic Hemipharyngolaryngectomy

The supraglottic hemipharyngolaryngectomy is a variant of the supracricoid hemipharyngolaryngectomy only in that both true vocal cords are conserved here. Furthermore, the functional results are better than with the supracricoid hemipharyngolaryngectomy. The indication for this operation is a tumor of the upper part of the piriform sinus extending to the aryepiglottic fold, particularly in cases with ulceration or infiltration.

The surgery begins with neck dissection. The infrahyoid muscles are transected from the lower border of the hyoid bone. Half of this hyoid horn is resected. The infrahyoid muscles are reflected inferiorly, and the thyroid cartilage is exposed. The ipislateral superior two-thirds of the thyroid cartilage is resected to allow exposure of the ipisilateral vocal cord. The larynx is entered through the vallecula, and the preepiglottic space and epiglottis are vertically transected. Resection is continued inferiorly above the floor of the ventricle, sparing the vocal cord. At this point, the lateral margin and the piriform sinus are visualized, and a vertical posterior resection is performed under direct vision. Superiorly, the pharynx is closed by suturing the remaining mucosa of the pharyngeal wall to the vallecula and to the medial laryngeal remnant, taking care not to suture the remaining half of the epiglottis. Then, the edges of the previously spared infrahyoid muscles are sutured externally to the constrictor muscles, medially to the contralateral infrahyoid muscles, and superiorly to the mylohoid muscle. Closure is achieved by apposing the mucosal edges or use of a subhyoid muscle flap.

During follow-up, the tracheotomy tube is plugged by the eighth postoperative day. The patient can begin to phonate after day 8, and oral feeding can begin by the tenth postoperative day.

A high local control rate (97.8%) was reported for a series of 45 patients who underwent this procedure in association with postoperative radiotherapy [6].

To avoid complications, follow these guidelines.

* At time of closure of the pharynx, stitches must be made without tension to avoid dysfunction of the cricopharyngeal muscle and aspiration.
* If radiotherapy is performed, it is better to keep the tracheotomy in place to avoid obstruction of the larynx due to edema.

References

1. Alonso JM (1951) La chirurgie conservatrice pour le cancer du larynx et de l'hypopharynx. Ann Otolaryngol Chir Cervicofac 68:689–696
2. Bouche J, Freche C (1965) L'hémilaryngectomie avec epiglottoplastie. Ann Otolaryngol Chir Cervico Fac 82:421–424
3. Brumund K, Gutierrez-Fonseca R (2005) Frontolateral vertical partial laryngectomy for invasive squamous cell carcinoma of the true vocal cord: a 25 year experience. Ann Otol Rhinol Laryngol 114:314–322
4. Castelijns JA, Gerritsen GJ (1998) Invasion of laryngeal cartilage by cancer: comparison of CT and MRI imaging. Radiology 167:199–206
5. Chevalier D, Piquet JJ (1994) Subtotal laryngectomy with cricohyoidopexy for supraglottic carcinoma: review of 61 cases. Am J Surg 168(5):472–473
6. Chevalier D, Watelet JB (1997) Supraglottic hemipharyngolaryngectomy plus radiation for the treatment of early lateral margin and pyriform sinus carcinoma. Head Neck 19:1–5
7. Chevalier D, Laccourreye O (1997) Cricohyoidoepiglottopexy for glottic carcinoma with fixation or impaired mobility of the true vocal cord: 5-year oncologic results with 112 patients. Ann Otol Rhinol Laryngol 106:364–369
8. Chevalier D, Fayoux P (1997) Endoscopic evaluation of glottic cancer. Ann Otolaryngol Chir Cervicofac (Paris) 114: 197–198
9. Giovanni A, Guelfucci B (2001) Partial frontolateral laryngectomy with epiglottic reconstruction in the management of early-stage glottic carcinoma. Laryngoscope 111:663–668
10. Kacker A, Wolden S (2003) Cancer of the larynx. In: Shah J (ed.) Head and neck surgery and oncology. Mosby, New York
11. Laccourreye H, Laccourreye O (1990) Supracricoid laryngectomy with cricohyoidoepiglottopexy: a partial laryngeal procedure for glottic carcinoma. Ann Otol Rhinol Laryngol 99: 421–426
12. Laccourreye H, Laccourreye O (1990) Supracricoid laryngectomy with cricohyoidopexy: a partial laryngeal procedure for selected supraglottic and transglottic carcinomas. Laryngoscope 100(7):735–741
13. Laccourreye O, Merite-Drancy A (1993) Supracricoid hemilaryngopharyngectomy in selected pyriform carcinoma. Laryngoscope 103:1373–1379
14. Lefebvre JL, Vankemmel B (1987) La cordectomie dans le traitement des cancers de corde vocale. A propos de 200 cas. J Français d'ORL 36:415–421
15. Lefebvre JL, Coche-Dequeant B (2004) Treatment of laryngeal cancer: the permanent challenge. Expert Rev Anticancer Ther 4:913–920
16. Majer H, Rieder A (1959) Technique de laryngectomie permettant de conserver la perméabilité respiratoire: la cricohyoido-pexie. Ann Otolaryngol Chir Cervicofac 76:677–683
17. Mallet Y, Chevalier D (2001) Near total laryngectomy with epiglottic reconstruction, our experience of 65 cases. Eur Arch Otorhinolaryngol 258:488–491
18. Naudo P, Laccourreye O (1997) Functional outcome and prognosis factors after supracricoid partial laryngectomy with cricohyoidopexy. Ann Otol Rhinol Laryngol 106(4): 291–296
19. Piquet JJ, Desaulty A (1974) Crico-hyoido-épiglotto-pexie. Technique opératoire et résultats fonctionnels. Ann Otolaryngol Chir Cervicofac 91:681–689
20. Piquet JJ (1976) Functional laryngectomy (cricohyoidopexy). Clin Otolaryngol 1:7–16
21. Piquet JJ, Chevalier D (1991) Subtotal laryngectomy with crico-hyoido-epiglotto-pexy for the treatment of extended glottic carcinoma. Am J Surg 162:357–361
22. Robert Y, Rocourt N (1996) Helical CT of the larynx a comparative study with conventional CT scan. Clin Radiol 51: 882–885
23. Tucker HM, Wood BJ (1979) Glottic reconstruction after near total laryngectomy. Laryngoscope 89:609–617
24. Silver CE, Moisa I (1993) Surgical therapy. In: Ferlito A (ed.) Neoplasm of the larynx. Churchill Livingstone, London

Total Laryngectomy

13e

Miquel Quer and Hans Edmund Eckel

Core Messages

> Total laryngectomy is the gold standard for the surgical treatment of advanced laryngeal tumors: is the standard against which the cure rates of other treatment modalities must be compared.

> The main indication for total laryngectomy is locally advanced tumors of the larynx or hypopharynx that are not suitable for open or endoscopic partial laryngectomy.

> Salvage total laryngectomy has an important role in nonsurgical organ preservation protocols.

> Prior to surgery, the patient must understand the indication and sign an informed consent, including realistic understanding of the total laryngectomy state and lifestyle modifications after surgery.

> The surgeon must have a very precise knowledge of the extension of the tumor prior to surgery (via fibroscopy, endoscopy, computed tomography/magnetic resonance imaging). This information can indicate the best way to remove the larynx and obtain free margins.

> For hypopharyngeal and subglottic primaries, unilateral or subtotal thyroid gland and paratracheal node resection may be necessary.

> Three main ways to remove the larynx can be used: above-downward approach, below-upward approach, and lateral approach. For every tumor, the surgeon must analyze the best way to remove the larynx. For endolaryngeal tumors, it is to use the above-downward approach; for extensions to valecula or when a mechanical closure of the pharynx, the best approach is below-upward; and for extensions to the piriform sinus the best approach is the lateral one.

> Obtain frozen section specimens of the margins if there is any doubt, especially in cases of salvage surgery after radiotherapy.

> There are many ways to reconstruct the pharynx. Surgeons should be familiar with primary closure of the defect and free flap reconstruction.

> The status of the quality of life after total laryngectomy is highly personal and subjective. In general, survivors have the perception of a good quality of life and most have a high level of satisfaction with their decision to undergo total laryngectomy.

13e.1 Indications

Total laryngectomy is the gold standard for surgical treatment of advanced laryngeal and hypopharyngeal tumors. That means that total laryngectomy remains the standard against which the cure rates of other treatment modalities must be compared. Total laryngectomy includes removal of all laryngeal and associated structures including strap muscles, from the hyoid bone and epiglottis superiorly to the tracheal rings inferiorly, with varying amounts of the hypopharynx and thyroid gland. It can be extended to the base of the

M. Quer (✉)
Professor of Otorhinolaryngology, Head of the Department of Otorhinolaryngology and Head and Neck Surgery, Hospital de la Santa Creu i Sant Pau, Universitat Autonoma de Barcelona, Barcelona, Spain
e-mail: mquer@santpau.cat

M. Remacle, H. E. Eckel (eds.), *Surgery of Larynx and Trachea,*
DOI: 10.1007/978-3-540-79136-2_13e, © Springer-Verlag Berlin Heidelberg 2010

tongue, pharynx, trachea, and prelaryngeal soft tissues including skin. Total laryngectomy has low cost, low mortality, and low morbidity with good oncology results. The main disadvantage of total laryngectomy is the permanent tracheotomy and loss of the laryngeal voice [3, 5, 7, 8, 10, 19, 22, 24, 25].

Laryngologists and radiation oncologists have been searching for alternatives to total laryngectomy to avoid this mutilation while preserving local control and cure rates documented for radical surgery [9, 10, 16, 18, 20]. Chemoradiation-based organ preservation protocols, laser surgery, and extended open partial surgery are attempts to achieve this goal. For advanced laryngeal and hypopharyngeal cancer, induction chemotherapy followed by radiotherapy in patients with objective responses has been shown to allow conservation of the larynx in nearly two-thirds of individuals without having an effect on survival. Concurrent chemoradiotherapy also provides high rates of laryngeal preservation, again without affecting survival; and induction chemotherapy followed by concurrent chemo radiotherapy is under investigation. Hence, evidence supports the use of larynx preservation approaches for appropriately selected patients without a compromise in survival; however, no larynx preservation approach offers a survival advantage compared with that of total laryngectomy and adjuvant therapy. Moreover, salvage total laryngectomy plays an important role in those preservation protocols in case of persistence or recurrence. Therefore, despite all efforts, total laryngectomy continues to be highly useful surgery for many patients, either as a primary treatment or as salvage surgery.

The main indication for total laryngectomy is a locally advanced tumor of the larynx in which partial conservative surgery is not feasible. For example, partial surgery may not be possible due to extension of the tumor or to the poor general conditions of the patient (age, cardiopulmonary condition). The locations in which partial surgery is often not recommended are the retrocricoid, the interarytenoid, and the posterior subglottis as well as multifocal affectation of the larynx (carcinomatosis). The indications for total laryngectomy differ among teams and surgeons. In general, total laryngectomy is indicated for most T3 and T4 tumors and for some T2 tumors with wide subglottal extension. Other indications for total laryngectomy are chondronecrosis; recurrent aspiration pneumonia that cannot be controlled with more conservative measures, especially when it is due to cerebrovascular accident; apraxia or degenerative neurological disease.

Contraindications for total laryngectomy include lesions too extensive to permit complete resection of local disease; when it is associated with unacceptable medical risks; and patient refusal.

13e.1.1 Summary of Indications

13e.1.1.1 Oncological Indications

- Advanced laryngeal or hypopharyngeal cancer not treatable with partial surgery
- Recurrence or persistence of advanced laryngeal or hypopharyngeal cancer after organ preservation protocol with any combination of chemotherapy and radiotherapy
- Recurrence or persistence of the cancer after radiotherapy or partial surgery, not treatable with partial surgery
- Patients with laryngeal or hypopharyngeal cancer appropriate for conservative surgery whose medical status, age, or personal preference does not permit temporary aspiration
- Massive thyroid cancer (usually recurrent) invading both sides of the larynx or the laryngotracheal junction
- Palliative local control for advanced, not curable (e.g., due to distant metastases) laryngeal or hypopharyngeal cancer

13e.1.1.2 Nononcological Indications

- Chondroradionecrosis with loss of laryngeal function
- Recurrent and severe aspiration pneumonia not responding to less aggressive treatment

13e.2 Preoperative Assessment

Total laryngectomy requires two basic preconditions.

1. The patient must be fit for general anesthesia and surgery.
2. The patient (and family) must understand the reason to opt for mutilating surgery and give informed consent, including realistic understanding of total laryngectomy and lifestyle modifications after surgery.

The workup required includes an anesthesia-related assessment of the patient's general health and specific assessment relevant to the oncological situation and planning the surgery. Clinically assessing the extension of the disease is important when planning surgery and should include transnasal fibreoptic or indirect laryngoscopic assessment of the disease and of vocal cord mobility; microlaryngoscopy with panendoscopy for histological verification of the diagnosis and to rule out synchronous secondary primaries; combination of laryngeal computed tomography (CT) with ultrasonography of the neck; or magnetic resonance imaging (MRI) of the neck. Positron emission tomography (PET) or PET-CT is useful for detecting subclinical lymph node metastasis and dissemination of the disease to distant sites, but it is not readily available throughout Europe and so remains optional to date.

Before surgery, physical examination with complete blood analysis, chest radiography, and electrocardiography are undertaken. In addition, if a neck dissection is to be performed, 1 or 2 units of typed and cross-matched blood should be made available.

The patient is not allowed to eat or drink anything for 8 hours before surgery. Antibiotic prophylaxis and local antiseptic washing of the oral cavity and the pharynx prior to surgery is compulsory. Many surgeons routinely advocate additional antibiotic treatment for 5–7 days after surgery.

13e.3 Surgical Technique for Endolaryngeal Tumors

13e.3.1 Patient Positioning

Patient positioning requires access to the anterior part of the neck for both surgeon and assistant. This is conveniently achieved by placing the patient on a table fitted with a head holder, allowing the head to be cantilevered out but well supported, or on a normal table, placing a rolled sheet underneath the shoulders to fully extend the neck.

In advance of the operation, airway management is planned with the anesthesiologist such that a common agreement is reached regarding the timing of tracheotomy and intubation. In the nonobstructed larynx, the anesthesiologist can pass an orotracheal tube with anesthesia induction, which is left until tracheal transection is performed at the end of the laryngectomy. With an obstructed airway, or in cases where intubation might displace malignant tissue into the lower airway, a preliminary tracheotomy with the patient under local anesthesia is performed. A precurved or flexible reinforced, cuffed tube is then passed into the trachea and adequate ventilation confirmed.

13e.3.2 Skin Incision

Although various options exist, the most used incision is a broad U-incision because it provides excellent exposure and permits comfortable treatment of the neck areas (Fig. 13e.1). The incision begins approximately 3–4 cm below the mastoid, descends to the posterior third of the sternocleidomastoid muscle, and curves to the midline approximately 3 cm above the internal third of the clavicle to pass parallel 2 cm above the sternal pitchfork. It is continued symmetrically toward the other side. If only a unilateral neck dissection is necessary, a J ("hockey stick") incision can be used. If no neck dissection is planned, a U-shaped incision starting at the level of the greater cornu of the hyoid bone and at the anterior margin of the sternocleidomastoid muscle is sufficient.

Another option, also widely used, is a curved horizontal neck incision from the sternocleidomastoid to the sternocleidomastoid muscle at or above the level of the cricoids such that a 2- to 3-cm bridge of skin is preserved between the main incision and the upper stoma verge. This configuration avoids diversion of pharyngeal contents away from the stoma should a pharyngocutaneous fistula complication occur. However, exposition of the surgical field is less extensive. In any case, the incision is carried through the skin, subcutaneous tissue, and platysma, taking care to avoid sectioning the anterior and external jugular veins [3, 5, 7, 19, 22, 24, 25].

13e.3.3 Flap Elevation

The upper skin flap is retracted superiorly with hooks or clamps and is elevated upward in the subplatysmal plane. It is carried superiorly past 2–3 cm of the upper edge of the hyoid bone in the middle and 2 cm below the mandible on the sides. The cervical superficial fascia, external and anterior jugular veins, and prelaryngeal

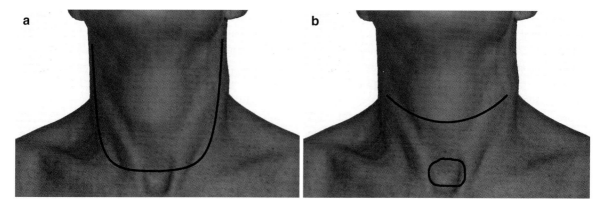

Fig. 13e.1. Two types of incision most often used. (**a**) Broad U-incision. (**b**) Two independent incisions

node must remain in place. The same is done inferiorly until 1–2 cm above the clavicles and sternum.

13e.3.4 Division of the Infrahyoid Muscles

If a neck dissection is necessary, it is performed before the total laryngectomy [3, 5, 7, 19, 22, 24, 25]. When neck dissection is not needed, the superficial fascia is divided in the anterior border or each sternocleidomastoid muscle. Then the sternocleidomastoid muscle is mobilized, and the internal jugular vein and carotid artery are repaired; the omohyoid muscle is clearly exposed and divided at the level of this tendon. The superficial fascia is open over the strap muscles in the supraesternal area, and the sternohyoid muscle is exposed (Figs. 13e.2 and 13e.3) and divided as distally as possible. The sternothyroid muscle then appears and is careful divided distally (taking care of the inferior thyroid veins) and softly separated from the thyroid gland. The surgeon must be aware of the relation between the external part of the sternothyroid muscle and the internal jugular vein (Figs. 13e.2 and 13e.3). Once all three muscles are divided, they are held superiorly to expose the thyroid gland and the cricoid and thyroid cartilages (Fig. 13e.3).

13e.3.5 Division of the Suprahyoid Muscles

After dividing and ligating the upper and lower extent of the external jugular veins, the body of the hyoid

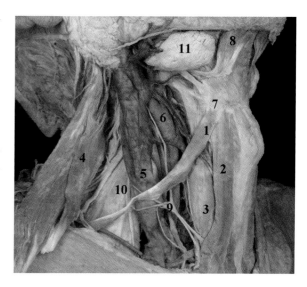

Fig. 13e.2. Anatomical preparation of the strap muscles, with their relations with the internal jugular vein and the carotid artery. Note that the inferior insertion of the sternocleidomastoid muscle has been cut and the muscle displaced posteriorly to expose the great vessels and the inferior part of the strap muscles. *1*, omohyoid muscle; *2*, sternohyoid muscle; *3*, thyrohyoid muscle; *4*, sternocleidomastoid muscle; *5*, internal jugular vein; *6*, carotid artery; *7*, hyoid bone; *8*, digastric muscle; *9*, hypoglossus ansa; *10*, scalenus muscle; *11*, submandibular gland

bone is grasped with a clamp and retracted anteroinferiorly. This tenses the suprahyoid musculature and exposes the superior surface of the hyoid bone, which is then skeletonized by detaching the mylohyoid muscle, geniohyoid muscle, digastric sling, and hyoglossus muscle in sequence in a medial to lateral direction. In addition, the stylohyoidal ligament is detached from the lesser cornu. Monopolar electrocautery is used for this division to limit troublesome bleeding. When detaching the hyoglossus muscle, one must be

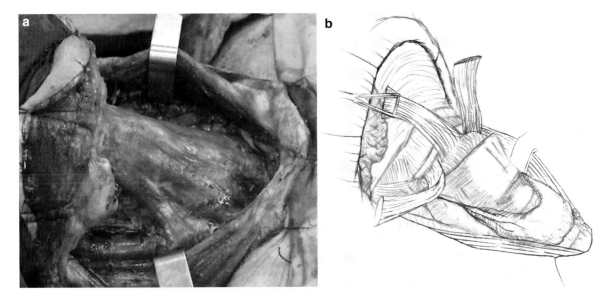

Fig. 13e.3. (**a**) Exposition of the inferior infrahyoid muscles and their relation to the vascular axis (superficial fascia has been removed). (**b**) After sectioning them, the thyroid gland became exposed

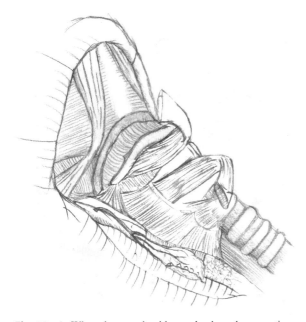

Fig. 13e.4. When the suprahyoid muscles have been sectionated and the thyroid gland separated of the larynx, the inferior constrictor muscle is well exposed (*right side*)

careful to avoid injuring the hypoglossus nerve and the lingual artery. The hyoid bone can now be resected away from the larynx. For extended supraglottic tumors, the sternohyoid and thyrohyoid muscle attachments on the lower border of the hyoid bone remain undisturbed, and the hyoid is excised with the larynx (Fig. 13e.4).

When the tumor invades the valecula, this division is done at the end of the resection, with the tumor under the vision of the surgeon (see below-upward approach resection).

13e.3.6 Separation of the Thyroid Gland

Regarding the thyroid gland, three situations can occur when performing total laryngectomy.

- The thyroid gland is completely preserved.
- The isthmus and the ipsilateral lobe are removed with the larynx, and the contralateral lobe is preserved.
- The entire gland must be removed with the larynx.

The surgeon must decide on the suitable strategy depending on the site and size of the tumor. In general, for large tumors [2, 3, 11] with subglottic extension and for hypopharyngeal carcinoma, the isthmus and the ipsilateral lobe with the paratracheal nodes are removed.

In the case of complete preservation of the gland, after division and ligation of the isthmus, both lobes are dissected away from the larynx and trachea from medial to lateral, preserving all of the blood supply, particularly the superior thyroid artery (Fig. 13e.4).

In the case where the isthmus and the ipsilateral lobe are removed, they are left attached to the larynx and trachea for en bloc resection. Therefore, the ipsilateral superior and inferior thyroid vascular pedicles are ligated and divided, as is the middle thyroid vein. After dividing the thyroid isthmus, the contralateral lobe is dissected away from the larynx and trachea from medial to lateral, thereby preserving the blood supply to the remaining thyroid and parathyroid parenchyma via superior or inferior thyroid vessels. If total thyroidectomy is indicated, two or more parathyroid glands should be removed from the thyroid and be replanted into a small pocket in a muscle (e.g., sternocleidomastoid muscle) to prevent postoperative and lifelong hypocalcemia.

13e.3.7 Division of the Inferior Constrictor Muscle

At this moment only the inferior constrictor muscle remains inserted in the larynx and must be divided. The posterior border of the thyroid cartilage lamina is rotated anteriorly by traction with a hook, allowing good exposure of the inferior constrictor muscle. Using scalpel or electrocautery, the inferior constrictor is incised 5 mm anterior to the posterior edge of the thyroid ala and cricoid cartilage (Fig. 13e.5). The muscle is then freed from the thyroid ala and cricoid cartilage, trying to preserve it for later reinforcement of the closure.

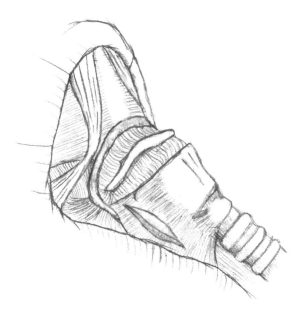

Fig. 13e.5. The inferior constrictor muscle fibers are incised along the posterior edge of the thyroid ala, exposing the piriform sinus mucosa underneath

If the tumor has not invaded the piriform sinus, the mucosa of the piriform sinus is separated from the thyroid cartilage using a blunt elevator (Tapia's maneuver) [3].

13e.3.8 Division of the Superior Laryngeal Pedicle

The superior laryngeal pedicle can be easily found between the cornu superior of the thyroid cartilage and the hyoid bone. First, the laryngeal branch of the superior thyroid artery is identified, ligated, and divided before it penetrates the thyrohyoid membrane (if the ipsilateral thyroid lobe is removed this is not necessary because the superior thyroid artery has been ligated). The same is done to the superior laryngeal vein and the internal laryngeal nerve. A ligature can be placed on the upper stump of the nerve to minimize the risk of a painful neuroma.

13e.3.9 Transection and Division of the Trachea

The trachea is usually transected between the second and third ring. In case of subglottal extension, tracheal resection must be extended up to obtaining a safe margin. In case of previous tracheotomy performed some days before, it is safe to completely excise the tracheostoma with the surrounding skin in order to reduce the risk of peristomal recurrence [11]. Once the trachea is open, and after looking into the subglottic space to make sure there is a sufficient inferior surgical margin, the trachea is intubated with a new, cuffed endotracheal tube that is inserted into the distal trachea for control of the airway. Only then the tracheal division is completed with the incision in the posterior tracheal wall that should curve upward slightly at its midpoint to optimize the mucosa remaining for tracheostomy.

13e.3.10 Removal of the Larynx

The larynx can be removed in several ways, depending on the locations of the tumor and the surgeon's preference.

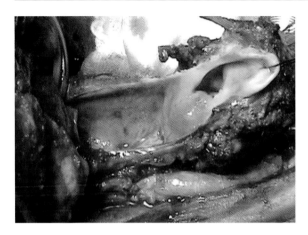

Fig. 13e.6. With the above-downward approach, the surgeon enters across the valecula, and removal of the larynx is continued along the external part of both arytenoepliglottic folds (*right-side view*)

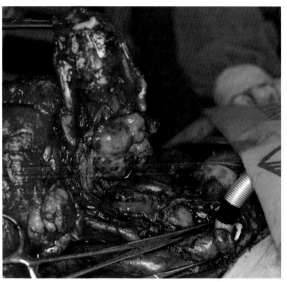

Fig. 13e.7. With the below-upward approach, the surgeon ends the resection in the valecula (*right-side view*)

We use three different ways: from above-downward (Gluck-Sœrensen's), from below-upward (Tapia), or via a lateral approach. In most cases, the easiest way is from above-downward because it is simpler and the surgeon has better control of the tumor. However, in cases where the tumor extends to the vallecula, it is advisable to use the below-upward approach; we use this approach also when a linear stapler will be used to close the pharynx. The lateral approach may be useful when the tumor extends to one piriform sinus [3, 5, 7, 19, 22, 24, 25].

Above-downward approach (Fig. 13e.6). With this approach, the surgeon enters across the vallecula glossoepiglottica. The hyoid bone is grasped with forceps and pulled forward. The space between the base of the tongue and the vallecula is then progressively dissected (usually with an electric knife). Palpating this area, the surgeon can note the tip of the epiglottis between his or her fingers. Finally, the mucosa of the vallecula is opened, and the epiglottis appears. The tip of the epiglottis is held with a suture to be pulled anteriorly and inferiorly, and a retractor is placed on the base of the tongue.

At that moment, the surgeon changes position (passes to the head of the patient) to have the best vision of the tumor. Removal of the larynx is continued along the external part of both aryepiglottic folds. When both sides are cut, arriving at the posterior arytenoid area, the two cuts are joined below the cricoarytenoid joint, where there is a good plane of cleavage on the postcricoid area. Dividing the trachea and the cricoid cartilage from the esophagus finally joins the above incision, and the superior part of the trachea and the larynx are excised.

Below-upward approach (Fig. 13e.7). After tracheal division, an easy plane of cleavage is found between the posterior wall of the trachea and the anterior wall of the esophagus. The dissection is carried up to the inferior edge of the cricoid cartilage, assuming that the subglottic carcinoma does not extend too close to this area. Then the blunt dissection continues superiorly, exposing the posterior cricoarytenoid muscle.

If a linear stapler will be used for closure, the pharynx is not opened, and the dissection is continued, freeing the mucosa of the piriform sinus and vallecula to leave only mucosa to be compressed and cut by the mechanical device.

In case the pharynx is entered, the point of entry is chosen so it is as far as possible from the tumor. Generally, the pharynx is opened through the interarytenoid area and to the piriform sinus on the least involved side. This is done by retracting the thyroid cartilage ala anteriorly with a double hook and placing a retractor gently in the mucosa of the piriform sinus so the surgeon can control the tumor. Then, progressively the surgeon uses scissors to cut the mucosa following the aryepiglottic folds and extend the cut though the vallecular mucosa by placing one blade of the scissors into the vallecula and the other blade on the outside of the specimen just above the hyoid bone. If there is carcinoma in the pharyngoepiglottic fold or

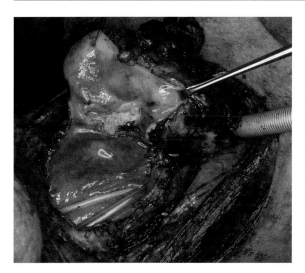

Fig. 13e.8. With the lateral approach, the final resection is done in the piriform sinus under good direct visual control (*right-side view*)

in the vallecula, the cut must be directed more laterally or cranially with at least 1 cm of surgical margins (preferably 2 cm).

Lateral approach (Fig. 13e.8). This approach is mainly used when the tumor extends to the piriform sinus. It is a combination of the two approaches just discussed. On the affected side, the thyroid lobe is left attached to the larynx, and the inferior constrictor muscle is not divided. The surgeon begins with the tracheal division and blunt dissection from below until exposure of the posterior cricoarytenoid muscle; then the dissection moves to the vallecula glosoepiglottica where the pharynx is open. Progressively, the surgeon cuts the aryepiglottic fold of the unaffected side until it reaches the arytenoid. At this moment, the surgeon is able to rotate the larynx-pharynx and clearly expose the tumor and the involved piriform sinus. The resection can thus be done under direct visual control, cutting not only the mucosa but also the constrictor muscles at the correct level, with a security margin of 2 cm if possible.

Finally, the specimen is inspected to confirm the location of the tumor and evaluate the security margins. When indicated, frozen section specimens of the margins are obtained.

Tracheoesphageal puncture, voice prosthesis placement, and cricopharyngeal myotomy can now be performed before the pharynx is closed or reconstructed.

13e.3.11 Repair of the Pharynx

Once the tumor removal is completed, it is time to irrigate the wound and perform meticulous hemostasis. With a conventional total laryngectomy, it is not a problem to close the pharynx; Traditionally, closure in three layers—mucosal, fascial, muscular—using inverting sutures for the mucosa has been the standard technique. Many surgeons now prefer to suture only two layers, the first being mucosal/fascial and the second being muscle.

With extended laryngectomy (for treatment of hypopharyngeal cancer), pharyngeal reconstruction must be performed. If direct closure of the pharynx is not feasible for oncological reasons (following circumferential pharyngectomy) or to prevent later pharyngeal stenosis, tissue transfer is needed to reconstruct the pharynx.

A direct repair may be horizontally or T-shaped in configuration. Selection of closure is based on an assessment of the shape and size of the anterior pharyngeal defect and simulated wound approximation before suturing. The least tensioned apposition of wound edges is the best.

A running or interrupted closure, according to the surgeon's preference, is used, in general trying to obtain inversion of the mucosal edges into the pharynx. Some surgeons use linear staplers for uncomplicated closure of the pharynx, whereas others prefer to rely on traditional suturing techniques.

Horizontal closure. A horizontal straight closure is the preferred way to close the pharynx for many surgeons. First, the mucosa of the tongue base is everted using resorbable material. The suture line then starts at both lateral edges and is done in two layers (mucosa and fascia). The surgeon then performs a third layer, suturing the constrictor muscles to the suprahyoid muscles. A tightly constricted muscular ring should be avoided. In some cases, the thyroid lobe can be used to reinforce closure when the muscles cannot be approximated.

T-suture (Fig. 13e.9). When is not possible to achieve a horizontal suture, the inferior part of the pharyngeal defect is closed vertically, forming a T. The same layers are used.

In some postirradiated cases, when the neck tissues are fibrotic and the resection is large, it is safe to use a salivary bypass tube into the pharynx to try to protect

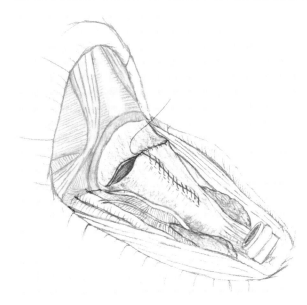

Fig. 13e.9. With the T-closure, a combination of horizontal and vertical straight lines are used to obtain a nontensioned wound. The constrictor muscle is used for reinforcement while avoiding a tightly muscular ring

the closure line. In some cases, to prevent complications pectoral muscular flap is used to protect the pharyngeal closure.

Mechanical closure. There are two ways to achieve mechanical closure: open and closed. With the open technique of stapling, after conventional excision of the larynx, the mucosal edges of the defect are aligned by evenly spaced holding sutures placed between the jaws of the stapler, and the device is activated. The open technique, other than time-saving, has no clear benefit over traditional suturing [1].

With the closed technique, the stapler is placed without opening the pharynx. The indications for the closed technique are endolaryngeal tumors without suprahyoid vallecular, piriform sinus, or postcricoid extension. Once the skeletonization of the larynx is properly completed, a single application of the 60- or 90-mm stapler suffices to close the pharyngeal defect without problems. The below-upward approach is used for applying mechanical sutures. It is good practice to transect the greater cornu of the hyoid bone and thyroid cartilage for easier application of the stapling device. Special attention is placed on complete visualization of the contour of the suprahyoid part of the epiglottis. When the laryngeal specimen remains connected only

to the hypopharynx by a thin mucosal-submucosal layer, the surgeon inserts a tracheal hook through the tracheal lumen into the larynx and grasps the epiglottis, thus everting it and preventing its disruption in the staple suture line. The stapler is then placed and activated, automatically forming a hemostatic double-row suture line, and the laryngeal specimen is separated. The specimen surgical margins are evaluated and frozen sections obtained if necessary. A second layer closure of the constrictor muscles is done as with the others types of closure.

The advantages of mechanical closure in the closed technique are simple, rapid application, watertight closure with good hemostasis, prevention of field contamination, and a lower fistula rate. Furthermore, the mechanical suture is nonstrangulating at the wound edges and permits vessels to pass through the staple loops with minimal tissue injury; finally, the mechanical suture reduces the operating time.

The main drawback of the technique is that the tumor itself is not visualized during resection, which carries a potential for oncological compromise if applied in unsuitable cases. Tumors that are not entirely endolaryngeal are evidently at risk for compromise with this technique.

13e.3.12 Tracheostoma and Closure

For tracheostoma and closure, the entire cartilaginous portion of the trachea is sutured to the inferior skin flap (with a U-incision) with interrupted sutures of 0 or 2-0 silk to widen the diameter of the tracheostoma. The suture line should provide support for the trachea and accurate skin-mucosa apposition without cartilage exposure. This is best achieved by a modified vertical mattress suture that traverses (1) skin (peripherally), (2) cartilaginous tracheal wall, and (3) skin (centrally). The inferior margin of the U-flap is sutured to the posterior (membranous) part of the trachea.

When two skin incisions are used, the permanent end tracheal stoma is created before or after pharyngeal repair. An appropriate shield-shaped skin button is removed from the lower neck flap in the midline, just above the sternal notch. Any excess adipose tissue or bulky sternocleidomastoid muscle/tendon is excised deep to the skin flap to minimize tracheal stenosis.

The tracheal end is then passed through the hole and secured with several stay stitches.

After placing suction drains, one on each side, the skin is closed in two planes. The platysma and subcutaneous tissue are reapproximated with 3-0 absorbable suture material. The skin is carefully approximated with interrupted dermal sutures or skin clips. Dressings are placed according to the preferences of the surgical team.

13e.4 Extended Total Laryngectomy

13e.4.1 Total Laryngectomy Extended to the Tongue Base

Total laryngectomy is an extension of the surgery to the tongue base for laryngeal tumors that compromise the vallecula or/and the base of the tongue. In those cases, we use the below-upward laryngeal resection, sectioning the suprahyoid muscles to see the tumor. Once the pharynx is open, the larynx is grasped up and ahead to expose the epiglottis and the base of the tongue. The resection is done trying to leave a free margin at least of 1 cm (ideally 2 cm). It is necessary to dissect the hypoglossal nerve and the lingual arteries carefully when the resection will be large. The pharyngeal defect can be large, and for this closure it is important to evert the lingual mucosa. For very large resections some type of flap reconstruction may be necessary.

13e.4.2 Total Laryngectomy Extended to the Hypopharynx

When the tumor originates in the hypopharynx or there is a clear hypopharyngeal extension of a supraglottic carcinoma, a partial or total laryngopharyngectomy may be needed. If the extension in the hypopharynx is limited, partial pharyngectomy is done, whereas with extensions of more than 50% of the hypopharynx it is advisable do a total (circular) pharyngectomy. For extension to the esophagus, total laryngopharyngectomy with esophagectomy can be performed [4, 24].

Total laryngectomy with partial pharyngectomy. The best approach for total laryngectomy with partial pharyngectomy is to remove the larynx using a combined lateral approach. The surgeon avoids cutting the constrictor muscle on the affected side, and opens the pharynx completely on the uninvolved side. The surgeon can now clearly see the tumor and excise it with the necessary mucosa and constrictor muscle.

The safety margin of 2 cm advisable. We perform frozen sections of tissues from the resection edges. The pharynx can be closed directly in cases of resection of less than 50% of the pharyngeal wall, or local pedicled flaps may be needed.

Total laryngectomy with total (circular) pharyngectomy. The initial dissection steps for total laryngopharyngectomy are the same as for total laryngectomy except that mobilization of the larynx, pharynx and cervical oesophagus as a unit is performed by extending the lateral dissection into the retropharyngeal and retroesophageal space. Careful observation is maintained for spread beyond the buccopharyngeal and prevertebral fasciae into the prevertebral muscles or vertebral bodies. The prevertebral fascia itself is a moderately resistant barrier to tumor spread but is resected in continuity with the specimen if necessary.

Once the pharynx, larynx, and upper cervical esophagus are circumferentially mobilized, the complete thyroid gland or one lobe (the ipsilateral) must be dissected free from its vascular pedicles to be removed with the specimen in continuity with the surrounding paratracheal nodes. The pharynx is entered above the hyoid contralateral to the site with the most superior spread. The pharyngeal mucosa cuts are then continued horizontally around and onto the posterior pharyngeal wall at least 2 cm above the highest extent of the lesion, such that the whole upper pharynx and larynx are now free. The trachea is then transected, followed by the cervical esophagus at the level appropriate to the tumor extent. If total esophagectomy is to be performed, blunt dissection of the esophagus continues from above-downward until the inferior esophageal dissection is encountered.

Reconstruction. An extensive history and voluminous surgical literature deals with reconstruction of circumferential pharyngeal defects. The most frequently used techniques are a tubed jejunum free flap, tubed or semitubed pectoralis major flap, and tubed forearm flap. If the esophageal resection extends below the thoracic inlet, a visceral transposition (usually gastric pull-up) is used, thus avoiding anastomoses in the mediastinum. Microvascular tubed jejunum flaps are now clearly the gold standard for hypopharyngeal reconstruction whenever this technique is feasible in the individual patient and experienced surgeons are available.

13e.4.3 Total Laryngectomy Extended to Prelaryngeal Tissues

Total laryngectomy extended to prelaryngeal tissues is indicated for laryngeal tumors with extralaryngeal extension to prelaryngeal musculature, subcutaneous tissues, and skin and usually extended across the thyroid cartilage or the cricothyroid membrane.

The technique consists in the conventional laryngectomy but removing with the larynx the skin and subcutaneous tissues of the anterior cervical area (Fig. 13e.10). Usually, the skin removed extends from the hyoid level to the suprasternal level and from sternocleidomastoid muscle level on each side.

For the nonirradiated neck with limited resection, reconstruction can be done with residual neck skin. With more extended resections, however, flap reconstruction (Fig. 13e.10) is needed (deltopectoral flap, major pectoral flap, free flap).

13e.4.4 Complications

General complications associated with total laryngectomy are those of any major operation, but the incidence of pulmonary embolism is low. Local complications are the following [6, 15, 21].

Early hematoma. Although rare, haematoma requires prompt intervention to avoid pressure separation of the pharyngeal repair and compression of the upper trachea. The patient is returned to the operating room, the clot is evacuated, and any detectable bleeding is controlled. New drains are inserted because blockage of the original ones with clots is inevitable.

Drain failure. Drains unable to hold a vacuum represent a threat to the wound. There is usually either a leak in the pharynx or the skin/stoma closure that must be detected and sealed.

Infection. Increasing erythema and edema of the skin flaps, usually at the third to fifth postoperative day, indicates a subcutaneous infection. Associated odor, fever, and elevated white blood cell count can

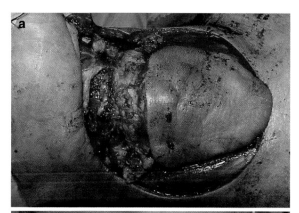

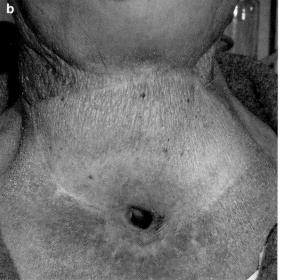

Fig. 13e.10. (**a**) Typical total laryngectomy extended to prelaryngeal tissues in a salvage situation. A major pectoral flap was used to reconstruct the defect. (**b**) Long-term result

occur. If an infected collection is present, the wound is opened under sterile conditions and the pus evacuated and cultured. Dead space between the neopharynx and skin flap is managed with repeated antiseptic gauze packing until healed. Antibiotic coverage is used according to culture results. A pharyngocutaneous fistula must be suspected if wound discharge continues or increases. A chylous fistula must be ruled out if neck dissection was performed.

Pharyngocutaneous fistula. This is the most frequent complication and the one that produces the most significant increase in the duration of hospitalization. Preoperative irradiation and large resections are associated with an increased risk of the incidence and severity of pharyngocutaneous fistula. Erythema and edema around the wound closure, which, on opening, drains purulent material and saliva, often heralds its existence. Such fistulas usually occur within the first 5–6 days postoperatively in nonirradiated patients, and within 10–11 days in irradiated patients. Communication with the pharynx can be confirmed by a methylene blue swallowing test. Initial management is conservative, by nonoral feeding and local measurements including antiseptic gauze fistula-track packing, and antibiotic therapy. The fistula eventually closes spontaneously. If the conservative approach is unsuccessful within 2 weeks in a nonirradiated patient or 3 weeks in an irradiated patient, operative closure should be considered. An excellent option for fistula closure before complete epithelialization is a pedicled muscle flap (pectoralis mainly) slipped between the pharyngeal and skin defects.

Bleeding. Bleeding that takes place 4 days to several weeks after the surgery can be attributed to rupture of an arterial or venous trunk due to infection, necrosis, or wound dehiscence. The most dangerous hemorrhage is due to carotid artery rupture with high rates of mortality and neurological morbidity. The risk factors include radical neck dissection, previous irradiation, and pharyngocutaneous fistula. The treatment can be by external surgery or by endovascular occlusion.

Wound dehiscence. Wound dehiscence may result from skin closure under tension, previous irradiation, wound infection, fistula, or poorly designed, ischemic neck flaps. Local wound care should suffice for healing by secondary intention; but if the carotid becomes persistently exposed, vascularized muscle flap coverage is advisable. The long-term complications include stomal stenosis, pharyngoesophageal stenosis, and hypothyroidism.

Stomal stenosis. Most patients have a stable tracheostoma for some time after surgery. If stomal stenosis occurs, one can consider, as a first option, the use of a cannula or a stoma button. If the stomal stenosis continues to be a source of problems, surgery is indicated.

Pharyngoesophageal stenosis/stricture. In the presence stenosis or stricture, tumor recurrence should be suspected; but once it is excluded by endoscopy and biopsy, outpatient dilation is usually effective. An adequate lumen is necessary not only for swallowing and nutrition but also for tracheoesophageal speech production. If dilation is unsuccessful, flap augmentation (e.g., pectoral major or jejunal free flap) may be necessary for successful rehabilitation.

Hypothyroidism. Preoperative or postoperative radiation therapy plus hemithyroidectomy is usually sufficient to induce a low thyroid state [17, 23]. Thyroid function tests every 6 months after completion of all treatment can indicate when supplemental thyroid medication is required.

13e.4.5 Recommendations for the Follow-up

Early postoperative care. This includes the general care of a patient undergoing major surgery. The patient is kept under observation in the postoperative unit for at least 4 hours to observe his/her general conditions. Tracheal secretions are suctioned as necessary. The drains and all the vital functions must be under control.

After the patient is returned to his regular room in the hospital, ambulation is started as early as possible. Nasogastric tube feeding begins once bowel sounds are present, beginning slowly with water. As soon as this is tolerated without nausea or vomiting, the intravenous line is removed. The drains are removed when output is less than 25 ml/day for two consecutive days.

Oral intake is usually started on the seventh to tenth postoperative day (in nonirradiated patients) if there is no sign of wound breakdown, tenderness, or flap elevation. In previously irradiated necks is advisable to wait until the 12th–14th day postoperatively to allow a longer healing time after the pharyngeal repair. Some authors have encouraged oral intake starting on the first postoperative day, avoiding temporary nasogastric tube feeding, but this is not the general practice.

The stomal sutures are removed on the ninth day. The nonirradiated patient can be discharged on the tenth day if there are no residual problems such as a fever, flap tenderness, or discharge.

Long-term care. Follow-up office visits should be scheduled at monthly intervals during the first year, lengthened to 2-month intervals the second year, 3-month intervals the third year, and 6-month intervals the fourth and fifth years. Follow-up is extended to yearly intervals after the fifth year to rule out recurrence of cancer in the hypopharynx or the neck, which might be effectively treated. The patient undergoes chest imaging once a year and a thyroid-stimulating hormone (TSH) assay every 6 or 12 months if the neck has been irradiated.

13e.4.6 Consequences of Total Laryngectomy and Quality of Life

The two must evident consequences of total laryngectomy are loss of the laryngeal voice (see Rehabilitation) and the permanent tracheostoma, but there are many others. First, permanent respiration for the tracheostoma changes the quality of the air inhaled: The air reaching the lungs is dryer and cooler. This may cause respiratory problems, with coughing, excessive phlegm production, forced expectoration, and dyspnea. For this reason, patients should learn how to take care of their stoma (periodic suctioning and cleaning, and use of a humidifier). Modern heat and moisture exchangers help diminish these problems.

Second, owing to the lack of glottis closure, there is decreased strength in the superior extremities and decreased of intrathoracic and intraabdominal pressure (less effective cough, tendency to constipation). Deterioration of the sense of smell is another consequence of total laryngectomy.

Deglutition is not impaired following standard laryngectomy. However, deglutition disorders may arise if flap reconstruction of the hypopharynx was used and/or postoperative irradiation was applied. Also, owing to the tracheostoma, patients cannot swim because of the risk of aspirating water via the tracheostoma.

Finally, there are psychological and social consequences; the most important is transient depression, which is found in half of the patients. In terms of working activity, around 50% of the patients stop work because of permanent disability. As a consequence of these factors, it is estimated than 50% of the patients have family problems with difficulties between the couple and their sons. Suicide is rare, however. Support groups comprising patients who have also had a laryngectomy can provide good help and information.

Despite the functional impairments, the self-assessment of the quality of life (QOL) using questionnaires answered by individuals who have undergone a laryngectomy indicates only limited QOL changes that go beyond speech and the stoma [26]. The largest QOL changes are seen during the first year after the diagnosis, with significant deterioration on finishing the treatment and slow recovery after that point. Long term, laryngectomy survivors have good global QOL when it is measured with general health instruments and compared with norms. Compared with other chronic diseases, patients with total laryngectomy score higher on QOL questionnaires than patients with diabetes, heart failure, hearing impairment, or other types of cancer. Of course, QOL is highly personal due to personal psychological adaptation and includes multiple variables that contribute to psychological distress.

13e.5 Results

It is not possible to present general results for a surgical technique used for so many different tumors and situations, but we can offer a short summary of our experience with total laryngectomy.

Complications. The overall surgical mortality rate for total laryngectomy is less than 0.5%. Around one-third of our patients developed a postoperative complication after total laryngectomy. Local complications are the most frequent (~25%) and pharyngocutaneous fistula is the most important one (~20% of patients).

Local control. For T3 glottic and supraglottic cancer treated by total laryngectomy as the primary treatment, local control is good, around 92% of local control in cases with free margins. For T4a laryngeal cancer, the local control is ~80%. The same data (~80% local control) are obtained for hypopharyngeal cancer (T3–T4a) with total laryngopharyngectomy and postoperative radiotherapy.

Regional failure. The neck failure is ~10% for laryngeal cancer and ~20% for hypopharyngeal cancer when treated by radical surgery.

Distant metastasis. Distant metastasis is rare for laryngeal cancer (5%) treated by total laryngectomy but more common (~ 25%) for hypopharyngeal cancer treated by radical surgery [13].

Survival. For laryngeal cancer the adjusted survival (disease-related survival) is 80% at 5 years for T3 tumors treated by total laryngectomy and 50% for T4a tumors treated also by total laryngectomy. The observed survival (all causes of death) is 60% for T3 tumors and 40% for T4a tumors. For hypopharyngeal cancer treated by radical surgery followed by radiotherapy, the adjusted survival at 5 years is ~50%, and the observed survival is ~35% [4, 8, 12, 14, 15].

13e.6 Tips and Pearls to Avoid Complications

- Take your time to be sure the patient understands the consequences of total laryngectomy for his/her quality of life and the alternative therapeutic options. He/she must sign an informed consent.
- Discuss voice rehabilitation options with the patient before surgery.
- Plan the airway management with the anesthesiologist before surgery (timing of tracheotomy and intubation), especially for advanced tumors.
- Prepare the strategy for resection, knowing accurately the extension of the tumor (endoscopy, CT, MRI).
- The incision must carry across the skin, subcutaneous tissue, and platysma. Avoid sectioning the anterior and external jugular vein at the time of the incision.
- When sectioning the infrahyoid muscles, be aware that the internal jugular vein is close to the external portion of the sternothyroid muscle.
- Pull up the hyoid bone anteroinferioly when detaching the suprahyoid muscles. This protects the hypoglossus nerve and the lingual artery.
- Plan what to do with the thyroid gland. For large tumors with subglottic extension and/or hypopharyngeal extension, at least the isthmus and the ipsilateral lobe with the paratracheal nodes should be removed.
- For removal of the larynx, try to choose the approach than gives you the best direct view of the tumor. Do not work blindly around corners; perform the removal work under direct vision.
- The specimen should be inspected to confirm the location of the tumor and to evaluate the safety margins.
- In case of any doubt, use the frozen section examination to determine the completeness of tumor resection before closing.
- Prior irradiation makes removal of a laryngeal tumor more difficult because of fibrosis and the lack of good definition. Therefore, during salvage surgery it is always good to use frozen section analysis.
- Selection of the closure method is based on an assessment of the shape and size of the pharyngeal defect and simulated wound approximation before suturing. The least tensioned apposition of wound edges is the best.
- In some irradiated necks with a lot of fibrosis associated with neck dissection (especially if radical), it is better to use a salivary bypass tube and a pectoralis muscular flap to protect the pharyngeal closure and prevent complications.
- Use mechanical closure with a stapler (closed technique) only in cases of endolaryngeal tumors without suprahyoid vallecular, piriform sinus, and postcricoid extension.

References

1. Bedrin L, Ginsburg G, Horowitz Z, Talmi YP (2005) 25-year experience of using a linear stapler in laryngectomy. Head Neck 27:1073–1079
2. Brennan JA, Meyers AD, Jafek BW (1991) The intraoperative management of the thyroid gland during laryngectomy. Laryngoscope 101:929–934
3. Burgués Vila J (1992) Laringectomia total. In: Abello P, Traserra J (eds) Otorrinolaringología. Doyma, Barcelona
4. Eckel HE, Staar S, Volling P, Sittel C, Damm M, Jungehuelsing M (2001) Surgical treatment for hypopharynx carcinoma: feasibility, mortality, and results. Otolaryngol Head Neck Surg 124:561–569
5. Dedo HH (1990) Surgery of the larynx and trachea. BC Decker, Philadelphia, PA/Toronto
6. Ganly I, Patel S, Matsuo J, Singh B, Kraus D, Boyle J, Wong R, Lee N, Pfister DG, Shaha A, Shah J (2005) Postoperative complications of salvage total laryngectomy. Cancer 103:2073–2081
7. Guerrier Y (1977) Traité de Technique Chirurgicale ORL et Cervico-Faciale. Tome III. Pharynx et Larynx. Masson, Paris
8. Hoffman HT, Porter K, Karnell LH, Cooper JS, Weber RS, Langer CJ, Ang KK, Gay G, Stewart A, Robinson RA (2006) Laryngeal cancer in the United States: changes in demographics, patterns of care, and survival. Laryngoscope 116(Suppl. 111):1–13
9. Lefebvre JL (2006) Laryngeal preservation in head and neck cancer: multidisciplinary approach. Lancet Oncol 7:747–755
10. Lefebvre JL, Coche-Dequeant B, Degardin M, Kara A, Mallet Y, Ton Van J (2004) Treatment of laryngeal cancer: the permanent challenge. Expert Rev Anticancer Ther 4:913–920
11. León X, Quer M, Burgués J, Abelló P, Vega M, De Andrés L (1996) Prevention of stomal recurrence. Head Neck 18:54–59
12. León X, Quer M, Diez S, Orús C, López-Pousa A, Burgués J (1999) Second neoplasm in patients with head and neck cancer. Head Neck 21:204–210
13. León X, Quer M, Orús C, Venegas MP, Montoro V (2000) Distant metastases in head and neck cancer patients who achieved loco-regional control. Head Neck 22:680–686
14. León X, Quer M, Orús C, Venegas MP (2001) Can cure be achieved in patients with head and neck carcinomas? The problem of second neoplasm. Expert Rev Anticancer Ther 1:125–133
15. León X, Quer M, Orús C, López M, Gras JR, Vega M (2001) Results of salvage surgery for local or regional recurrence after larynx preservation with induction chemotherapy and radiotherapy. Head Neck 23:733–738

16. León X, Quer M, Orús C, Morán J, Recher K (2002) Results of an organ preservation protocol with induction chemotherapy and radiatiotherapy in patients with locally advanced sinus carcinoma. Eur Arch Otorhinolaryngol 259:32–36

17. León X, Gras JR, Pérez A, Rodríguez J, Andrés L de, Orús C, Quer M (2002) Hypothyroidism in patients treated with total laryngectomy: a multivariate study. Eur Arch Otorhinolaryngol 259:193–196

18. Leon X, Lopez-Pousa A, De Vega M, Orus C, De Juan M, Quer M (2005) Results of an organ preservation protocol with induction chemotherapy and radiotherapy in patients with locally advanced laryngeal carcinoma. Eur Arch Otorhinolaryngol 262:93–98

19. Montgomery WW (1999) Surgery of the upper respiratory system, 2nd ed. Lea &Febiger, Philadelphia, PA

20. Pfister DG, Laurie SA, Weinstein GS, Mendenhall WM, Adelstein DJ, Ang KK, Clayman GL, Fisher SG, Forastiere AA, Harrison LB, Lefebvre JL, Leupold N, List MA, O'Malley BO, Patel S, Posner MR, Schwartz MA, Wolf GT (2006) American Society of Clinical Oncology clinical practice guideline for the use of larynx-preservation strategies in the treatment of laryngeal cancer. J Clin Oncol 24:3693–3704

21. Schwartz SR, Yueh B, Maynard C, Daley J, Henderson W, Khuri SF (2004) Predictors of wound complications after laryngectomy: a study of over 2000 patients. Otolaryngol Head Neck Surg 131:61–68

22. Stell PM (1991) Total laryngectomy. In: Silver CE (ed.) Laryngeal cancer. Thieme Medical Publishers, New York.

23. Smolarz K, Malke G, Voth E, Scheidhauer K, Eckel HE, Jungehulsing M, Schicha H (2000) Hypothyroidism after therapy for larynx and pharynx carcinoma. Thyroid 10:425–429

24. Silver AE, Smith RV (1999) The larynx and hypopharynx. In: Silver CE, Rubin JS (eds) Atlas of head and neck surgery, 2nd ed. Churchill Livingstone, New York

25. Tucker HM (1987) The larynx. Thieme Medical Publishers New York

26. Vilaseca I, Chen Ay, Backscheider AG (2006) Long-term quality of life after total laryngectomy. Head Neck 28:313–320

Voice Restoration

13f

Frans J. M. Hilgers, Alfons J. M. Balm,
Michiel W. M. van den Brekel, and I. Bing Tan

Core Messages

> Surgical prosthetic voice restoration is the best possible option for patients to regain oral communication after total laryngectomy. It is considered to be the present "gold standard" for voice rehabilitation of laryngectomized individuals.

> Surgical prosthetic voice restoration, in essence, is always achievable in patients fit enough to tolerate total laryngectomy and motivated to regain optimal oral communication.

> Surgical prosthetic voice restoration requires a multidisciplinary team approach (physician, speech therapist, oncology nurse) to obtain optimal results.

> If a good prosthetic voice deteriorates, the underlying problem most likely requires prompt clinical consultation, and patients should be instructed accordingly.

> Most of the problems with prosthetic voice restoration are relatively simple and immediately solvable.

> If there is no immediate explanation for the inability to voice, a further search more often than not clarifies the cause and shows the way to solve the problem.

> Reconstruction of the pharynx with, for example, free revascularized or pedicled flaps does not preclude surgical prosthetic voice restoration.

F. J. M. Hilgers (✉)
Department of Head and Neck Oncology and Surgery,
The Netherlands Cancer Institute,
Antoni van Leeuwenhoek Hospital, Plesmanlaan 121,
1066 CX Amsterdam, The Netherlands
e-mail: f.hilgers@nki.nl

13f.1 Indication

This chapter is not intended to discuss the indication(s) for total laryngectomy (TLE) but to discuss the main surgical option for voice restoration once the patient is scheduled for total laryngectomy. Ever since its successful start in 1980 with the work of Singer and Blom [51], tracheoesophageal voice restoration using one of the presently commercially available voice prostheses can be considered to be the "gold standard." The main reason for this is that any voice prosthesis, essentially a one-way valve implanted in a surgical puncture in the tracheoesophageal (TE) party wall, enables controlled diversion of pulmonary air into the pharynx and prevents aspiration. The pulmonary air produces mucosal waves in the pharyngoesophageal (PE) segment and thus sound, which subsequently is transformed into understandable speech in the speech canal. Pulmonary driven tracheoesophageal speech resembles laryngeal voicing most closely and outperforms the traditional esophageal and electrolarynx voice in many aspects.

Esophageal voice, which is achieved by injecting air into the esophagus and subsequently ejecting this column of air into the pharynx is characterized by a short phonation time as only 60–80 ml of air is available for voicing. It is difficult to learn, and it often times takes many months to develop a useful voice. Electrolarynx voicing, in contrast, is much easier to learn but lacks the variation in tone required to be as naturally perceived as laryngeal or pharyngeal voicing. The latter two voice rehabilitation techniques are still relevant as backup methods, and patients should be motivated to try to acquire at least one of them. However, they are not further discussed here, and the interested reader is referred to the relevant speech/language pathology literature.

13f.2 Specific Assessment/Preoperative Workup

Basically, any patient able to tolerate total laryngectomy can also tolerate primary surgical voice restoration. Prior to total laryngectomy, aside from the regular medical preoperative workup and surgical and nursing counseling, patients especially need counseling by the speech therapist and a laryngectomized patient counselor. The various possibilities of postlaryngectomy voice rehabilitation (prosthetic, esophageal, electrolarynx voice) should be discussed, and the motivation of the patient should be assessed if prosthetic voice restoration is chosen. The patient has to understand that a voice prosthesis is a semipermanent implant that requires regular replacement. Also, the difference between indwelling (clinician handled) and nonindwelling (patient handled) devices should be explained. If the choice is made to apply a nonindwelling device, it is important to establish whether the dexterity of the patient is good enough to guarantee its successful application. Also, the patient has to understand that using a nonindwelling device makes the start more uncomfortable and requires more long-term self-activation than indwelling prostheses.

Voice prostheses can also be employed in a secondary fashion (i.e., some time after total laryngectomy and, if necessary, postoperative radiotherapy). This can be a matter of the surgeon's preference (although there is not much justification for that), being indicated by surgical circumstances during the laryngectomy (e.g., the need to resect the trachea very low, leading to a suboptimal stoma), or if the patient has chosen to try one of the other options first and the results are unsatisfactory. In this case, preoperative counseling is the same as for primary voice restoration, but during this workup it is important to establish the anatomy of the pharynx and stoma to anticipate possible impeding factors, such as pharyngoesophageal stricture, hypertonicity of the constrictor muscles, or stomal stenosis.

To predict the success of secondary tracheoesophageal puncture (TEP) voice restoration, some authors advocate carrying out a so-called insufflation test [52]. This test consists of inserting a tube and insufflating air into the pharynx to determine if a sound can be produced. The air is supplied from the patient him/herself, by connecting the tube with the stoma, or by the examiner who uses an outside source or blows him/herself into the tube. A positive test (i.e., production of sound), is predictable for success, whereas a negative test is not (the tube might

irritate or is in the way just enough to block airflow) [13]. Hence, this test is not recommended. If the patient after a secondary puncture cannot vocalize immediately, mostly because of hypertonicity or spasm of the constrictor muscles, that is the proper moment for a diagnostic workup.

13f.3 Surgical Techniques

13f.3.1 Primary Prosthetic Voice Rehabilitation

Primary prosthetic voice restoration, meaning TEP, and immediate insertion of a voice prosthesis at the time of total laryngectomy (TLE) is presently the method of choice for many experienced medical professionals [28]. The optimal technique to achieve this is to use an indwelling prosthesis (e.g., Groningen or one of the Provox prostheses) because such a device has the required shape and robustness for reliable retention in the freshly created by the TEP [22, 27, 46]. This enables the easiest, most comfortable voice rehabilitation because the patient is still under general anesthesia when the first prosthesis is inserted. Moreover, no stenting of the fistula with a nasogastric feeding tube is needed as the device itself is used to stabilize the puncture site [30]. Advocates of using a feeding tube in the fistula and inserting the first prosthesis after removing the feeding tube after 10–12 days underestimate the burden this poses on the patient. Realizing that the same patient was under general anesthesia just some days before should be reason enough not to continue this questionable and unfounded custom. Immediate insertion of the prosthesis has a good track record, and its reliability and low complication rate has been substantiated in many publications [5, 22, 27, 42, 43, 56].

Additionally, the psychological advantage of the possibility to start voicing immediately after removal of the feeding tube hardly can be overestimated. Furthermore, there is a tendency to start oral intake soon after the surgery, in some clinics after 24–48 hours, which would require inserting the prosthesis even earlier postoperatively [6]. Timing of the TEP almost always can be primary, even if most or all of the pharyngeal circumference has to be reconstructed, so long as the esophagus is still present at the level of the trachea [25]. Only when the proximal esophagus is dissected off the trachea, as for a gastric pull-up, is the TEP best delayed 4–5 weeks. In those cases, secondary TEP is performed after completion of wound healing and prior to possible postoperative radiotherapy (see also the role of radiotherapy below).

13f.3.2 Specific Recommendations for Surgical Refinements

Prosthetic voice restoration should be compatible with standard TLE, and little adjustment of the usual surgical techniques and standards is necessary to ensure optimal worldwide acceptance and applicability. With the presently available voice prostheses this is possible indeed: wherever in the world TLE is executed, voice prostheses (if available and affordable [17, 45, 53, 61]) can be applied, irrespective the method of closure of the pharyngeal mucosa and pharyngeal constrictor muscle defect. However, with a few refinements in the surgery of TLE several postlaryngectomy problems can be avoided or diminished—more specifically, hypertonicity of the pharyngoesophageal (PE) segment, a too narrow stoma, and a too deep stoma.

13f.3.2.1 Prevention of Hypertonicity of the PE Segment

Hypertonicity of the PE segment is the most frequent reason for failure to develop fluent prosthetic speech (and for that matter also esophageal speech) [9, 15]. The cause is too high muscle tonicity in the constrictor pharyngeus muscles forming the wall of the PE segment. This tonicity increases after inflation of air and blocks the flow of air through the pharynx, preventing mucosal vibrations and thus sound production. Although there are several surgical solutions described in the literature, the best option to prevent this problem is

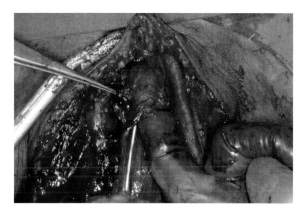

Fig. 13f.1. Myotomy of the cricopharyngeus muscle prevents hypertonicity of the pharyngoesophageal segment

to perform a short anterior myotomy of the circular proximal upper esophageal sphincter (cricopharyngeus) muscle (see Fig. 13f.1) in every patient unless palpation during surgery reveals that this muscle is completely relaxed [48]. After this myotomy (and prosthesis insertion), the surgeon can still close the pharynx (mucosa and constrictor muscles) in the preferred manner.

13f.3.2.2 Prevention of a Too Narrow Stoma

Ideally, the patient has a stable stoma of the same size as the trachea or only slightly narrower, providing easy access to the voice prosthesis and to avoid the need for a tracheal cannula to keep the stoma open wide enough for comfortable breathing. The causes of stomal stenosis are dehiscence of the trachea from the skin due to local infection and traction, disruption of the integrity of the cartilage of the proximal trachea "ring," or contraction of the scar between the trachea and the skin.

The best technique, in our hands, is to suture the trachea into a separate fenestra in the lower skin flap (see Fig. 13f.2) [19]. The fenestra should be approximately

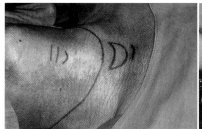 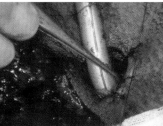 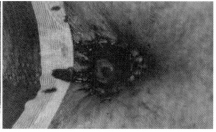

Fig. 13f.2. *Left* Outline of incisions for TLE and stoma creation. *Middle* Creation of a stoma in a separate fenestra in the lower skin flap, with subsequent meticulous skin-to-mucosa suturing, covering the exposed but intact tracheal cartilage. *Right* End result

the same size as the trachea, and the proximal tracheal "ring" must stay intact. This is the most important aspect of stoma creation: The collagen fibers in the trachea cartilage are distributed in such a manner that the cartilage acts as a "spring," trying to widen the trachea [49]. If the cartilage is cut, these "spring" forces are lost and the trachea collapses, with stoma shrinkage as a result. Obviously, meticulous suturing of the skin to the tracheal mucosa, optimally covering the exposed trachea cartilage, is important to prevent local infection and thus scarification and potential stenosis. The small strip of skin (8–10 mm) cranially is surprisingly vital and only rarely breaks down, even in irradiated patients. An additional advantage of this method is that there are no trifurcations in the wound, which is unavoidable if the stoma is created in the TLE skin incision itself. Obviously, in some cases in which the trachea has to be sectioned deeply, the remaining trachea is not long enough to be sutured in a separate fenestra, and the entire inferior skin flap is needed to be able to form a stoma. Even in these cases, however, with an intact tracheal ring it should be possible to get the patient through surgery without a tracheal cannula, which is our preferred method. The absence of a cannula is beneficial as well because there is less irritation of the trachea and stoma and thus less coughing, diminishing the need for sedation and limiting the chance of suture line damage and infection and thus potential stomal stenosis.

13f.3.2.3 Prevention of a Too Deep (Recessed) Stoma

A deep stoma is problematic for the later application of additional rehabilitation devices that potentially rely on peristomal attachment, such as a heat and moisture exchanger (HME) or an automatic speaking valve (ASV). Stomas that are called (too) deep can be the result of traction of the trachea in a caudal direction in case the trachea is cut very inferiorly but can also be caused by the fact that the sternal heads of the sternocleidomastoid muscles (SCMM) are protruding relative to the stomal level. An easy solution is to leave as much trachea as oncologically safe and to cut the sternal attachment of the SCMM, leaving it to sink into the neck before skin closure (see Fig. 13f.3). This generally results in a flatter stoma without any noticeable functional deficits from the resected SCMM, making peristomal attachment of external devices considerably easier.

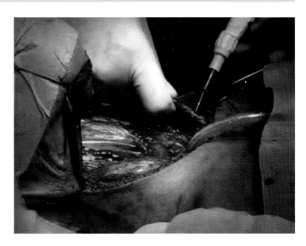

Fig. 13f.3. *Left* Cutting the sternal attachment of the sternocleidomastoid muscle. *Right* Completed section

13f.3.3 Secondary Prosthetic Voice Rehabilitation

Secondary TEP is a simple endoscopic technique using a rigid esophagoscope and a trocar and immediate insertion of a voice prosthesis (also in this case the method of choice). The method is essentially unchanged since the first description of Singer and Blom [51], although some new instruments (e.g., the Provox trocar and guidewire) have made the technique even simpler [22]. When the Provox system is used, in most cases an 8-mm prosthesis is long enough for the first insertion, although sometimes a longer device is required. Palpation in the stoma with the rigid scope in situ easily reveals whether the standard 8-mm or longer device is needed. In any case, one should avoid inserting a too short prosthesis because it induces edema by too high pressure of the flanges on the tissues and potentially tissue necrosis.

Relative to further prevention of problems with secondary TEP, there are three issues worthwhile mentioning. If the patient is a failed esophageal speaker, there is a chance that the cause for this failure is hypertonicity of the PE segment [15]. This means that the medical professional and the patient have to anticipate further treatment before optimal fluent voicing can be achieved (see below regarding secondary hypertonicity treatment). With respect to the technique, it is important to ensure that the puncture is made high in the trachea (5–10 mm from the mucocutaneous border). This makes daily maintenance by the patient (cleaning with a brush and/or flushing device) and replacement by the medical professional in the out patient clinic easier. Finally, to prevent local infection, as with all "clean-contaminated" head and neck surgery, broad-spectrum antibiotic prophylaxis should be applied during TEP.

13f.3.4   Prosthetic Voice Restoration and Radiotherapy

Many surgeons have an understandable reluctance of applying TEP in patients needing TLE for a recurrence after (chemo)radiotherapy or in patients with advanced disease needing postoperative radiotherapy. Especially in the radiation failures the incidence of complications, particularly fistula development, is possibly increased (the data in the literature are controversial), and then there is an obvious bias for creating a fistula oneself. Nevertheless, there is enough evidence in the literature that this controlled fistula formation does not increase the incidence of wound healing complications; therefore, TEP with immediate insertion of a voice prosthesis is a safe, reliable method [5, 24, 42, 47]. The only warning to be given is that after radiotherapy one should wait 6 weeks to let the radiation side effects heal before performing a TEP. Otherwise, the fistula is created in a too vulnerable, not yet completely healed area, and undoubtedly the risk of complicated healing of the TEP is too high.

13f.3.5   Recommendations for Follow up (Postoperative Care)

In case of primary prosthetic voice restoration and immediate prosthesis insertion, it is important to check the puncture site daily. If the length of the prosthesis chosen is sufficiently long, the prosthesis can easily be seen. If there is excessive edema, making the prosthesis too short for the elongated puncture tract, either corticosteroids can be given or the prosthesis has to be changed for a longer version. This latter solution might be difficult and, in the authors' experience, has never been necessary. During the postoperative period, the nursing staff can start familiarizing the patient with the daily maintenance (brush cleaning or cleaning with a flushing device) and teach the patient to use a plug to prevent possible (later) leakage through the device, something that is useful to learn early on. Voice rehabilitation instruction by the speech pathologist can start after 10–12 days, if wound healing is sufficient and oral intake has been fully restored.

In case of secondary puncture with immediate prosthesis insertion, speech therapy can start the same day, as can oral intake.

13f.4   Prosthesis Replacement

13f.4.1   Indications

Silicon rubber voice prostheses, irrespective of the brand applied, are semipermanent devices that do not have an unlimited lifespan. The life spans of prostheses show considerable variation; and in the literature mean device lives are 4–5 months in the Western world but much longer (10–18 months) in the Mediterranean areas and the United States [4, 7, 12, 14, 16, 24, 35, 47, 50, 56, 58]. However, it is more important to look at the *median* device life, which is a better reflection of clinical practice, as the *mean* is often considerably influenced by a limited number of patients with an unusual long survival of their prosthesis (sometimes even several years, with two champions in our institution with a device life of 11.5 years) [47].

The main reason for replacement is leakage of fluids through the prosthesis, which signals incompetence of the valve. Although patients can temporarily apply a plug into the prosthesis to prevent aspiration, eventually replacement is necessary. It is an outpatient procedure that is easy enough nowadays with the availability of anterograde replacement procedures. The reason a valve starts to leak is mostly the growth of *Candida* species on the valve mechanism, preventing its proper closure [40]. Measures to limit this *Candida* growth (e.g., by antifungal drugs such as nystatin or diflucan) have been debated, but there is limited clinical evidence about their effectiveness [41, 59]. A better option is to check the diet of the patient and advise consumption of probiotics, such as certain yoghurts, which have been proven to be effective in both at vitro and in vivo studies [10, 11, 18, 57].

There is a second reason for early prosthesis failure: inadvertent opening of the valve due to an underpressure created in the esophagus during deep breathing and swallowing. Especially during deep breathing an underpressure is created inside the thorax and thus also inside the esophagus. Normally, this is of no consequence because the upper esophageal sphincter is preventing the flow of air into the esophagus. But with a voice prosthesis present under the level of the sphincter, the valve can open and air can be drawn in. Consequently, these patients often complain of disturbing aerophagia. The easier opening of the valve, maybe in conjunction with its delayed closure, makes leakage occur more readily. Increasing the airflow resistance of the valve could limit this problem but would create a voicing problem. Recently a special voice prosthesis (Provox ActiValve) became available that eliminates both the problem of *Candida* growth on the valve mechanism and the inadvertent opening by underpressure [29]. This has been accomplished by creating a valve mechanism made of Teflon-like material, which is insensitive to *Candida* growth, with built-in magnets to counteract the underpressure in the esophagus. With this valve a significant (3–39 times, mean 14 times) prolongation of the device life could be achieved in a selected group of patients with a mean device life of 30 days and a median device life of 25 days [29].

Internal blockage of the valve itself preventing proper voicing is a rare problem, and blockage is mostly caused by interference of the mucosa with valve function. This issue and other indications for prosthesis replacement, such as leakage around the device and local fistula problems, are discussed below.

13f.4.2 Valve Incompetence: Leakage through the Valve

If cleaning the valve with a brush or flushing device does not solve leakage through the prosthesis, simple anterograde replacement of the device is required [4, 27]. The preventive action to be taken with any replacement is that the length of the valve always should be checked carefully, even if there is no sign of leakage around it. By gently pulling at the tracheal flange with a hemostat it is easy to see whether the length is still good or if the prosthesis has become too long in relation to the

mostly gradually decreasing length of the fistula. A discrepancy up to 2–3 mm is tolerable because there is little or no pressure of the flanges on the mucosa. More than 3 mm discrepancy is an indication to downsize the prosthesis by one size (e.g., from 8 mm to 6 mm). Care should be taken not to create a too tight fit, causing pressure of the flanges on the mucosa leading to edema and an even tighter fit, possibly followed by tissue necrosis. In patients needing frequent replacements (on the order of only weeks up to 2 months) one could consider application of a Provox ActiValve, as described above.

13f.4.3 Valve Discrepancy: Leakage Around a Too Long Prosthesis

Valve-fistula discrepancy leads to leakage around the prosthesis. In most instances, it is a result of the natural gradual decrease in the thickness of the TE party wall. Subsidence of the surgical edema and tissue inflammation leads to a shorter fistula tract, and a once well fitting prosthesis becomes too long. This can result in pistoning of the prosthesis inside the fistula and, hence, squeezing of fluids around the prosthesis. Because subsidence of edema and inflammation is part of a normal healing process, we do not consider this a complication and the solution is simply to insert a shorter prosthesis [47]. In our experience, one should avoid downsizing more than one size at a time to prevent a too tight fit, which as mentioned above and further discussed below, would cause problems of its own.

13f.5 Results (Author's Experience)

Assessment of the long-term clinical results is important to gain insight in the advantages and disadvantages of any surgical method. This is also true for postlaryngectomy prosthetic voice rehabilitation [4, 22, 24, 47]. Retrospective clinical analysis of 318 patients with consistent use of indwelling voice prostheses (Provox and Provox2) in a comprehensive national cancer center setting was published in 2000 [47]. There were 261 men and 57 women with a mean age of 62 years treated over slightly more than 10 years. Standard wide-field total laryngectomy was carried out in 287 patients and total laryngectomy with a circumferential pharyngeal resection in 31 patients. During the study period there were 2700 prosthesis replacements. Prostheses were in situ for an accumulative period of 364,339 days or 1000 patient-years. The main outcome measures were device life, indications for replacement (device- or fistula-related), adverse events, and voice quality. The median patient–device follow-up was 67 months. The mean actuarial device life for all replacement indications was 163 days (median 89 days). The main indications for replacement were device-related—i.e., leakage through the prosthesis (73%) and obstruction (4%)—or fistula-related—i.e., leakage around the prosthesis (13%) and hypertrophy and/or infection of the fistula (7%). Adverse events occurred in 10.7% of all replacements in one-third of the patients, mostly solvable by a shrinkage period, adequate sizing, and/or antibiotic treatment. Definitive closure of the TE fistula tract occurred in 5% of the patients. Significant clinical factors for increased device life were no radiotherapy ($p = 0.03$) and age > 70 years ($p < 0.02$). Success rate with respect to voice quality (i.e., fair-to-excellent rating) was 88%, which was significantly influenced by the extent of surgery ($p < 0.001$). The conclusion of this study is that the consistent use of indwelling voice prostheses shows a high success rate of prosthetic vocal rehabilitation in terms of the percentage of long-term users (95%) and of fair-to-excellent voice quality (88% of the patients). Furthermore, adverse events, occurring in one-third of the patients and in 1 of 9–10 replacements, are easily manageable in most cases (see next paragraphs).

13f.6 Tips and Pearls to Troubleshoot Adverse Events

As with any surgical and prosthetic method, complications and adverse events must be taken into account. Straightforward diagnostics and solutions can solve most of the presently known problems. Patients with voice prosthesis problems, which often develop gradually, tend to postpone the visit to the clinic until "the last minute." Therefore, it is important for any clinic seeing these TLE patients to have a comprehensive straightforward protocol for dealing with all the known complications and adverse events. If such a protocol is "in place," taking care of these occasional problems is

hardly more time-consuming than dealing with the regular replacement procedure needed for a leaking valve. It is important to instruct patients that they seek attention at the clinic as soon as they notice a change in their voicing and not to wait too long because the sooner a problem is handled the easier it is to correct.

13f.7 Most Important Adverse Events and Issues to Discuss

- Atrophy of the fistula/party wall
- Infection of the fistula
- Hypertrophy of the fistula
- Partial prosthesis extrusion
- Hypertonicity of the PE segment
- Hypotonicity of the PE segment
- Pulmonary rehabilitation and voice restoration

13f.7.1 Atrophy of the Fistula/Party Wall

Atrophy of the party wall occurred in our data in 3% of the prosthesis replacements in 18% of the patients, ultimately leading to temporary fistula closure in 6% and to a permanent closure in 1 of 318 patients [47]. Gradual thinning of the TE tissues is a natural process and in only a small number of cases leads to such a short fistula tract that the shortest voice prosthesis (4.5 mm length) is still too long to ensure proper sealing of the fistula. Thus, most problems of leakage around the prosthesis occur in patients with a 4.5-mm prosthesis although sometimes in longer fistula tracts. The following algorithm is used by the authors.

13f.7.2 Algorithm to Solve Atrophy/ Leakage Around the Prosthesis

1(a). Shrinkage. Nowadays shrinkage is seldom applied because it is cumbersome for the patient. After removing the prosthesis, most fistulas shrink in a few days, but a feeding tube and a cuffed cannula is needed to prevent aspiration.

1(b). Silicon sealing ring. A thin ring (outer diameter 18 mm, inner diameter 7.5 mm, thickness 0.5 mm) is punched out from a larger piece of silicone sheeting using a tailored punch, and this ring is placed behind the tracheal flange and around the shaft of the prosthesis with the help of two hemostats (like pulling a button through a buttonhole). The sealing ring is not intended to compensate for a too long prosthesis but to adhere to the mucosa by surface tension; hence, it should not be thicker than 0.5 mm.

2. Purse-string suture. A purse-string suture using 3×0 atraumatic Vicryl can be an effective and quick physician's solution. After removal of the prosthesis, the suture is started at 12 o'clock with the needle curving submucosally at a distance of 1–2 mm from the edged of the fistula until 6 o'clock; and from there it curves submucosally on the other side until 12 o'clock. After placing the suture, a new prosthesis is inserted, and the suture is gently tightened to pull the mucosa against the prosthesis. This procedure is always successful for the short term; and by letting the suture degrade spontaneously, it can have a tissue-augmenting effect, solving the problem also long term.

3. Augmentation of the party wall. Permanent augmentation of the party wall with a nondegradable product such as Bioplastique is highly successful and has been described in several articles [38, 39]. The same effect can be achieved with injection of, for example, autologous fat or glutaraldehyde crosslinked (GAX) collagen, but in our experience Bioplastique gives the best permanent effect and is safe to use in everyday clinical practice [8, 36]. Another option is the use of granulocyte-macrophage colony stimulating factor (GM-CSF) to induce a sterile inflammation to augment the fistula tract [44].

4. Fistula closure and later secondary puncture. If all of the previous measures fail or in case there is a too wide fistula with a lack of tissue to be tightened around the prosthesis or to be augmented, fistula closure is unavoidable. Because most fistulas after some time (> 6 months) are completely epithelialized, they have to be dissected and closed in three tissue layers. This can best be achieved by approaching the fistula from above, separating the esophagus and trachea until just caudal to the fistula, sectioning the fistula, closing the esophageal side in two layers and the tracheal side in one, and closing the skin also in layers. If the tissues are markedly atrophic, one can consider swinging the sternal head of the SCMM muscle in between the

trachea and esophagus or use a dermal graft to enforce the esophageal and tracheal suture lines. Generally, repuncture with immediate prosthesis insertion can be carried out after 6 weeks. Larger fistulas sometimes cannot be closed in this way, and some tissue augmentation has to be performed using a properly tailored pectoralis major muscle–fascia flap, with occasionally using a split skin graft fixed with tissue glue for coverage on the tracheal side. Only seldom is more extensive surgery required (e.g., free radial forearm flap or gastric pull-up). There is no standard procedure for these situations, which always require a tailored approach.

13f.7.3 Infection of the Fistula

Local infection is seen in approximately 10% of the patients, and the treatment is mostly simple. Because local infection leads to swelling of the tissues, it is important to decrease the pressure of the flanges on the mucosa. If the prosthesis originally was fitted well, this means that in such a case the prosthesis has to be replaced for a longer device. In contrast to the down-sizing at least between advice of one shaft length, one should upsize it with and two steps (e.g., 6 to 10) to allow proper fitting in the infected fistula. In case of a local infection, removal of the prosthesis should be avoided because it would likely lead to permanent closure of the TEP, leaving the patient unnecessarily "speechless" for a period of time. Broad-spectrum antibiotic treatment in most cases eliminates the infection. It usually takes several months for the tissue swelling to subside, making the prosthesis too long and potentially prone to leakage around it; but by that time the prosthesis likely has to be replaced for leakage through it anyway.

13f.7.4 Hypertrophy of the Fistula

There are two forms of hypertrophy of the fistula's tissues.

Anterior hypertrophy is a mostly fibromatous or granulating mucosa excess, potentially leading to complete overgrowth of the tracheal flange. This is most often seen in patients requiring a trachea cannula exerting constant pressure on the prosthesis or in case of a too short prosthesis, which is drawn inward. Obviously, the prosthesis should be of the correct size, and use of a cannula should be avoided; if the latter is not possible, a stoma plasty should be considered [60]. Sometimes it is necessary to remove the excess tissue because it bulges too far forward into the trachea, decreasing the airway too much. This can be done with any form of electrocautery or (laser) resection.

Posterior hypertrophy or esophageal pocket (sometimes incorrectly called separation of the party wall) is a more important problem in daily practice because it is less obvious and the diagnosis is often delayed. These patients typically complain of deterioration of their voice (more strained) and seeing some blood on the brush while cleaning the inside of the prosthesis. Sometimes even an overt esophageal pocket is formed, with eventually complete mucosa overgrowth on the backside of the prosthesis. Once this problem is suspected, it is easy to diagnose by careful inspection of the fistula with a thin (flexible) endoscope through the prosthesis, or after removal of the prosthesis it can often be seen directly. The solution is also simple: Insert a longer prosthesis (usually at least two sizes longer) that encompasses the excess tissue in between the flanges; this immediately "gives the patient the voice back" and leads to "fistulizing" the excess tissue. Anterograde insertion can be accomplished in most cases, but it is wise to "overshoot" the device (i.e., push the complete prosthesis into the esophagus and then pull the tracheal flange in situ with a hemostat to ensure the proper position of the esophageal flange on the backside). Only rarely does the traditional retrograde insertion method [21] have to be applied, and even more seldom is this procedure carried out under general anesthesia (only when the fistula tract cannot be found atraumatically).

13f.7.5 Partial Prosthesis Extrusion

The potentially most risky complication is (partial) extrusion of the prosthesis. This adverse event has been seen only when a too short prosthesis is exerting too much pressure on the tissues, leading to local necrosis. This too short prosthesis can be the result of a too rapid downsizing or a local infection. In any case, the too short prosthesis must be removed and a longer prosthesis inserted, which usually solves the problem. The new prosthesis covers the thickened fistula tract,

and in all cases we encountered complete spontaneous healing. Sometimes some excess tissue had to be removed to ensure proper fit of the new, longer prosthesis. A course of broad-spectrum antibiotics has always been prescribed. Thus, although potentially dangerous because of the risk of aspirating the device "on its way out," pressure necrosis with partial prosthesis extrusion can be solved by replacing the too short prosthesis with a properly sized, longer device.

If the prosthesis is completely extruded and the patient cannot indicate its whereabouts, it is important to check whether dislodgment has occurred toward the trachea or into the esophagus. In this situation, flexible endoscopy of the trachea and/or radiological examination (thorax and/or abdomen overview) is indicated. If the prosthesis is trapped in the bronchial tree it must be removed endoscopically. If the device is located in the alimentary tract, spontaneous passage can be awaited in most cases.

13f.8 Non-Prosthesis-Related Problems

13f.8.1 Hypertonicity of the PE Segment

Hypertonicity, although not a "complication" of prosthetic voicing, is still worth mentioning here because it is considered to be the most important reason for failure to develop fluent speech. As already described, performing a short myotomy of the upper esophageal sphincter is probably the most effective preventive measure to be taken during TLE [48]. However, if hypertonicity is still present, and intensive speech therapy is not capable of solving it, the condition warrants treatment. The easiest and least invasive option presently available is chemodenervation with botulinum toxin [20, 33, 37, 54]. After proper identification of the hypertonic PE segment with video-fluoroscopy, marking the segment on the skin, 100 MU of Botox (the equivalent dose for the other brand, Dysport, is 400 MU) is injected into the constrictor pharyngeus muscle area, preferably through using a hollow electromyography (EMG) needle. Interestingly, the effect is long-lasting if not forever, in contrast to other clinical conditions in which Botox is used. Apparently, once the patient has experienced fluent speech, through some kind of biofeedback, the effect is maintained. This phenomenon sometimes is seen even after temporary "denervation" with lidocaine injection, advocated to be used as a "diagnostic procedure" in all cases of hypertonicity. Since Botox has become available, surgical myotomy is rarely necessary, although it is still an option. If still indicated, care should be taken to perform a myotomy of the complete middle and inferior constrictor and cricopharyngeus muscle groups and obviously avoid fistula formation, especially in irradiated patients.

13f.8.2 Hypotonicity of the PE Segment

Although also not a "complication" of the use of voice prostheses, hypotonicity of the PE segment can be a disturbing condition because the patient is not able to produce a good sound and only has a whispering, aphonic voice. Mostly, there is no pitch detectable at all in the voice of patients with this condition. The sometimes extreme distension of the PE segment is caused by inadvertent complete denervation of the constrictor muscles. Until recently, only through application of some external pressure (digital or with a special pressure band) this problem could be "treated" to some extent [15, 47]. However, recently we have described an interesting surgical technique in which we have successfully applied a sternocleidomastoid muscle sling to form an internal "pressure band" [32]. This resulted in clear improvement in the voice, especially through an increase of the maximum phonation time and the dynamic range.

13f.8.3 Pulmonary Rehabilitation and Voice Restoration

Although seemingly not a directly relevant issue in this chapter on problem solving during prosthetic voice rehabilitation, it is still essential to make a few remarks on the importance of pulmonary rehabilitation after total laryngectomy. TLE disrupts normal pulmonary physiology, and the best option to correct this (in part) is the consequent application of a heat and moisture exchanger (HME) [1, 22, 62]. All of the HMEs described in the literature help decrease pulmonary complaints and diminish the increased phlegm production [2, 26, 23]. There is also an indication that regular HME use leads to decreased pulmonary infections [34].

Additionally, and relevant to this chapter on voice restoration, in several studies it was demonstrated that consequent HME use improves voice quality [3, 55]. Because an HME is applied through special adhesive with peristomal attachment or a specialized cannula, it prevents direct digital contact with the stoma and the voice prosthesis, making voicing also more hygienic.

13f.9 Concluding Remarks

As with any surgical method, the highly successful method of surgical prosthetic voice restoration requires special considerations to obtain optimal results. This chapter has outlined the basic surgical techniques and refinements, the daily maintenance aspects, and solutions for the commonly encountered adverse events. To obtain optimal results (90% success rate should be the norm) a multidisciplinary approach to this important form of rehabilitation of laryngectomized individuals is indispensable and a proper protocol to deal with these adverse events should be in place in every clinic supporting TLE patients.

References

1. Ackerstaff AH, Hilgers FJM, Aaronson NK, Balm AJM, Van Zandwijk N (1993) Improvements in respiratory and psychosocial functioning following total laryngectomy by the use of a heat and moisture exchanger. Ann Otol Rhinol Laryngol 102:878–883
2. Ackerstaff AH, Hilgers FJM, Aaronson NK, de Boer MF, Meeuwis CA, Knegt PPM, Spoelstra HAA, Van Zandwijk N, Balm AJM (1995) Heat and moisture exchangers as a treatment option in the post-operative rehabilitation of laryngectomized patients. Clin Otolaryngol 20:504–509
3. Ackerstaff AH, Hilgers FJM, Balm AJM, Tan IB (1998) Long term compliance of laryngectomized patients with a specialized pulmonary rehabilitation device, Provox® Stomafilter. Laryngoscope 108:257–260
4. Ackerstaff AH, Hilgers FJM, Meeuwis CA, Van der Velden LA, Van den Hoogen FJA, Marres HAM, Vreeburg GCM, Manni JJ (1999) Multi-institutional assessment of the Provox®2 voice prosthesis. Arch Otolaryngol Head Neck Surg 125:167–173
5. Annyas AA, Nijdam HF, Escajadillo JR, Mahieu HF, Leever H (1984) Groningen prosthesis for voice rehabilitation after laryngectomy. Clin Otolaryngol Allied Sci 9:51–54
6. Aprigliano F (1990) Use of the nasogastric tube after total laryngectomy: is it truly necessary? Ann Otol Rhinol Laryngol 99:513–514

7. Aust MR, McCaffrey TV (1997) Early speech results with the Provox voice prosthesis after laryngectomy. Arch Otolaryngol Head Neck Surg 123:966–968

8. Brasnu D, Strome M, Laccourreye O, Weinstein G, Menard M (1991) Gax-Collagen as an adjunctive measure for the incontinent myomucosal shunt. Arch Otolaryngol Head Neck Surg 117:767–768

9. Brok HAJ, Stroeve RJ, Copper MP, Schouwenburg PF (1998) The treatment of hypertonicity of the pharyngo-oesophageal segment after laryngectomy. Clin Otolaryngol 23:302–307

10. Busscher HJ, Bruinsma G, Van Weissenbruch R, Leunisse C, Van Der Mei HC, Dijk F, Albers FWJ (1998) The effect of buttermilk consumption on biofilm formation on silicone rubber voice prostheses in an artificial throat. Eur Arch Otorhinolaryngol 255:410–413

11. Busscher HJ, Free RH, Van Weissenbruch R, Albers FWJ, Van Der Mei HC (2000) Preliminary observations on influence of diary products on biofilm removal from silicon rubber voice prostheses in vitro. J Diary Sci 83:641–647

12. Callanan V, Baldwin D, White-Thompson M, Beckinsale J, Nennett J (1995) Provox valve use for post-laryngectomy voice rehabilitation. J Laryngol Otol 109:1068–1071

13. Callaway E, Truelson JM, Wolf GT, Thomas-Kincaid L, Cannon S (1992) Predictive value of objective esophageal insufflation testing for acquisition of tracheoesophageal speech. Laryngoscope 102:704–708

14. Carpentier JWd, Ryder WDJ, Grad IS, Saeed SR, Woolford TJ (1996) Survival times of Provox valves. J Laryngol Otol 110:37–42

15. Cheesman AD, Knight J, McIvor J, Perry A (1986) Tracheo-oesophageal "puncture speech." An assessment technique for failed oesophageal speakers. J Laryngol Otol 100:191–199

16. Chung RP, Patel P, Ter Keurs M, van Lith Bijl JT, Mahieu HF (1998) In vitro an in vivo comparison of the low-resistance Groningen and the Provox tracheoesophageal voice prostheses. Rev Laryngol Otol Rhinol 119:301–306

17. Fagan JJ, Lentin R, Oyarzabal MF, Isaacs S, Sellars SL (2002) Tracheoesophageal speech in a developing world community. Arch Otolaryngol Head Neck Surg 128:50–53

18. Free RH, Van Der Mei HC, Dijk F, Van Weissenbruch R, Busscher HJ, Albers FWJ (2000) Biofilm formation on voice prostheses: influence of diary products in vitro. Acta Otolaryngol 120:92–99

19. Gregor RT, Hassman E (1984) Respiratory function in post-laryngectomy patients related to stomal size. Acta Otolaryngol 97:177–183

20. Hamaker RC, Blom ED (2003) Botulinum neurotoxin for pharyngeal constrictor muscle spasm in tracheoesophageal voice restoration. Laryngoscope 113:1479–1482

21. Hilgers FJM, Schouwenburg PF (1990) A new low-resistance, self-retaining prosthesis (Provox®) for voice rehabilitation after total laryngectomy. Laryngoscope 100:1202–1207

22. Hilgers FJM, Ackerstaff AH, Aaronson NK, Schouwenburg PF, Van Zandwijk N (1990) Physical and psychosocial consequences of total laryngectomy. Clin Otolaryngol 15:421–425

23. Hilgers FJM, Aaronson NK, Ackerstaff AH, Schouwenburg PF, Van Zandwijk N (1991) The influence of a heat and moisture exchanger (HME) on the respiratore symptoms after total laryngectomy. Clin Otolaryngol 16:152–156

24. Hilgers FJM, Balm AJM (1993) Long-term results of vocal rehabilitation after total laryngectomy with the low-resistance, indwelling Provox® voice prosthesis system. Clin Otolaryngol 18:517–523

25. Hilgers FJM, Hoorweg JJ, Kroon BBR, Schaeffer B, de Boer JB, Balm AJM (1995) Prosthetic voice rehabilitation with the Provox system after extensive pharyngeal resection and reconstruction. In: Algaba J (ed.) 6th International Congress on Surgical and Prosthetic Voice Restoration after Total Laryngectomy, Exerpta Medica International Congress Series, San Sebastian, pp. 111–120

26. Hilgers FJM, Ackerstaff AH, Balm AJM, Gregor RT (1996) A new heat and moisture exchanger with speech valve (Provox® Stomafilter). Clin Otolaryngol 21:414–418

27. Hilgers FJM, Ackerstaff AH, Balm AJM, Tan IB, Aaronson NK, Persson J-O (1997) Development and clinical evaluation of a second-generation voice prosthesis (Provox®2), designed for anterograde and retrograde insertion. Acta Otolaryngol (Stockh) 117:889–896

28. Hilgers FJM, Ackerstaff AH, Van As CJ (1999) Tracheoesophageal puncture: prosthetic voice management. Curr Opin Otolaryngol Head Neck Surg 7:112–118

29. Hilgers FJM, Ackerstaff AH, Balm AJM, Van den Brekel MWM, Tan IB, Persson J-O (2003) A new problem-solving indwelling voice prosthesis, eliminating frequent candida- and "under-pressure"-related replacements: Provox ActiValve. Acta Otolaryngol (Stockh) 123:972–979

30. Hilgers FJM, Balm AJM, Tan IB, Gregor RT, Van den Brekel MWM, Scholtens BEGM, Van As CJ, Ackerstaff AH (2003) A practical guide to postlaryngectomy rehabilitation, including the Provox system. The Netherlands Cancer Institute/Antoni van Leeuwenhoek Hospital, Amsterdam

31. Hilgers FJM, Balm AJM, Van de Brekel MWM, Tan IB (2006) Problembehandlung bei der prothetischen Stimmrehabilitation nach (totaler) Laryngektomie. DPGW J 33:41–51

32. Hilgers FJM, van As-Brooks C.J., Polak MF, Tan IB (2006) Surgical improvement of hypotonicity in tracheoesophageal speech. Laryngoscope 116:345–348

33. Hoffman HT, Fischer H, VanDenmark D, Peterson KL, McCulloch TM, Hynds Karnell L, Funk GF (1997) Botulinum neurotoxin injection after total laryngectomy. Head Neck 3:92–97

34. Jones AS, Young PE, Hanafi ZB, Makura ZG, Fenton JE, Hughes JP (2003) A study of the effect of a resistive heat moisture exchanger (trachinaze) on pulmonary function and blood gas tensions in patients who have undergone a laryngectomy: a randomized control trial of 50 patients studied over a 6-month period. Head Neck 25:361–367

35. Laccourreye O, Ménard M, Crevier-Buchman L, Couloigner V, Brasnu D (1997) In situ lifetime, causes for replacement, and complications of the Provox® voice prosthesis. Laryngoscope 107:527–530

36. Laccourreye O, Papon JF, Brasnu D, Hans S (2002) Autogenous fat injection for the incontinent tracheoesophageal puncture site. Laryngoscope 112:1512–1514

37. Lewin JS, Bishop-Leone JK, Forman AD, Diaz EM (2001) Further experience with botox injection for tracheoesophageal speech failure. Head Neck 23:456–460

38. Lorincz BB, Lichtenberger G, Bihari A, Falvai J (2004) Therapy of periprosthetical leakage with tissue augmentation using bioplastique around the implanted voice prosthesis. Eur Arch Otorhinolaryngol 261:381–385

39. Luff DA, Izzat S, Farrington WT (1999) Viscoaugmentation as a treatment for leakage around the Provox2 voice rehabilitation system. J Laryngol Otol 113:847–848

40. Mahieu HF, Van Saene HKF, Rosingh HJ, Schutte HK (1986) Candida vegetations on silicone voice prostheses. Arch Otolaryngol Head Neck Surg 112:321–325

41. Mahieu HF, Van Saene JJM, Den Besten J, Van Saene HKF (1986) Oropharynx decontamination preventing Candida vegetations on voice prostheses. Arch Otolaryngol Head Neck Surg 112:1090–1092

42. Manni JJ, Broek Pvd, Groot AHd, Berends E (1984) Voice rehabilitation after laryngectomy with the Groningen prosthesis. J Otolaryngol 13:333–336

43. Manni JJ, Broek Pvd (1990) Surgical and prosthesis related complications using the Groningen button voice prosthesis. Clin Otolaryngol 15:515–523

44. Margolin G, Masucci G, Kuylenstierna R, Bjorck G, Hertegard S, Karling J (2001) Leakage around voice prosthesis in laryngectomees: treatment with local GM-CSF. Head Neck 23:1006–1010

45. Mehta AR, Sarkar S, Mehta SA, Bachher GK (1995) The Indian experience with immediate tracheoesophageal puncture for voice restoration. Eur Arch Otorhinolaryngol 252:209–214

46. Nijdam HF, Annyas AA, Schutte HK, Leever H (1982) A new prosthesis for voice rehabilitation after laryngectomy. Arch Otorhinolaryngol 237:27–33

47. Op de Coul BMR, Hilgers FJM, Balm AJM, Tan IB, Van den Hoogen FJA, Van Tinteren H (2000) A decade of postlaryngectomy vocal rehabilitation in 318 patients: a single institution's experience with consistent application of indwelling voice prostheses (Provox). Arch Otolaryngol Head Neck Surgery 126:1320–1328

48. Op de Coul BMR, Van den Hoogen FJA, Van As CJ, Marres HAM, Joosten.FBM, Manni JJ, Hilgers FJM (2003) Evaluation of the effects of primary myotomy in total laryngectomy on the neoglottis using quantitative videofluoroscopy. Arch Otolaryngol Head Neck Surg 129:1000–1005

49. Roberts CR, Rains JK, Pare PD, Walker DC, Wiggs B, Bert JL (1998) Ultrastructure and tensile properties of human tracheal cartilage. J Biomech 31:81–86

50. Schafer P, Klutzke N, Schwerdtfeger FP (2001) Voice restoration with voice prosthesis after total laryngectomy. Assessment of survival time of 378 Provox-1, Provox-2 and Blom-Singer voice prosthesis. Laryngorhinootologie 80:677–681

51. Singer MI, Blom ED (1980) An endoscopic technique for restoration of voice after laryngectomy. Ann Otol Rhinol Laryngol 89:529–533

52. Singer MI, Blom ED (1981) Selective myotomy for voice restoration after total laryngectomy. Arch Otolaryngol 107:670–673

53. Staffieri A, Mostafea BE, Varghese BT, Kitcher ED, Jalisi M, Fagan JJ, Staffieri C, Marioni G (2006) Cost of tracheoesophageal prostheses in developing countries. Facing the problem from an internal perspective. Acta Otolaryngol 126:4–9

54. Terrell JE, Lewin JS, Esclamado R (1995) Botulinum toxin injection for postlaryngectomy tracheoesophageal speech failure. Otolaryngol Head Neck Surg 113:788–791

55. Van As CJ, Hilgers FJM, Koopmans-van Beinum FJ, Ackerstaff AH (1998) The influence of stoma occlusion on aspects of tracheoesophageal voice. Acta Otolaryngol (Stockh) 118:732–738

56. Van den Hoogen FJA, Oudes MJ, Hombergen G, Nijdam HF, Manni JJ (1996) The Groningen, Nijdam and Provox Voice Prostheses: a prospective clinical comparison based on 845 replacements. Acta Otolaryngol (Stockh) 116:119–124

57. Van Der Mei HC, Free RH, Elving GJ, Van Weissenbruch R, Albers FWJ, Busscher HJ (2000) Effect of probiotic bacteria on prevalence of yeasts in oropharyngeal biofilms on silicon rubber voice prostheses in vitro. J Med Microbiol 49:713–718

58. Van Weissenbruch R, Albers FWJ (1993) Vocal rehabilitation after total laryngectomy using the Provox voice prosthesis. Clin Otolaryngol 18:359–364

59. Van Weissenbruch R, Bouckaert S, Remon J-P, Nelis HJ, Aerts R, Albers FWJ (1997) Chemoprophylaxis of fungal deterioration of the Provox silicone tracheoesophageal prosthesis in postlaryngectomy patients. Ann Otol Rhinol Laryngol 106:329–337

60. Verschuur HP, Gregor RT, Hilgers FJM, Balm AJM (1996) The tracheostoma in relation to prosthetic voice rehabilitation. Laryngoscope 106:111–115

61. Vlantis AC, Gregor RT, Elliot H, Oudes M (2003) Conversion from a non-indwelling to a Provox2 indwelling voice prosthesis for speech rehabilitation: comparison of voice quality and patient preference. J Laryngol Otol 117:815–820

62. Zuur JK, Muller SH, de Jongh FH, Van Zandwijk N, Hilgers FJ (2006) The physiological rationale of heat and moisture exchangers in post-laryngectomy pulmonary rehabilitation: a review. Eur Arch Otorhinolaryngol 263:1–8

Neurolaryngology

14

Orlando Guntinas-Lichius and Christian Sittel

Core Messages

> Neurolaryngology: definition and applications
> Laryngeal electromyography: when and how
> Beyond electromyography: more electrodiagnostic tests
> Neurolaryngological disorders: systematic overview
> Laryngeal dystonia: clinical classification
> Botulinum toxin: a practical guide

Neurolaryngology is a challenge for otolaryngologists. Laryngeal neurophysiology depends on neuromuscular forces acting on a framework of cartilage, soft tissue, and vocal cords. Understanding its pathophysiology requires knowledge of specific neurological processes that affect voice and airway regulation. It is essential that the practitioner becomes familiar with the basics of electromyography (EMG) as it is the most important diagnostic tool in neurolaryngology. This chapter opens with practical guidelines on how to use this essential method. The technical approach is explained in detail. The clinical significance and the limits of the method are pinpointed. Thereafter, a review is given of the most frequent neurolaryngological disorders. The most important diseases in daily practice, vocal cord paralysis and laryngeal dystonia, are described in detail. Many practitioners are not aware that many central nervous disorders may cause laryngeal disease. Hence, great importance is attached to explaining the relation between central nervous diseases and laryngeal pathology. Finally, we discuss the important role of botulinum toxin therapy for neurolaryngeal disorders and offer some practical guidelines for using this medication in neurolaryngology.

14.1 Electromyography

14.1.1 Definition

Laryngeal electromyography (LEMG) comprises a set of electrophysiological procedures for diagnosis, prognosis, and treatment of laryngeal movement disorders including laryngeal dystonias, vocal fold paralysis, and other neurolaryngological disorders. It is performed by otolaryngologists, often in collaboration with a neurologist. LEMG requires special skills and equipment as well as considerable experience, although no formal education exists so far for the laryngeal electromyographer. LEMG may provide useful information that cannot be obtained by other techniques, although it is still not a routine examination available at every ENT department in Europe. Although LEMG has been the subject of much investigation over the past decades for the management of various laryngological disorders, up to today there is much variability in the opinions on the use of LEMG among otolaryngologists for management of unilateral vocal fold immobility [14].

14.1.2 Technique

Electromyography evaluates the integrity of the motor system by recording action potentials generated in the muscle fibers. Principally all five major laryngeal muscles

O. Guntinas-Lichius (✉)
Department of Otolaryngology, Friedrich-Schiller-University
Jena, D-07740 Jena, Germany
e-mail: orlando.guntinas@med.uni-jena.de

M. Remacle, H. E. Eckel (eds.), *Surgery of Larynx and Trachea*,
DOI: 10.1007/978-3-540-79136-2_14, © Springer-Verlag Berlin Heidelberg 2010

(thyroarytenoid muscle, lateral cricoarytenoid muscle, posterior cricoarytenoid muscle, interarytenoid muscle, cricothyroid muscle) lend themselves to electrophysiological examination, with the thyroarytenoid muscle being investigated most frequently. This muscle may be approached in the awake patient either transcutaneously or transorally. For the transcutaneous approach bipolar concentric needle electrodes are passed through the cricothyroid membrane; then the tip of the needle is angled to the affected side laterally and superiorly 30°–45°. If the patient coughs, indicating penetration of the airway space, the needle is withdrawn and repositioned. Increased LEMG activity while the patient is phonating validates correct electrode position. If no muscle activity is detectable, electrode displacement cannot be discriminated from complete vocal fold paralysis using the transcutaneous technique.

For transoral LEMG, bipolar hooked-wire electrodes are available. The hooks at the end of these thin flexible wires act as barbs, keeping the electrode in place once positioned in the muscle. Electrodes are positioned using a special device for application, which is inserted into the endolarynx under endoscopic guidance with the needle tip being secured in the applicator. Surface anesthesia of the oropharynx and endolarynx prior to the procedure is mandatory. When the applicator is positioned correctly above the mediodorsal aspect of the vocal fold, the tip of the needle is pushed into the thyroarytenoid muscle. Because of the hooks at the distal end of the wire, the electrode remains in position when the applicator is withdrawn. Although this technique allows better control over electrode positioning, it is more time-consuming, significantly more expensive, and technically more difficult.

LEMG recordings are made visible on a monitor and made audible through a loudspeaker.

14.2 Other Techniques

Spontaneous needle LEMG provides useful information regarding the innervation status of a muscle but cannot yield quantitative data for several reasons. Sampled recordings from a single site in a muscle may not reflect the overall status of innervation of the muscle. Recordings from a single site may be influenced by many variables, such as the size and shape of the electrodes, slight changes in electrode position relative

to each motor unit in a muscle, or the variation in voluntary effort among trials and among subjects.

In theory, these shortcomings can be overcome by employing nerve stimulation instead of voluntary effort to evoke a muscular response. In so doing, consistent responses in repeated trials would be warranted, and maximum stimulation could ensure that all motor units comprising the muscle would be activated and potentially contribute to the recorded response. This should give a far more representative picture of the innervation status of a large portion of the muscle during the initial phase of degeneration or the subsequent phase of reinnervation, allowing a more accurate diagnosis and prognosis. Recent animal investigations showed the potential value of the technique [53]. There have been attempts to establish transcutaneously evoked LEMG as a routine tool in humans [48–50], but these techniques lack reliability and reproducibility. Applying a sufficient electrical stimulus to the recurrent laryngeal nerve in a way acceptable to patients is still an unsolved problem. Invasive direct stimulation is not an option for diagnostic use for obvious reasons. Transcutaneous stimulation requires considerably high voltage to elicit a response from the deeply hidden recurrent laryngeal or vagal nerve, making the procedure inaccurate and uncomfortable for the patient. Magnetic stimulation is not sufficiently focalized to activate a target nerve with certainty.

In addition to these technical considerations, an alleged superiority of evoked LEMG over spontaneous LEMG is far from evident. Both techniques are well comparable to facial nerve electroneurography (evoked) and needle-EMG of facial muscles (spontaneous). Among the abundance of investigations over the last decades, yielding often confusing results, there are strong arguments casting some shadow on the reliability and accuracy of evoked EMG techniques in the facial nerve [41, 42].

14.3 Clinical Significance

14.3.1 Diagnosis

When reduced or absent abductor or adductor movement of the true vocal fold is observed on laryngeal examination, laryngeal paresis is suspected, and LEMG becomes an important diagnostic tool, especially if performed within 6 months of the onset of the voice problem. Normal electrical activity patterns on LEMG suggests arytenoid fixation [35], whereas abnormal electrical activity, including patterns of denervation or reinnervation, suggests unilateral vocal fold paresis/paralysis [22].

Abnormal activity can include the presence of fibrillation potentials, insertional fibrillations (insertional activity), complex repetitive discharges, sharp positive waves, and nascent and polyphasic motor unit potentials. Specifically, *fibrillation potentials* are defined as low-amplitude, short-duration units; and *insertional activity* is defined as mechanical discharge associated with repeated needle movement in a muscle. *Polyphasic units* are large-amplitude units with five or more baseline crossings of increased duration compared with normal units, whereas *nascent units* are defined as low-amplitude units with increased number of baseline crossings and do not meet the amplitude or duration criteria of polyphasic units. Abnormal activity can also be manifested as decrements in the number of normal motor unit potentials and a reduction in recruitment during volitional activity. *Recruitment* is defined as activation of motor units with increasing strength of voluntary muscle contraction and reflects the number of motor unit potentials identifiable during increasing activation during voicing tasks.

Interpretation of electrophysiological findings is based on the following criteria: LEMG allows distinction between the normal silent resting potential, voluntary motor unit potential, spontaneous fibrillation potential, and polyphasic reinnervation potential. The absence of any electrical activity either on electrode insertion or on attempted voluntary motion is called *electrical silence*. Normal voluntary action potentials are diphasic or triphasic and are extremely variable in amplitude (Figs. 14.1 and 14.2). *Spontaneous fibrillation activity* is defined as involuntary potentials generated by a single muscle fiber, indicating axonal degeneration (Fig. 14.3). However, this symptom of degeneration does not appear earlier than 10–14 days after injury. Polyphasic motor units have four or more phases and are heralding nerve regeneration (Fig. 14.4).

For routine clinical use, it is convenient to classify electrophysiological findings, according to Seddon [38], into neurapraxy, axonotmesis, or neurotmesis. For *neurapraxy* the diagnostic criteria in LEMG are detection of a rarefied recruitment pattern or single action

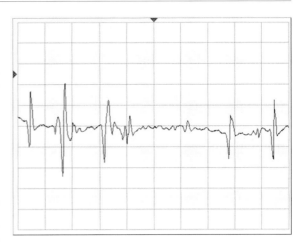

Fig. 14.1. Neurapraxy. Note the extremely rarefied firing pattern on phonation but no spontaneous activity at rest

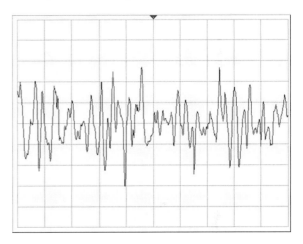

Fig. 14.2. Neurapraxy. Note the slightly reduced recruitment on phonation, with no spontaneous activity at rest

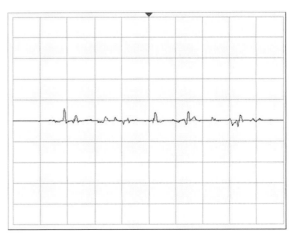

Fig. 14.3. Axonotmesis. Spontaneous fibrillation activity at rest, with minimal recruitment on voluntary action

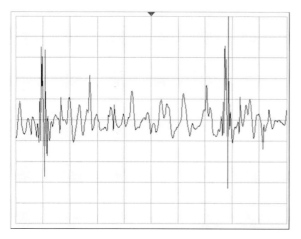

Fig. 14.4. Polyphasic, prolonged action potentials with giant amplitudes, indicating reinnervation 4 months after nerve injury

potentials on voluntary action without fibrillation activity and without spontaneous positive sharp waves. *Axonotmesis* is suspected when spontaneous activity, indicating neural degeneration, can be detected. Usually this is the case not earlier than 10–14 days after onset of paralysis. There is an inherent statement on prognosis in this classification [32] as neurapraxy is most likely to recover completely within 8–12 weeks whereas axonotmesis is thought to have only a poor chance of recovery to a functional level. If reinnervation occurs following axonotmesis, usually it is associated with sequelae such as synkinesis due to neuronal misdirection [3, 20, 37]. The result is simultaneous activation of adducting and abducting intrinsic laryngeal muscles. For the same situation in facial nerve disorder, the apposite term autoparalytic syndrome has been coined [44]. *Neurotmesis*, representing complete destruction of the whole nerve structure over its full diameter, apparently cannot be expected to recover at all.

14.3.2 Prognosis

The clinical use of LEMG has been advocated for diagnosis and prognostication of vocal fold palsy for more than two decades [7, 10, 37, 40, 48]. Surprisingly, there are only a few reports on the usefulness of this technique in terms of reliability and prognostic accuracy. Min et al. [29] reported a prognostic accuracy of an impressive 89% in patients with unilateral vocal

fold palsy. This study is seriously flawed for at least two reasons: First, the study population comprised only14 individuals. Second, criteria for prognostication were defined very generously: A positive prognosis for laryngeal recovery was assumed when motor unit waveform morphology was normal and significant persistent overall EMG activity as well as no electrical silence during voluntary tasks could be found. Obviously, this combination of favorable findings should be considered more an indication of a discrete lesion than an actual prognosis. Another study investigating 18 patients [34] was not truly focused on the prognostic accuracy of LEMG. The authors of that study concluded cautiously that LEMG may be of prognostic value.

A more recent study [43] suggested that detection of neural degeneration by LEMG allows the prediction of poor functional outcome with high reliability during an early phase of the disease process: LEMG had been used in 98 patients with 111 paralyzed vocal folds: 39 patients had been diagnosed with neurapraxy, and 72 laryngeal palsies had been characterized as axonotmesis. Neurotmesis was found in no case. Based on these data, a positive predictive value (PPV) of 94% for the event "defective recovery," defined as the absence of completely free vocal fold mobility, was calculated. For the event "complete recovery," the prognosis was accurate in only 12.8% of the cases. The quite accurate prognosis of the unfavorable event "defective recovery" at a comparatively early stage of the disease process can be valuable for the timing of a definitive surgical intervention, most of all in cases of bilateral recurrent nerve paralysis.

In a study on patients suffering from bilateral vocal fold palsy conducted by Eckel [8], the routine use of LEMG was helpful for deciding on posterior cordectomy (for widening the glottic chink) at an comparatively early stage. As a consequence, tracheotomy was required in only 21% of the study population. On the other hand, the absence of degenerative signs may not lead to the assumption that complete recovery is to be expected automatically. On the basis of data available today, it seems safe to say that in patients suffering from vocal fold palsy of lower motoneuron-type the detection of well defined signs of neural degeneration by LEMG allows the prediction of poor functional outcome with high reliability at an early phase of the disease process. In the presence of signs of neural degeneration detected by LEMG the decision for definitive surgical interventions such as thyroplasty or vocal fold augmentation during unilateral or partial cordectomy in bilateral vocal fold paralysis can be made safely at an earlier stage of the disease process. Thus, LEMG can be helpful for significantly shortening the process of voice rehabilitation. However, the absence of degenerative alterations in LEMG does not necessarily indicate recovery to a normal or near-normal functional level. Hypothetically, these findings may reflect secondary fibrosis of the cricoarytenoid joint following prolonged vocal fold immobility of primarily neurogenic etiology.

In summary, LEMG is a valuable tool in the workup of patients suffering from vocal fold palsy. Because the prognostic accuracy for favorable results is comparatively low, LEMG cannot replace clinical monitoring over at least 6 months or until complete recovery has been reached.

14.4 Neurolaryngological Disorders

Laryngeal physiology depends on dynamic neuromuscular forces acting on a basic framework of cartilage and specialized soft tissues, the vocal folds. Specific neurological processes may affect voice, swallowing, or airway regulation. Neuromuscular impairment continues to be a dominant topic in the study of neurolaryngological disorders [46]. Table 14.1 gives an overview about the most common neurolaryngological disorders and their characteristics. Perhaps the most common neuromuscular impairment of the larynx is vocal cord paralysis. In most cases this paralysis is caused by a lesion of the recurrent or vagal nerve. In these cases, the typical signs of a lower motor neurons disease are found in the larynx: peripheral neuropathy, isolated

Table 14.1. Characteristics of the most common neurolaryngological disorders

Disease	Laryngoscopic features	Electrodiagnostic features
Lower motor neuron vocal cord paralysis (recurrent or vagal nerve lesion)	Vocal cord paralysis	Spontaneous activity in thyroarytenoid muscle starts 10–14 days after lesion for about 2–3 months. Reduced or no voluntary activity. In vagal nerve lesions: also features of superior laryngeal nerve lesion
Vocal cord synkinesis	Vocal cord paralysis	Polyphasic reinnervation potentials in thyroarytenoid muscle during phonation. No spontaneous activity
Isolated lesion of the superior laryngeal nerve	Normal vocal cord movement but bowing during phonation	Spontaneous activity in cricothyroid muscle starts 10–14 days after lesion for about 2–3 months. Reduced or no voluntary activity
Upper motor neuron vocal cord paralysis	Vocal cord paralysis	No spontaneous activity
Adductor spasmodic dysphonia	Symmetrical glottic compression during phonation. Normal vocal cord mobility	Abnormal bursts of activity in the thyroarytenoid muscle during phonation. Some patients show enlarged or polyphasic potentials
Abductor spasmodic dysphonia	Incomplete glottic opening during phonation. Normal vocal cord mobility	Abnormal bursts of activity in the posterior cricoarytenoid muscle during phonation. Some patients show enlarged or polyphasic potentials
Essential voice tremor	No action-induced spasms. Rhythmic, periodic glottic spasms	Spontaneous activity in thyroarytenoid and/or lateral cricoarytenoid muscle tremor bursts in thyroarytenoid and/or lateral cricoarytenoid muscle
Parkinson's disease	Vocal cord bowing during phonation. Delayed movements	Decreased voluntary activity in thyroarytenoid muscle. Single-fiber EMG may show increased variability of the interspike interval of single motor units.
Stroke	Signs of lower and/or upper motor neuron vocal cord paralysis	Signs of lower and/or upper motor neuron vocal cord paralysis

flaccid paralysis, decreased agility, muscle atrophy, but normal coordination of the laryngeal muscles. In the rare case of a disorder of the neuromuscular junction, fatigability and fluctuating abnormalities are common signs of laryngeal movement. However, vocal cord paralysis or other vocal manifestations are frequently the primary modes of presentation for neurological disease.

The typical signs of an upper motor neuron disease can be found, as in other central nervous diseases, in the larynx: Spastic paralysis of muscles groups and decreased agility are symptoms of cerebral diseases. Disorders affecting the basal ganglia present with a resting tremor, dystonia, or rigidity of the laryngeal muscles. In cerebellar diseases, intention tremor and dysdiadokinesis are seen during laryngoscopy. Myoclonus and choreatic movement in the larynx are unspecific signs of an upper motor neuron disease. The most important movement disorders affecting the larynx are presented here.

The major components of the neurolaryngological examination of all patients are a detailed history, evaluation of the voice, stroboscopy, and EMG of the larynx [27].

14.4.1 Vocal Cord Paralysis of the Lower Motor Neuron Type: Recurrent and Vagal Nerve Lesions

The potential causes of vocal cord paralysis are manifold [15, 33]. Surgical trauma has long been recognized as the most common cause of unilateral and bilateral vocal cord paralysis. Thyroid surgery still is the major risk factor. Carotid endarterectomy or neck dissection is seen as another underlying cause. Other causes are neoplasms in the neck and mediastinum and traumatic and idiopathic conditions. Various neurological disorders, including poliomyelitis, Guillain-Barré syndrome, and multiple sclerosis, could lead to direct damage of the vagal nerve [17]. Lower motor neuron lesions could also be affected by diseases in the brain stem, leading to direct damage of the motor neurons in the vagal nuclei. Typical examples are Wallenberg syndrome, bulbar polio, amyotrophic lateral sclerosis, syringomyelia, multiple sclerosis, and encephalitis. When the reasons for unilateral and bilateral vocal cord paralysis are compared, there are no significant differences [15].

The major symptom indicating a lower motor neuron lesion of the recurrent or vagal nerve is unilateral or bilateral vocal cord paralysis. The lesions are caused by injuries directly affecting the recurrent nerve or the vagal nerve. Localized lesions of the myelin sheath (neurapraxy) regenerate without functional deficits. Axonal lesions (axonotmesis) or combined damage of axons and myelin sheaths (neurotmesis) induces Wallerian degeneration of the distal nerve stump to the peripheral target muscle. Axon sprouting starts at the first Ranvier node proximal to the lesion site on the axon. In consequence, the regeneration time depends mainly on the site of the lesion. The first clinical signs of nerve regeneration after peripheral damage of the vagal nerve or the recurrent nerve are typically not seen before 3 months after the trauma. The axonal sprouting leads to misdirected reinnervation of the laryngeal muscles. Therefore, retrieval of muscle tone (e.g., in the vocal cords) is observed after some months, but movement does not come back because of simultaneous movements of antagonistic laryngeal muscles caused by the misdirected reinnervation. Severe lesions in the brain stem and some forms of peripheral toxic lesions lead to degeneration of the related motor neurons at the nuclear level in the brain stem. The reduced driving motor neuron pool results in decreased muscle strength and limited movements. The therapeutic possibilities for transient and permanent vocal cord paralysis are described in Chapter ??.

Information on the integrity of the recurrent nerve can by obtained by laryngeal EMG of the thyroarytenoid muscle [22, 47]. The superior laryngeal nerve is analyzed by EMG of the cricothyroid muscle. The posterior cricoarytenoid muscle has to be analyzed in special situations. Reduced insertion potentials indicate muscle wasting and atrophy. A loss of nerve function demonstrates a decrease or absence in frequency of firing in the muscle action potential. If some fibers remain intact, the amplitude of the muscle action potential is normal. Axonal damage leads to Wallerian degeneration of the distal nerve fibers. In consequence, fibrillation potentials are seen about 10–14 days later and can persist for some weeks. The detection of neural degeneration by laryngeal EMG allows the prediction of poor functional outcome [43]. Polyphasic reinnervation potentials indicate an old lesion with definitive misdirected reinnervation. The laryngeal synkinesis is directly demonstrable by EMG [25]. Depending on the site of the lesion, polyphasic reinnervation potentials are not seen before 2–3 months after axonal lesion.

Increased polyphasic reinnervation potentials are typically seen up to 6–12 months after the lesion.

Electromyograpy is also an important tool for monitoring the reinnervation and to determine the outcome after surgical reconstruction of the recurrent nerve by direct nerve anastomosis, cross-anastomosis with the ansa cervicalis, or use of a nerve-muscle pedicle. Reinnervation and maturation of the voluntary action potential are typically seen by EMG over the first 1½ years [25].

If the site of the lesion is proximal to the recurrent or vagal nerve (i.e., the lesion is affecting the first motor neuron or complex cortical structures), spontaneous activity is absent during EMG recording despite clinically evident vocal cord paralysis. If the vocal cord immobility was caused by cricoarytenoid joint fixation or interarytenoid scar formation, laryngeal EMG shows completely normal activity of the laryngeal muscles.

14.4.2 Vocal Cord Paralysis of the Upper Motor Neuron Type

In infants and children, bilateral vocal cord paralysis is most often congenital [12]. About half of the congenital cases are associated with other anomalies. Even many acquired cases are secondary to underlying congenital anomalies, particularly meningomyeloceles, midbrain or brain stem dysgenesis, Arnold-Chiari malformation, and hydrocephalus [17]. Patients with co-morbid factors, especially severe neurological abnormalities, often require tracheotomy to manage the child's airway [30]. After laryngomalacia, vocal cord paralysis is the second most common cause of stridor in children. Onset of paralysis in children may not be immediate. Age of onset may range from birth to 6–8 weeks of age. Unilateral paralysis is more common than bilateral paralysis. Recovery can be expected in only 20–30% of the congenital cases. Other reasons for vocal cord paralysis in children are birth trauma, surgical trauma, or congenital infection. The acquired cases show a higher recovery rate of up to 50–60% [9]. If an older child does not present other symptoms, the vocal cord dysfunction could be confused with exercise-induced asthma because the disease tends to be triggered by exercise [51]. Management of vocal cord paralysis in children should be directed toward establishing a secure airway and treating the underlying disease. Whereas tracheotomy is normally not required for unilateral paralysis, the rate of tracheotomies is high for bilateral disease. The techniques for airway management are described in detail in Chapter ??. The same is valid for upper motor type vocal cord paralysis in adults. The various diseases are described below in more detail. As explained above, EMG is an important tool for differentiating an upper motor neuron type lesion from a lower motor neuron lesion as the latter shows typical EMG alterations.

14.4.3 Laryngeal Dystonia: Adductor and Abductor Spasmodic Dysphonia

Laryngeal dystonia, or spasmodic dysphonia, is a form of dystonia, a chronic neurological disorder of central motor processing characterized by task-specific action-induced muscle spasms. Dystonia may be generalized or limited to one functional group of muscles. Laryngeal dystonia is usually focal. A strained, strangled quality to the voice with effortful voicing and voice fatigue is typical. Approximately four of five affected individuals have adductor spasmodic dysphonia, which causes inappropriate glottal closure and consequently strangled breaks in connected speech. A subentity is termed adductor breathing dystonia (or breathing dystonia) if the patient develops adductor spasms during breathing, producing paradoxical vocal cord motion [11]. EMG demonstrates bursts of glottic compression in the thyroarytenoid muscle during phonation at unpredictable intervals. Abductor spasmodic dysphonia, in contrast, causes inappropriate glottal opening in one of five patients that produces hypophonia and breathy breaks. Hence, EMG shows bursts of muscle activity in the posterior cricoarytenoid muscle. Because of compensatory maneuvers or mixed dystonic features, the voice patterns encountered clinically may not always be typical or easy to discern [46].

Electromyography is important for treatment planning. It shows the major muscular source of the dystonia. Only EMG detects the rare cases where the lateral cricoarytenoid muscle, the interarytenoid muscle, or the cricothyroid muscle is the major focus of the dystonia [16, 21]. Spasms typically do not occur during singing. The most important differential diagnoses that can cause voice breaks are essential voice tremor, muscle tension dysphonia, and a functional disorder. As spasmodic dystonia is a disorder of the central nervous system rather than of the larynx, interventions at the end organ do not offer a definitive cure.

Botulinum toxin (BTX) therapy is the treatment of choice. There is a report of 90% overall improvement after BTX therapy for adductor spasmodic dysphonia. The results of BTX for abductor spasmodic dysphonia have been less favorable. Only 20–40% of these patients improve after BTX treatment [45]. The BTX application technique is described in detail below. Voice therapy may be useful in addition to BTX therapy. In patients with contraindications for BTX or if BTX fails, surgical treatment should be discussed with the patient. Lateralization thyroplasty is an easy but mechanical approach to help patients with refractory adductor spasmodic dysphonia [18]. Long-term results are often disappointing. Alternatively, selective section of the distal branches of the recurrent nerve leading to the thyroarytenoid and sometimes the lateral cricoarytenoid muscle, with immediate reinnervation using a nonlaryngeal nerve, generally the sternohyoid branch of the ansa cervicalis, is proposed. This was done in an attempt to prevent reestablishment of abnormal central motor control by connecting the laryngeal musculature to a nerve supply not affected by the disorder [1, 46]. In patients with refractory abductor spasmodic dysphonia, bilateral medialization thyroplasty could be helpful [2, 31]. Recently it was shown that unilateral posterior cricothyroid myoplasty (i.e., unilateral desertion of the muscle) could improve the effect of medialization thyroplasty [39].

14.4.4 Stroke

Stroke is a highly prevalent disease that has significant potential to affect the voice and swallowing adversely. Expressive aphasia due to stroke in the frontal cortex (Broca area) and receptive aphasia due to stroke in the temporal cortex (Wernicke area) are well known clinical signs of a stroke. However, the corticobulbar tract and cranial nerves themselves could also be affected directly by the cerebrovascular accident. Isolated vocal paralysis is an uncommon manifestation of stroke. Most often, multiple cranial nerves are involved. Clinically, voice quality and speech production are affected. Of course, perhaps more common than these direct effects of the stroke

on voice production are the multitude of indirect effects on the voice from the general neurological characteristics of stroke patients. Hoarseness and chronic laryngitis can go along with vocal cord paralysis. Chronic laryngitis is the result of the laryngopharyngeal reflux and/or prolonged nasogastric feeding. Therefore, otolaryngological management of most stroke patients is dictated by the urgent problems of protecting the airway, controlling respiration, and finally phonation. The need for prolonged ventilation should be recognized early. The patient may be converted appropriately to tracheotomy. Down-sizing the tracheotomy tube when appropriate facilitates speech therapy for voice and communication.

14.4.5 Essential Voice Tremor

Essential tremor is an idiopathic disorder of involuntary movement. The classification of voice tremor is controversial. The tremor has also been characterized as a separate subtype of laryngeal dystonia [26]. The tremor is believed to originate from disordered cerebellar control of vocal cord length and tension. Patients generally report slowly worsening symptoms over months to years. Voicing worsens with anxiety or stress and is especially troublesome under more demanding acoustical conditions, such as speaking against background noise. Laryngeal tremor often is not restricted to the intrinsic muscles of the larynx. The other muscles of the phonatory apparatus are often and variably involved. Tremor in the larynx characteristically is seen as bilateral, symmetrical, involuntary, rhythmic, periodic spasms of the laryngeal, supraglottic, or pharyngeal muscles. The reliable periodicity of the spasms, similar to the ticking of a clock, is the key feature of tremor. The tremor frequency has been documented between 3 and 6 Hz. Tremors can occur at rest or with intention, which in the larynx is seen during sustained phonation. Action-induced spasms, which are typical for spasmodic dysphonia, are not seen here. The larynx may be normal at rest. Myoclonus is differentiated from tremor in that the spasms seen during myoclonic activity are jerky and arrhythmic. EMG shows spontaneous activity at rest. Typically, EMG exhibits signs of tremor in all laryngeal muscles during phonation. The thyroarytenoid and the lateral cricoarytenoid muscle are most often involved [26].

Propranolol (a β-adrenergic blocker) and primidone (a neuroleptic) are the mainstays of treatment. BTX treatment does not alleviate the essential tremor in any case; generally, it only decreases the amplitude of the tremor. The result is severe breathiness of the patient, although many patients are content with BTX treatment [27]. BTX injections are most effective if the dominating tremor muscles (shown by EMG) are treated [26].

14.4.6 Parkinson's Disease

Most patients with Parkinson's disease complain of voice problems characterized by vocal tremor, decreased volume, and hoarseness [5]. Vocal fold bowing is a common finding during laryngoscopy. The source of this bowing has not been fully elucidated, but some patients show dyskinesia of the intrinsic laryngeal muscles that might be the result of defective basal ganglia control. Often vocal cord closure is slowed or delayed. Tremor associated with Parkinson's disease present is evident at rest. Most important, the speech, although often breathy and of low intensity, does not demonstrate the characteristics in a rhythmic fashion as in patients with essential tremor. Rather, the characteristic hypophonia is relatively constant. The extrinsic laryngeal muscles (strap muscles) could also be affected. The result is a significant slowing of vertical laryngeal excursion during deglutition [23]. Additionally, poor breath support may be present as a result of chest wall rigidity. The disease is often exacerbated by articulatory difficulties and sometimes by cognitive and articulatory problems. Other findings are pooled hypopharyngeal secretions, decreased sensation, diminished cough reflex, and aspiration. Laryngeal EMG demonstrates a decreased firing rate and, in older male Parkinson's patients, increased variability of the interspike interval of single motor units [24].

Efficient therapy of the dysphonia in Parkinson's patients is difficult. Vocal fold augmentation is often not effective in severely affected patients [19]. Standard Parkinson's treatment with L-DOPA, deep brain stimulation, or neurosurgical interventions have shown only limited results with the dysphonia. Only behavioral therapy has shown sustained beneficial effect on voice and speech functions of patients with Parkinson's disease [52].

14.4.7 Other Central Nervous Diseases

Patients with amyotrophic lateral sclerosis display several laryngological symptoms. Adductor type spasmodic dysphonia has been described as a feature of the central motor neuron degeneration [36]. Multiple system atrophy encompasses three neurodegenerative syndromes (striatonigral degeneration, olivopontocerebellar atrophy, and Shy-Drager syndrome). In addition to the typical symptoms of autonomic, cerebellar, and pyramidal dysfunction, stridor occurs in multiple system atrophy at different stages. Severe respiratory insufficiency sometimes requires tracheotomy. The cause of stridor in multiple system atrophy is dystonia of the vocal cords. In most cases, laryngoscopy reveals normal bilateral movements of the vocal cords. EMG during quiet breathing shows persistent tonic activity in both abductor and adductor vocal cord muscles [28]. Botulinum toxin injection into the adductor muscles can be offered to patients to reduce the tonic EMG activity.

14.4.8 Botulinum Toxin Treatment in the Larynx

Botulinum toxin has been used successfully in otolaryngology for more than 20 years to treat an increasing number of diseases [4]. BTX blocks the release of acetylcholine from nerve terminals and thereby causes flaccid paralysis of the muscle starting about 48 hours after injection. Its effect is transient and nondestructive. Recovery starts after about 28 days and is complete after about 90 days, a length of time that correlates with the clinically observed duration of effect. Two serotypes of BTX, serotype A and B, are available for clinical use. Three compounds of BTX type A (Botox, Dysport, Xeomin) and a type B compound (NeuroBloc) are commercially available (Table 14.2). To date, BTX treatment in the larynx is still "off-label" use; but due to the large experience with the drug in the larynx, the AAO-HNS considers the laryngeal treatment safe and effective. The dosage is measured in mouse units (MU). A unit is defined by the median lethal intraperitoneal dose (LD_{50}) in Swiss Webster mice. It is important to be aware that a unit of Botox is not equivalent to a unit of Dysport, Xeomin, or NeuroBloc. Botox, Dysport, and Xeomin require rehydration with normal saline prior to

Table 14.2. Comparison of the four licensed botulinum toxin formulations

	Botox	Dysport	Xeomin	NeuroBloc[a]
Company	Allergan, Irvine, CA 92612, USA	Ipsen Biopharm, UK-Wrexham LL13 9UF, UK	Merz Pharmaceuticals GmbH, 60048 Frankfurt, Germany	Solstice Neuroscience, South San Francisco, CA 94080, USA
Neurotoxin type	A	A	A	B
Mouse units per vial	100	500	100	2500/5000/10,000
2°–8°C	2°–8°C	2°–8°C	2°–8°C	2°–8°C
Durability	36 months	24 months	36 months	24 months
Solvent	0.9% saline	0.9% saline	0.9% saline	Premanufactured solution
Labeled therapeutic indications	Blepharospasm in adults, spasmodic torticollis in adults, hemifacial spasm in adults, dynamic equines foot deformity due to spasticity in children > 2 years, focal hand spasticity of adults after stroke, axillary hyperhidrosis, wrinkles[b]	Blepharospasm in adults, spasmodic torticollis in adults, hemifacial spasm in adults, dynamic equines foot deformity due to spasticity in children older than 2 years, axillary hyperhidrosis	Blepharospasm and spasmodic torticollis in adults	Cervical dystonia in adults

[a]Named MyoBloc in the United States
[b]The commercial name for treatment of wrinkles is Botox Cosmetic in the United States and Vistabel in Switzerland.

usage. NeuroBloc is directly delivered by the company as a solution. We recommend using the BTX type A formulation for first-line treatment. BTX type B should be reserved for patients with secondary treatment failure of BTX type A [13]. The concentration may be varied depending on the physician's need, the involved muscles, and prior experience with the individual patient. Treating the small muscles of the larynx, Botox (5 MU/0.1 ml), Dysport (20 MU/0.1 ml), Xeomin (5 MU/0.1 ml), or NeuroBloc (500 MU/0.1 ml) may be used. A higher concentration may be useful in some patients if side effects are seen as the result of diffusion of the toxin from the target muscle to adjacent muscles.

In general, multiple small-volume injections may have a better effect with less risk of side effects. The clinical effect is dose-related, but the range of effective doses among patients with the same disease may vary to the extreme [6]. The physician finds the correct dose only through experience with each individual case. BTX should not be used in pregnant women because teratogenicity and safety has not yet been established. It has been used for a long time in children, suggesting that its efficacy and side effects are the same as in adult patients. In general, BTX should be used carefully in patients with neuromuscular disease because of the higher risk of systemic muscle weakness. Aminoglycoside antibiotics interfere with BTX and may potentiate its effect. Therefore, BTX therapy should be avoided during such antibiotic treatment.

The amount of toxin used in the larynx is low. Hence, an overdose has never been described. Moreover, the risk of acquired resistance to BTX by a patient's production of antibodies against the drug is low. To our knowledge, immunoresistance in patients with laryngeal treatment have not been described. The development of immunoresistance seems to occur more often in patients treated with large doses and short treatment intervals. We recommend starting treatment with the smallest effective dose, avoid booster injections, and maximize intertreatment intervals.

If possible, we prefer endoscopy-assisted transoral injections of BTX into the intrinsic laryngeal muscles. If the transcutaneous approach is used, EMG is recommended to prove precisely the placement of BTX. The target muscle is identified by the EMG needle first, as described above, and the BTX is injected parallel to the EMG needle to deliver the toxin into the muscle. Alternatively, the BTX is delivered directly through a

Table 14.3. Recommended botulinum toxin injection technique for neurolaryngological disorders

Disorder	Injection site and doses	Comment
Adductor spasmodic dysphonia	Thyroarytenoid muscle bilateral: 1–5 MU Botox/1–5 MU Xeomin/10–40 MU Dysport per side	In some patients unilateral treatment is sufficient
Abductor spasmodic dysphonia	Posterior cricoarytenoid muscle unilateral or bilateral: 2.5–5.0 MU Botox/2.5–5..0 MU Xeomin/20–40 MU Dysport per side	The risk of dyspnea is less after unilateral treatment of the most active side (as shown by EMG)
Essential voice tremor	Thyroarytenoid muscle or lateral cricothyroid muscle unilateral or bilateral: 2.5 MU Botox/2.5 MU Xeomin/20 MU Dysport per side	Selection of the target muscles by EMG is important
Bilateral vocal cord paralysis	Thyroarytenoid muscle bilateral: 2.5–5.0 MU Botox/2.5–5.0 MU Xeomin/20–40 MU Dysport per side	Only in selected cases as an adjuvant treatment to surgery

Teflon-coated needle attached to the EMG machine. If both methods, transoral and transcutaneous, fail to induce an effect, we recommend reevaluating the indication. If the indication remains, we recommend repeating the transoral injection under general anesthesia. Guidelines for BTX dosages and injection sites for the most frequent indications in patients with neurolaryngological disorders are presented in Table 14.3.

14.4.9 Tips and Pearls

- Differential diagnosis between vocal fold paralysis and arytenoids fixation using laryngeal electromyography is reliable
- Laryngeal electromyography is the method of choice for assessment of neural damage
- Prognosis vocal fold paralysis can be assessed reliably within 2 weeks after onset
- Botulinum toxin therapy is the treatment of choice for laryngeal dystonia

References

1. Berke GS, Blackwell KE, Gerratt BR, Verneil A, Jackson KS, Sercarz JA (1999) Selective laryngeal adductor denervation-reinnervation: a new surgical treatment for adductor spasmodic dysphonia. Ann Otol Rhinol Laryngol 108:227–231
2. Blitzer A, Brin MF, Stewart CF (1998) Botulinum toxin management of spasmodic dysphonia (laryngeal dystonia): a 12-year experience in more than 900 patients. Laryngoscope 108:1435–1441
3. Blitzer A, Jahn AF, Keidar A (1996) Semon's law revisited: an electromyographic analysis of laryngeal synkinesis. Ann Otol Rhinol Laryngol 105:764–769
4. Blitzer A, Sulica L (2001) Botulinum toxin: basic science and clinical uses in otolaryngology. Laryngoscope 111:218–226
5. Blumin JH, Pcolinsky DE, Atkins JP (2004) Laryngeal findings in advanced Parkinson's disease. Ann Otol Rhinol Laryngol 113:253–258
6. Boutsen F, Cannito MP, Taylor M, Bender B (2002) Botox treatment in adductor spasmodic dysphonia: a meta-analysis. J Speech Lang Hear Res 45:469–481
7. Crumley RL (1994) Unilateral recurrent laryngeal nerve paralysis. J Voice 8:79–83
8. Eckel HE, Thumfart M, Wassermann K, Vossing M, Thumfart WF (1994) Cordectomy versus arytenoidectomy in the management of bilateral vocal cord paralysis. Ann Otol Rhinol Laryngol 103:852–857
9. Emery PJ, Fearon B (1984) Vocal cord palsy in pediatric practice: a review of 71 cases. Int J Pediatr Otorhinolaryngol 8:147–154
10. Ford CN (1998) Laryngeal EMG in clinical neurolaryngology Arch Otolaryngol Head Neck Surg 124:476–477
11. Grillone GA, Blitzer A, Brin MF, Annino DJ, Jr., Saint-Hilaire MH (1994) Treatment of adductor laryngeal breathing dystonia with botulinum toxin type A. Laryngoscope 104:30–32
12. Grundfast KM, Harley E (1989) Vocal cord paralysis. Otolaryngol Clin North Am 22:569–597
13. Guntinas-Lichius O (2003) Injection of botulinum toxin type B for the treatment of otolaryngology patients with secondary treatment failure of botulinum toxin type a. Laryngoscope 113:743–745
14. Halum SL, Patel N, Smith TL, Jaradeh S, Toohill RJ, Merati AL (2005) Laryngeal electromyography for adult unilateral vocal fold immobility: a survey of the American Broncho-Esophagological Association. Ann Otol Rhinol Laryngol 114:425–428
15. Hillel AD, Benninger M, Blitzer A, Crumley R, Flint P, Kashima HK, Sanders I, Schaefer S (1999) Evaluation and management of bilateral vocal cord immobility. Otolaryngol Head Neck Surg 121:760–765
16. Hillel AD, Maronian NC, Waugh PF, Robinson L, Klotz DA (2004) Treatment of the interarytenoid muscle with botulinum

toxin for laryngeal dystonia. Ann Otol Rhinol Laryngol 113: 341–348

17. Holinger LD, Holinger PC, Holinger PH (1976) Etiology of bilateral abductor vocal cord paralysis: a review of 389 cases. Ann Otol Rhinol Laryngol 85:428–436

18. Isshiki N, Haji T, Yamamoto Y, Mahieu HF (2001) Thyroplasty for adductor spasmodic dysphonia: further experiences. Laryngoscope 111:615–621

19. Kim SH, Kearney JJ, Atkins JP (2002) Percutaneous laryngeal collagen augmentation for treatment of parkinsonian hypophonia. Otolaryngol Head Neck Surg 126:653–656

20. Kirchner JA (1982) Semon's law a century later. J Laryngol Otol 96:645–657

21. Klotz DA, Maronian NC, Waugh PF, Shahinfar A, Robinson L, Hillel AD (2004) Findings of multiple muscle involvement in a study of 214 patients with laryngeal dystonia using fine-wire electromyography. Ann Otol Rhinol Laryngol 113: 602–612

22. Koufman JA, Postma GN, Whang CS, Rees CJ, Amin MR, Belafsky PC, Johnson PE, Connolly KM, Walker FO (2001) Diagnostic laryngeal electromyography: The Wake Forest experience 1995–1999. Otolaryngol Head Neck Surg 124: 603–606

23. Leopold NA, Kagel MC (1997) Laryngeal deglutition movement in Parkinson's disease. Neurology 48:373–376

24. Luschei ES, Ramig LO, Baker KL, Smith ME (1999) Discharge characteristics of laryngeal single motor units during phonation in young and older adults and in persons with parkinson disease. J Neurophysiol 81:2131–2139

25. Maronian NC, Robinson L, Waugh P, Hillel AD (2004) A new electromyographic definition of laryngeal synkinesis. Ann Otol Rhinol Laryngol 113:877–886

26. Maronian NC, Waugh PF, Robinson L, Hillel AD (2004) Tremor laryngeal dystonia: treatment of the lateral cricoarytenoid muscle. Ann Otol Rhinol Laryngol 113:349–355

27. Merati AL, Heman-Ackah YD, Abaza M, Altman KW, Sulica L, Belamowicz S (2005) Common movement disorders affecting the larynx: a report from the neurolaryngology committee of the AAO-HNS. Otolaryngol Head Neck Surg 133:654–665

28. Merlo IM, Occhini A, Pacchetti C, Alfonsi E (2002) Not paralysis, but dystonia causes stridor in multiple system atrophy. Neurology 58:649–652

29. Min YB, Finnegan EM, Hoffman HT, Luschei ES, McCulloch TM (1994) A preliminary study of the prognostic role of electromyography in laryngeal paralysis. Otolaryngol Head Neck Surg 111:770–775

30. Miyamoto RC, Parikh SR, Gellad W, Licameli GR (2005) Bilateral congenital vocal cord paralysis: a 16-year institutional review. Otolaryngol Head Neck Surg 133:241–245

31. Postma GN, Blalock PD, Koufman JA (1998) Bilateral medialization laryngoplasty. Laryngoscope 108:1429–1434

32. Pototschnig C, Thumfart WF (1997) Electromyographic evaluation of vocal cord disorders. Acta Otorhinolaryngol Belg 51:99–104

33. Richardson BE, Bastian RW (2004) Clinical evaluation of vocal fold paralysis. Otolaryngol Clin North Am 37:45–58

34. Rodriquez AA, Myers BR, Ford CN (1990) Laryngeal electromyography in the diagnosis of laryngeal nerve injuries. Arch Phys Med Rehabil 71:587–590

35. Rontal E, Rontal M, Silverman B, Kileny PR (1993) The clinical differentiation between vocal cord paralysis and vocal cord fixation using electromyography. Laryngoscope 103:133–137

36. Roth CR, Glaze LE, Goding GS, Jr., David WS (1996) Spasmodic dysphonia symptoms as initial presentation of amyotrophic lateral sclerosis. J Voice 10:362–367

37. Sasaki CT, Horiuchi M, Ikari T, Kirchner JA (1980) Vocal cord positioning by selective denervation. Old territory revisited. Ann Otol Rhinol Laryngol 89:541–546

38. Seddon H (1943) Three types of nerve injury. Brain 66: 237–288

39. Shaw GY, Sechtem PR, Rideout B (2003) Posterior cricoarytenoid myoplasty with medialization thyroplasty in the management of refractory abductor spasmodic dysphonia. Ann Otol Rhinol Laryngol 112:303–306

40. Simpson DM, Sternman D, Graves-Wright J, Sanders I (1993) Vocal cord paralysis: clinical and electrophysiologic features. Muscle Nerve 16:952–957

41. Sittel C, Guntinas-Lichius O, Streppel M, Stennert E (1998) Variability of repeated facial nerve electroneurography in healthy subjects. Laryngoscope 108:1177–1180

42. Sittel C, Stennert E (2001) Prognostic value of electromyography in acute peripheral facial nerve palsy. Otol Neurotol 22:100–104

43. Sittel C, Stennert E, Thumfart WF, Daput U, Eckel HE (2001) Prognostic value of laryngeal electromyography in vocal fold paralysis. Arch Otolaryngol Head Neck Surg 127: 155–160

44. Stennert E (1994) Why does the frontalis muscle "never come back"? Functional organization of the mimic musculature. Eur Arch Otorhinolaryngol S91–S95

45. Stong BC, DelGaudio JM, Hapner ER, Johns MM, III (2005) Safety of simultaneous bilateral botulinum toxin injections for abductor spasmodic dysphonia. Arch Otolaryngol Head Neck Surg 131:793–795

46. Sulica L (2004) Contemporary management of spasmodic dysphonia. Curr Opin Otolaryngol Head Neck Surg 12: 543–548

47. Sulica L, Blitzer A (2004) Electromyography and the immobile vocal fold. Otolaryngol Clin North Am 37:59–74

48. Thumfart WF (1981) Elektrodiagnostik bei Läsionen des N. recurrens. Arch Otorhinolaryngol 231:483–505

49. Thumfart WF (1998) Endoscopic electromyography and neuromyography. In: Samii M, Jannetta PJ (eds) The cranial nerves, vol 597–606. Springer, Heidelberg

50. Thumfart WF, Pototschnig C, Zorowka P, Eckel HE (1992) Electrophysiologic investigation of lower cranial nerve diseases by means of magnetically stimulated neuromyography of the larynx. Ann Otol Rhinol Laryngol 101:629–634

51. Tilles SA (2003) Vocal cord dysfunction in children and adolescents. Curr Allergy Asthma Rep 3:467–472

52. Trail M, Fox C, Ramig LO, Sapir S, Howard J, Lai EC (2005) Speech treatment for Parkinson's disease. NeuroRehabilitation 20:205–221

53. Zealear DL, Swelstad MR, Fortune S, Rodriguez RJ, Chung SM, Valyi-Nagy K, Billante MJ, Billante CR, Garren K (2005) Evoked electromyographic technique for quantitative assessment of the innervation status of laryngeal muscles. Ann Otol Rhinol Laryngol 114:563–572

Swallowing Disorders

15

Hans Edmund Eckel and Gerhard Friedrich

Core Messages

> The three main symptoms of dysphagia are obstruction (impaired bolus transport), aspiration (inhalation of food particles or saliva), and globus sensation.

> Functional endoscopic evaluation of swallowing is the most important diagnostic tool in the practice of laryngology.

> For the treatment of most types of deglutition disorders, rehabilitation therapy is the basis of therapeutic management.

> Functional rehabilitation uses compensatory strategies to reduce the risk of aspiration.

> For patients with isolated cricopharyngeal achalasia without diverticulum, endoscopic cricopharyngeal myotomy or localized injection of botulinum toxin can be used.

> The treatment of Zenker's diverticulum has become an established domain of laser surgery, but open cricopharyngeus myotomy combined with diverticulectomy through a left-sided open approach is still an established surgical alternative.

> The most common procedure for controlling aspiration is tracheostomy and use of a cuffed tracheostomy tube.

> For severe aspiration, total laryngectomy, closure of the larynx, or tracheoesophageal diversion may be needed.

15.1 Anatomical and Physiological Background

The larynx has two major functions. It acts as a sphincter to close the lower airway during deglutition, preventing aspiration of food and saliva; and it serves secondarily as the organ of voice. The larynx also stabilizes the thorax by preventing exhalation and helps to compress the abdomen during coughing. Phylogenetically, airway protection is the oldest and most essential function of the larynx. Failure to protect the lower airway is a potentially life-threatening condition because it results in chronic aspiration and subsequent pneumonia.

To fulfill these physiological needs adequately, laryngeal function relies on afferent (sensory) and efferent (motor) innervation. The nerve supply to the larynx and pharynx is comprised of branches of the vagus nerve (cranial nerve X), which exits the skull through the jugular foramen and then bilaterally branches off the pharyngeal nerve, the superior laryngeal nerve, and the recurrent laryngeal nerve. The pharyngeal nerve enters the pharynx and divides into the pharyngeal plexus to supply all of the muscles (m.) of the soft palate and the pharynx except for the m. tensor veli palatini and the m. stylopharyngeus (which are innervated by cranial nerves V and IX, respectively). The superior laryngeal nerve innervates

H. E. Eckel (✉)
Department of Oto-Rhino-Laryngology,
A.ö. Landeskrankenhaus Klagenfurt, HNO, St. Veiter Str. 47,
A-9020 Klagenfurt, Austria
e-mail: hans.eckel@kabeg.at

M. Remacle, H. E. Eckel (eds.), *Surgery of Larynx and Trachea,*
DOI: 10.1007/978-3-540-79136-2_15, © Springer-Verlag Berlin Heidelberg 2010

the cricothyroid and the inferior constrictor muscles. The recurrent laryngeal nerves supply all of the intrinsic muscles of the larynx except the m. cricothyroideus. On the right, the recurrent laryngeal nerve twines itself round the subclavian artery and then turns upward again to the larynx, whereas the left recurrent laryngeal nerve passes under the aortic arch and then returns upward to the larynx. Parasympathetic fibers of the X cranial nerve also innervate smooth muscles of the airway and esophagus, providing signals to open the airway during respiration, produce bronchoconstriction, and induce peristalsis of the esophagus.

15.2 Clinical Classification of Deglutition Disorders

Difficulty swallowing (dysphagia) is a common complaint in the overall population. It is reasonable to expect that, with the growing percentage of older individuals in Europe, the numbers will further increase in the future.

Dysphagia may present with any one of three main symptoms.

- Obstruction (impaired bolus transport)
- Aspiration (inhalation of food particles or saliva)
- Globus sensation (vague feeling of fullness in the throat, often perceived subjectively as "difficult swallowing" although solid foods and fluids are still swallowed normally)

Surgical treatment is an option only for obstruction or aspiration-related dysphagia. No sound rationale exists for the operative treatment of globus sensation.

15.3 Obstruction

Swallowing of food may be obstructed by various factors.

- Mass lesions in the oral cavity, oropharynx, hypopharynx, or esophagus
- External compression of the alimentary tract
- Disturbed neuromuscular regulation, especially absent or delayed opening of the upper (cricopha-

ryngeus muscle) and/or lower esophageal sphincter during swallowing

Pharyngeal masses leading to dysphagia may be due to hyperplasia of the lymphatic Waldeyer ring (hyperplasia of the tonsils or lymphatic tissue at the base of the tongue) or benign and malignant tumors of the oral cavity, larynx, pharynx, and esophagus. Cervical osteophytes may cause dysphagia by compressing the pharynx, particularly in the elderly.

15.4 Zenker's Diverticulum

Esophageal diverticula occur at the pharyngoesophageal junction, in the middle esophagus, and immediately proximal to the lower esophageal sphincter. Whereas true diverticula contain all structural layers of the pharyngeal/esophageal wall, typical Zenker's diverticula lack a muscular layer and should therefore be considered false diverticula. They result from endoluminal pressure and structural weakness of the posterior pharyngeal wall at the point of Killian's dehiscence in the hypopharynx, proximal to the cricopharyngeal muscle. It is an acquired lesion that predominantly affects persons over 60 years of age. It results from delayed relaxation of the cricopharyngeal muscle during deglutition. These diverticula develop and grow slowly over months and years. The typical signs are regurgitation of food and obstruction of the alimentary tract.

15.5 Cricopharyngeus Motility Disorders without Diverticula

Delayed relaxation of the cricopharyngeus muscle during swallowing occasionally leads to dysphagia, often accompanied by secondary aspiration. A diverticulum is not (yet) demonstrable in these cases. As with Zenker's diverticulum, the disorder is more common in older individuals. Video-cinematography is generally necessary to make a diagnosis. Unlike a conventional oral contrast examination, the temporal resolution of this technique is high enough to demonstrate the underlying functional disorder. As for

Zenker's diverticula, the recommended treatment is endoscopic myotomy.

15.6 Aspiration

Aspiration is defined as entry of material into the airway below the level of the true vocal cords. *Silent aspiration* is defined as aspiration occurring in the absence of acute symptoms (i.e., lack of cough or gag reflex as the food or liquid bolus passed into the trachea). *Penetration* is the term used to describe the entry of material into the larynx but not below the glottic level.

Pulmonary aspiration is a serious cause of morbidity and mortality in patients with a depressed sensorium, those with neuromuscular incoordination, or patients having a structural disorder of the upper aerodigestive tract. It is a leading cause of nosocomial infection. The most common manifestations of pulmonary aspiration are pneumonia, pleuropulmonary infection, and acute airway obstruction. Aspiration may result from loss of substance, especially in the larynx (e.g., after supraglottic partial laryngectomy), or it may have a neurological cause (e.g., lesions of the superior laryngeal nerve or vagus nerve).

Disorders of the laryngeal nerve supply lead to a variety of phonatory, respiratory, and deglutition disorders resulting from impaired sensitivity of the larynx, movement disorders of the vocal cords, or impaired pharyngoesophageal bolus transport during deglutition. Neurological aspiration usually results from the loss of laryngeal sensitivity or loss of cough and swallow reflexes.

15.7 Aspiration Due to Anatomical Defects

Aspiration frequently occurs in patients following larynx-sparing surgical treatment for laryngeal or pharyngeal tumors. It is most frequently related to impaired sensation but may also be caused by a lack of substance, particularly at the level of the arytenoid cartilages or the aryepiglottic folds. In contrast, resection of the epiglottis may lead to temporary aspiration but is usually righted by compensatory movements of the base of the tongue, ventricular folds, and vocal cords.

15.8 Aspiration Following Neurological Disorders

Vagus nerve paralysis or dysfunction of its laryngeal and pharyngeal branches results in loss of vocal cord abduction or adduction and in uncoordinated bolus transport during deglutition. It may affect phonation and respiration; and food, fluids, and saliva may be aspirated into the trachea. It may result from lesions in the central nervous system (nucleus ambiguous and its supranuclear tracts) or the main trunk of the vagus and its two laryngeal branches (inferior, or "recurrent," laryngeal nerve and superior laryngeal nerve). Intracranial tumors or hemorrhage and demyelinating diseases cause central paralysis. Neoplasms at the base of the skull and trauma to the neck cause vagus paralysis. Isolated paralysis of the inferior or superior laryngeal nerve is caused by cervical or thoracic lesions.

Paralysis of the vagus nerve or, more commonly, the inferior laryngeal nerve most frequently occurs after surgical procedures in the neck (particularly thyroidectomy) and upper mediastinum. It may also be caused by malignant tumors invading the larynx, hypopharynx, esophagus, thyroid, or tracheobronchial tree and other malignant neoplasms in the lower neck or upper mediastinum. Neurogenic laryngeal stenosis may also develop during the course of viral inflammation or as a result of central nervous system processes (cerebral or skull-base tumors, injuries, surgical procedures at the lateral skull base). Preoperative recognition of concomitant unilateral superior laryngeal nerve paralysis is important because it is a contraindication for surgical measures (especially arytenoidectomy) that could result in increased aspiration.

Previous surgery, mostly thyroid surgery, is the most common cause of laryngeal nerve paralysis. Revision thyroidectomy bears a particularly high risk for inferior and superior laryngeal nerve trauma. The rate of immediate postoperative unilateral recurrent laryngeal nerve paresis following primary thyroid surgery for benign disease is approximately 2–7%, and the rate of permanent paralysis has been reported to range from 0.5% to 4.0%. During revision surgery and operations for malignant conditions of the thyroid gland, unilateral recurrent laryngeal nerve paresis occurs in some 10–20% of the interventions. Bilateral vocal fold paralysis is seen far less frequently. Surgery of the cervical spine via an anterior approach as well as surgery of the larynx, pharynx, cervical esophagus, upper mediastinum, and carotid artery surgery can typically result in laryngeal nerve or even vagus nerve injury. Other conditions causing laryngeal nerve palsies include the following.

- Lesions of the brain stem
- Neurovascular disorders (stroke) and other central nervous disorders
- Demyelinating disorders of the peripheral nervous system (Guillain-Barré syndrome)
- Lateral skull base lesions (trauma, tumor)
- Sequel of skull base surgery
- Cervical spine injury or surgery
- Degenerative motor unit disorders (e.g., amyotrophic lateral sclerosis)
- Infectious diseases of the affected nerves
- Neurotoxins (e.g., lead)
- Primary neurogenic tumours (e.g., schwannoma)
- Malignant tumors of the thyroid, larynx, pharynx, trachea, esophagus, bronchus, and thymus; other malignant tumors of the neck and mediastinum
- Traumatic lesions of the neck
- Aortic aneurysm

If despite a complete diagnostic workup no etiological factor can be found, the paralysis is labeled idiopathic. Viral neuronitis probably accounts for most cases of idiopathic vocal cord paralysis. However, a complete diagnostic workup is needed if the etiology of laryngeal nerve impairment cannot readily be derived from the patient's history or obvious medical findings.

15.9 Symptoms

Symptoms of deglutition disorders in aware patients are easily recognized and freely communicated by the patient. In patients with depressed sensorium, impaired deglutition is not readily detectable and requires close clinical observation. Symptoms of impaired swallowing in these patients include the following.

- Weight loss
- Unexplained fever > 38.0°C
- Coughing
- Bronchitis/pneumonitis
- Impaired voice
- Witnessed regurgitation/aspiration event at the bedside accompanied by coughing, choking, and/or expectoration of material
- Prolonged oral feeding
- Aversion for oral intake of liquids and solids
- Disturbed bolus transport
- Frequent postural changes during oral intake
- Regurgitation

If such conditions are observed in previously intubated or neurological patients, a fiberoptic endoscopic evaluation of swallowing (FEES) should be undertaken to assess the impaired deglutition.

15.10 Diagnosis

In most patients presenting with laryngeal palsies, the underlying condition is obvious from the patient's history (e.g., recurrent laryngeal nerve paresis following thyroidectomy). In patients with unclear etiology of the underlying condition, a complete diagnostic workup is compulsory. The diagnostic protocol for these patients includes indirect mirror laryngoscopy, zoom laryngoscopy and/or transnasal flexible laryngoscopy, lung function tests (expiratory peak flow, resistance), voice analysis, laryngeal electromyography (EMG), tracheobronchoscopy and suspension laryngoscopy with tactile assessment of arytenoid cartilage mobility.

Nonspecific methods to assess aspiration are usually subjective and inaccurate. Videofluoroscopy has traditionally been accepted as the "gold standard" for evaluating a swallowing disorder because of the comprehensive information it provides (Fig. 15.1). However, it is not readily accessible in certain clinical and practical situations.

FEES is the most important diagnostic tool in the practice of laryngology (Fig. 15.2). It is a portable examination, easily performed at the bedside in intensive care units. Because these patients are usually bedridden, the examination is performed with the head of the bed elevated to approximately 70° or with the patient sitting on a chair. A fiberoptic laryngoscope is

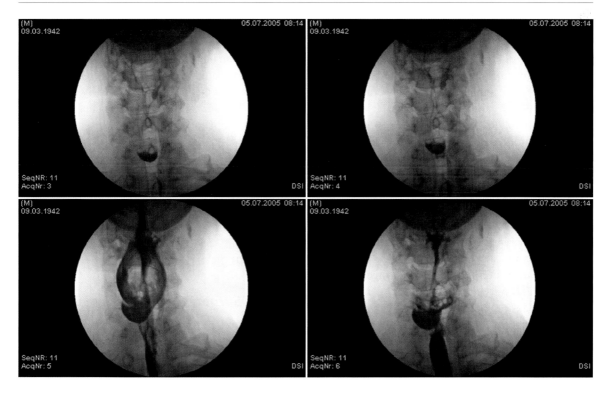

Fig. 15.1. Videofluoroscopy shows a small Zenker's diverticulum and prestenotic dilatation of the hypopharynx

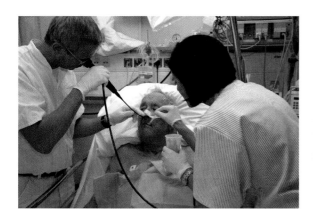

Fig. 15.2. Functional endoscopic evaluation of swallowing (FEES) performed at bedside

passed transnasally to the oropharynx, where the larynx and surrounding structures can then be visualized. Patients are led through various tasks to evaluate the sensory and motor status of the pharyngeal and laryngeal mechanism. Stained liquid and semiliquid boluses are given to assess pharyngeal deglutition. The larynx is examined for evidence of food penetration in the laryngeal vestibule and aspiration of food below the true vocal folds before and after each swallow. Endoscopic assessment includes looking for structural changes in the larynx and pharynx as well as noting the timing and direction of movement of the bolus through the pharynx, the ability to protect the airway and to uphold airway protection, the capability to clear the bolus during deglutition, the presence of pooling and residue of material in the hypopharynx, and the timing of bolus flow and laryngeal closure [1].

If the etiology of the condition remains unclear, a comprehensive diagnostic workup of the thyroid gland is undertaken, including [^{99m}Tc]-pertechnetate scintiscanning, ultrasonography of the neck, and related laboratory tests [thyroid-stimulating hormone (TSH) assay]. If the thyroid assessment remains inconclusive, chest computed tomography (CT) scans and a barium swallow with fluoroscopy should be done. If additional signs of neurogenic disorders are present, magnetic resonance imaging (MRI) studies of the brain and additional laboratory tests (including a complete blood count and cerebrospinal fluid examination) should be considered. In patients with a suspected inflammatory nerve disorder or joint disease, additional laboratory tests include white blood cell and differential counts; determination of an acute phase indicator (usually C-reactive protein); Lyme disease antibodies; tests for rheumatoid factor, antinuclear antibodies, anti-neutrophil cytoplasmatic antibodies (c-ANCA); and renal, liver, and electrolyte studies are sometimes helpful.

The use of laryngeal EMG has been advocated to classify the severity of neural damage, establish a prognosis for nerve recovery, and differentiate neurogenic palsy from vocal fold immobility caused by arytenoid fixation. Although it has been helpful in many cases, it is not considered a routine diagnostic tool by many laryngologists. Its prognostic accuracy is limited to cases of neurotmesis.

Delayed relaxation of the cricopharyngeus muscle during swallowing occasionally leads to dysphagia, which often is accompanied by secondary aspiration. A diverticulum is not (yet) demonstrable in all cases. The disorder is more common in older individuals. Video-cinematography is generally necessary to make a diagnosis.

15.11 Therapy

15.11.1 Nonsurgical Treatment

Rehabilitation therapy is the basis of management for most deglutition disorders [2]. Following the placement of a nasogastric feeding tube or percutaneous endoscopic or open gastrostomy, logopedic rehabilitation uses compensatory strategies to reduce the risk of aspiration.

- Oral feeding with consistency modifications (thickened liquids increase oropharyngeal control and decrease difficulties with mastication).
- Modifying the volume and tempo of food presentation.
- Head rotation (the ipsilateral pharynx is closed, forcing the food bolus to the contralateral pharynx while cricopharyngeal pressure is decreased).
- Anteroflexion of the head (chin down) during deglutition, narrowing the airway entrance.
- Supraglottic swallow. This technique uses simultaneous swallowing and breath-holding, closing the vocal cords and protecting the airway. The patient

thereafter can cough to eject any residue in the laryngeal vestibule.
- Mendelsohn maneuver. This is a form of supraglottic swallow in which the patient mimics the upward movement of the larynx by voluntarily holding the larynx at its maximum height to increase the duration of the cricopharyngeal opening.

Additional exercises are used to increase muscle tone and to improve coordination and strengthening of muscles of the jaw, lips, cheek, tongue, soft palate, and vocal cords.

15.12 Surgical Treatment

15.12.1 Surgery for Obstructive Disorders

Obstruction of the alimentary tract by tonsillar hyperplasia can be treated medically (for acute inflammation) or surgically (tonsillectomy). In children, laser tonsillotomy may be appropriate if the goal is to reduce the volume of the tonsils while preserving tonsillar remnants for immunological reasons. Obstruction related to neoplastic disease is treated by resecting the tumor or using nonsurgical oncological approaches. Temporary percutaneous endoscopic or open gastrostomy may be required to maintain adequate feeding during treatment.

Hypertrophic cervical osteophytes (Morbus Forestier) can be removed via a left-sided anterolateral extrapharyngeal approach or with a transoral, transpharyngeal procedure. The open approach carries the risk of recurrent laryngeal nerve paresis, hematoma, and Horner's syndrome, whereas the endoscopic intervention carries the risk of fistulas and local infections of the prevertebral space and the vertebrae.

The treatment of Zenker's diverticulum has become an established domain of laser surgery during recent years. Until a few years ago, open cricopharyngeus myotomy combined with diverticulectomy through a left-sided open approach was the standard surgical treatment for Zenker's diverticula (Fig. 15.3). Although endoscopic myotomy (division of the posterior part of the annular cricopharyngeus muscle) was described as early as 1917, the endoscopic approach was abandoned later due to excessive complications. Van Overbeek showed that endoscopic cricopharyngeal myotomy

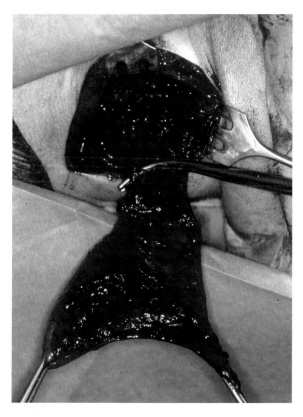

Fig. 15.3. Large Zenker's diverticulum. Open cricopharyngeus myotomy combined with diverticulectomy through a left-sided open approach is performed

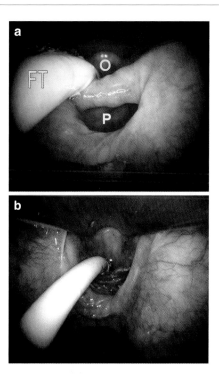

Fig. 15.4. Zenker's diverticulum treated by endoscopic myotomy (division of the posterior part of the annular cricopharyngeus muscle). (**a**) Endoscopic view of the hypopharyngeal pouch (*P*), esophagus (*O*), and feeding tube (*FT*). (**b**) Anatomical situation following complete transection of the posterior part of the cricopharyngeus muscle

could be done safely using CO_2 laser [3]. According to the literature, the complications and results of endoscopic myotomy appear to be comparable to or better than those achieved with open surgery [4]. In any case, endoscopic myotomy obviates the need for an external neck incision and practically eliminates the risk of recurrent nerve paralysis (Fig. 15.4a, b). Generally, the myotomy can be done without difficulty when a special diverticuloscope (Dohlman type) is used. There is disagreement as to whether patients should be fed through a temporary nasogastric tube (placed preoperatively and carefully protected during laser use) or by temporary parenteral nutrition. Opinions also vary as to the timing of the initial feeding after endoscopic myotomy. An interval of 2–7 days is most commonly recommended. In all cases, oral contrast examination with a water-soluble medium should be done before the resumption of oral intake to exclude paravasation into the upper mediastinum. Although endoscopic myotomy is technically straightforward, it should be

emphasized that this procedure is by no means without risks. Any complete cricopharyngeal myotomy opens the upper mediastinum and consequently carries the risk of mediastinitis. This underscores the urgent need for preoperative antibiotic prophylaxis. Local mucosal antisepsis in the region of the hypopharynx and diverticular sac may also help lower the risk of infection. Mild wound pain, leukocytosis, and temperature elevation are common after the operation, especially during the first night. If fever persists beyond the first day or does not respond promptly to antipyretic agents, and if the patient has respiration-dependent back pain, neck emphysema, or other manifestations of a septic systemic process, appropriate imaging studies (CT) should be done at once to assess the need for surgical intervention (opening the upper mediastinum through a left cervical incision, oversewing an esophageal perforation, local irrigation, and drainage). The surgeon should take note of the potential risks and be prepared to manage them.

A number of alternatives to laser surgery are available for the treating Zenker's diverticulum and cricopharyngeal dysfunction. Endoscopic myotomy with a stapler has been recommended in recent years. A special stapler has been developed for treatment of Zenker's diverticula and can be introduced and operated through a diverticuloscope. It divides the common wall between the diverticular sac and esophagus, simultaneously closing the wound surfaces on both sides with staples. This technique is supposed to prevent leakage into the mediastinum. Because of the way the stapler is designed, part of the wound always remains open at the lowest point of the incision.

Open myotomy is available as an alternative to endoscopic myotomy in cases where it is important to avoid opening the pharynx. The surgery is done through a left transcervical approach, like the classic operation for treating Zenker's diverticulum. Following meticulous division of the cricopharyngeus muscle, the diverticulum is not resected, and the pharynx remains unopened. There is virtually no risk of infection under these conditions (with proper attention to surgical asepsis). The procedure can thus provide an alternative to endoscopic myotomy and the classic open operation for Zenker's diverticula in all patients considered to be at increased risk for mediastinitis (patients with multiple morbidities, older patients).

For patients with isolated cricopharyngeal achalasia without a diverticulum, endoscopic cricopharyngeal myotomy has been described as a safe technique that does not incur a complication rate higher than that following endoscopic treatment of Zenker's diverticulum. The operative technique is the same as that used for Zenker's diverticulum [5].

An elegant, minimally invasive treatment option is to paralyze the cricopharyngeus muscle temporarily with a localized injection of botulinum toxin [6]. The advantage of this method is that it is practically free of complications when carried out correctly. The disadvantage is that its effect lasts only a few months, at which time the treatment may have to be repeated (generally necessitating brief general anesthesia). Thus, botulinum toxin injection is not a permanent treatment option. It does, however, provide an ideal test method in equivocal cases to determine if the proposed surgical division of the cricopharyngeus muscle can improve the patient's symptoms. If the symptoms diminish following transient paralysis of the muscle with botulinum toxin and then worsen again after the effect has subsided, the patient can be scheduled for a definitive cricopharyngeal myotomy.

15.13 Surgery for Aspiration Disorders

Aspiration resulting from anatomical defects following laryngeal surgery or unilateral neurological conditions (disorders of the superior laryngeal nerve, vagus nerve, unilateral lower motor neuron of the brain stem, or lower cranial nerves) frequently requires surgical treatment in addition to functional management. Nonoral enteral feeding options are required for patients unable to ingest adequate quantities of liquids and nutrients. Nasogastric feeding tubes and endoscopically or surgically placed gastrostomy or jejunostomy tubes are available. The most common procedure for controlling aspiration is tracheostomy and use of a cuffed tracheostomy tube. An epithelialized tracheostomy should always be placed to facilitate daily changes of the tube and care of the lower airway.

Laryngeal suspension procedures aim at correcting impaired laryngeal elevation during deglutition. Nonabsorbable sutures are used to sew the thyroid cartilage to the hyoid bone and the thyrohyoid complex to the anterior mandible (Fig. 15.5a, b). The procedure increases the pharyngeal opening and protection of the laryngeal inlet during deglutition [7].

Vocal fold medialization or augmentation is used to restore glottic closure during deglutition. Basically, the same surgical techniques that are used for phonosurgery can be applied. Medialization techniques are generally more effective than augmentation [8].

Cricopharyngeal myotomy is used to reduce the functional obstruction of the alimentary tract induced by delayed or inadequate opening of the cricopharyngeal muscle during deglutition. The procedure consists of incising the cricopharyngeus muscle (usually including the upper inferior portion of the constrictor pharynges muscle and the superior part of the esophageal musculature in the midline) down to the level of the mucosa, resulting in permanent, complete relaxation of the cricopharyngeus muscle and improved bolus transport from the hypopharynx into the esophagus [9]. For most patients, some or all of these procedures have to be combined to restore deglutition, and additional functional treatment is invariably required before the tracheotomy can be closed again.

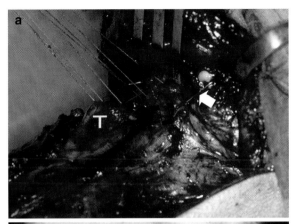

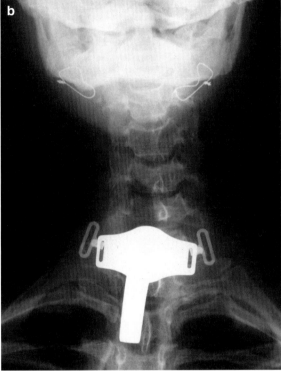

Fig. 15.5. (a-b) Laryngeal suspension procedure. (**a**) Anatomical situation following fixation of the thyroid cartilage to the hyoid bone and the thyrohyoid complex to the anterior mandible (wire sutures). (**b**) Radiographic view after laryngeal suspension (wire slings indicate suspension of the thyrohyoid complex to the mandible)

For severe aspiration (e.g., following mass lesions of the brain stem or bilateral paralysis of the lower cranial nerves), surgery is needed to separate the airway from the alimentary tract. Surgical procedures that may be used in this context include total laryngectomy, closure of the larynx, and tracheoesophageal diversion.

Total laryngectomy effectively separates the airway from the alimentary tract. It prevents aspiration completely and is generally considered a reliable, reproducible standard technique with a low incidence of severe complications. The loss of glottic phonation is frequently of little importance to the patients whose severe neurological disease is the cause of aspiration. Separation of the airway from the alimentary tract is irreversible.

Laryngeal closure and tracheoesophageal diversion are potentially reversible. However, laryngeal closure is technically difficult and frequently results in some kind of residual aspiration. Tracheoesophageal diversion is separation of the larynx from the trachea at about the fourth tracheal ring. The proximal tracheal stump is anastomosed in an end-to-side manner with the esophagus, allowing drainage of aspirates from the larynx into the esophagus. The distal end is anastomosed to the skin and forms a tracheostomy. Complications include tracheocutaneous fistulas, wound infections, stenosis at the tracheostomy site, and perioperative mortality [10]. As with laryngectomy, phonation is not possible with these procedures. With regard to the poor prognosis of severe neurological function impairment in most patients, total laryngectomy remains the gold standard for the surgical treatment of this condition.

15.14 Tips and Pearls

- When performing endoscopic surgery for Zenker's diverticulum, place a nasogastric tube at the beginning of the intervention under direct vision and avoid inserting it through the open wound at the end of the procedure.
- Administer local antiseptics to the oral cavity and pharyngeal pouch as well as perioperative antibiotic prophylaxis.
- Perform videofluoroscopy on day 2 or 3 following surgery to rule out paravasation from the cervical esophagus. A diverticular sac following endoscopic myotomy is frequently seen radiologically.
- Fever, pain in the back, and emphysema of the neck may be indicative of mediastinitis. When in doubt, obtain a CT scan of the mediastinum and be prepared to perform open drainage of the upper mediastinum.

- In patients undergoing tracheotomy for severe aspiration, dilatation tracheotomy is not adequate. A completely epithelialized tracheostomy should always be performed.

References

1. Langmore SE, Schatz K, Olson N (1991) Endoscopic and videofluoroscopic evaluations of swallowing and aspiration. Ann Otol Rhinol Laryngol 100:678–681
2. Bigenzahn W, Denk DM (1999) Oropharyngeale dysphagien. Thieme, Stuttgart
3. van Overbeek JJ (2003) Pathogenesis and methods of treatment of Zenker's diverticulum. Ann Otol Rhinol Laryngol 112:583–593
4. Lippert BM, Folz BJ, Gottschlich S, Werner JA (1997) Microendoscopic treatment of the hypopharyngeal diverticulum with the CO_2 laser. Lasers Surg Med 20:394
5. Lawson G, Remacle M (2006) Endoscopic cricopharyngeal myotomy: indications and technique. Curr Opin Otolaryngol Head Neck Surg 14:437–441
6. Schneider I, Thumfart WF, Pototschnig C, Eckel HE (1994) Treatment of dysfunction of the cricopharyngeal muscle with botulinum a toxin: Introduction of a new, noninvasive method. Ann Otol Rhinol Laryngol 103:31
7. Edgerton MT, Mc KD (1959) Reconstruction with loss of the hyomandibular complex in excision of large cancers. AMA Arch Surg 78:425–436
8. Schneider B, Denk DM, Bigenzahn W (2003) Functional results after external vocal fold medialization thyroplasty with the titanium vocal fold medialization implant. Laryngoscope 113:628–634
9. Ey W, Denecke-Singer U, Ey M, Guastella C, Onder N (1990) [surgical treatment of dysphagia of the pharyngoesophageal transition] chirurgische behandlung der dysphagien im bereich des pharyngoosophagealen uberganges. Arch Otorhinolaryngol Suppl 1:107
10. Zocratto OB, Savassi-Rocha PR, Paixao RM, Salles JM (2006) Laryngotracheal separation surgery: outcome in 60 patients. Otolaryngol Head Neck Surg 135:571–575

Nerve Reconstruction

16

Jean-Paul Marie

Core Messages

> Trunk-to-trunk anastomosis of a recurrent laryngeal nerve (RLN) does not allow recovery of vocal cord mobility.

> Vocal cord mobility is not necessary to achieve good voice results.

> Nonselective reinnervation is the optimal treatment of unilateral RLN lesion. It can be performed at the time of the injury, or it can be delayed.

> Dissection of the distal portion of the RLN is always possible by the retrograde intralaryngeal approach.

> Ansa hypoglossi- to-RLN anastomosis is the optimal technique for unilateral vocal cord paralysis.

> Nerve transfers have to be long enough to follow the laryngeal movements during swallowing.

> Superior laryngeal nerve (SLN) lesions can be sutured with good recovery of laryngeal sensation.

> In bilateral RLN lesion, with vocal cord in adductory position, treatments must respect the vocal cord integrity.

> New techniques of bilateral motor selective reinnervation of the larynx should be considered only in cases when the arytenoids remain passively mobile.

> Phrenic nerve is the optimal nerve supply for posterior cricoarytenoid muscle reinnervation. Preservation of some of its roots can spare some diaphragm innervation and function.

J.-P. Marie
Service d'ORL & Chirurgie Cervico faciale, Hopital Ch Nicolle, CHU Rouen, F-76031, Laboratoire de Chirurgie Expérimentale UPRES EA 3830 GRHV, IFRMP 23, Université de Rouen, France
e-mails: Jean-Paul.Marie@chu-rouen.fr
jean-paul.marie4@wanadoo.fr

16.1 Introduction

Laryngeal nerve lesions are a common occurrence, and they have medical or surgical etiologies. Depending on the level of the lesion and the unilaterality or bilaterality, the presentation is different as is the treatment.

With unilateral vocal cord paralysis, dysphonia is the major problem encountered. Swallowing problems are present at the onset of the disease, and they can increase pulmonary pathology, especially because the cough is not efficient.

With bilateral paralysis, vocal cords are usually in a paramedian position, which may result in inspiratory dyspnea. However, phonation is satisfactorily preserved. Classic modes of treatment for bilateral paralysis are aimed at enlarging the glottis (described in other chapters); unpredictable hoarseness and some lack of protective closure result with some of the treatment modalities. Laryngeal reinnervation can theoretically solve these problems.

Laryngeal reinnervation is not a new idea, but it is a challenging option. Numbers of animal experiments have been performed in the past, but human applications have been limited. We present techniques that have had substantial clinical application. Nevertheless, some of them have not been used extensively and must be compared to passive palliative techniques.

M. Remacle, H. E. Eckel (eds.), *Surgery of Larynx and Trachea,*
DOI: 10.1007/978-3-540-79136-2_16, © Springer-Verlag Berlin Heidelberg 2010

16.2 Anatomical Landmarks and Prerequisites

The intrinsic laryngeal muscles, with the exception of the cricothyroid (CT) muscle, are all innervated by the recurrent laryngeal nerve (RLN). The cricothyroid muscle is innervated by the external branch of the superior laryngeal nerve (SLN). The RLN and SLN are both branches of the vagus nerve. After a thoracic or cervical route, the RLN enters the larynx. It always proceeds posteromedially to the cricothyroid joint, which is an important landmark for its identification. Intralaryngeally, it divides into its motor branches. Roughly, the posteromedial bundle runs to the posterior cricoarytenoid muscle (PCA) and the interarytenoid muscles. The anteromedial bundle (adductor branch) innervates the remaining intrinsic laryngeal muscles with the exception of the cricothyroid muscle. One branch of the RLN, usually branching extralaryngeally forms a junction with the SLN (the ansa galeni). The precise intralaryngeal anatomy is variable and has been studied by several authors [28, 38, 53, 59]. The intralaryngeal RLN branch for the PCA is sometimes unique and sometimes multiple, originating from the common branch of the adductor muscles. The main trunk of the RLN carries motor fibers to both the intrinsic laryngeal adductor and abductor muscles and contains 500–1000 myelinated nerve fibers. The ratio of adductor and abductor fibers is approximately 3:1.

The intraneural structure of the RLN forms no topographical separation of the adductor and abductor fibers. Sunderland and Swaney, in serial sections from humans, found a constantly changing pattern with frequent communication between fascicles [63]. This plexifom disposition of the axons inside the nerve trunk explains the failure of direct nerve anastomosis: misdirected regeneration of the axons to the antagonist muscles (synkinesis) and subsequent lack of recovery of the vocal cord mobility.

The motor units of the adductor muscles are small and have 2–20 muscle fibers per motor unit; and the muscle fibers have mainly fast contraction times. The abductor muscle (PCA) has much larger motor units, with 200–250 muscles fibers per motor unit; these are mainly fibers with a slower contraction time. Characteristics of a muscle fiber (fast or slow contraction time) are determined by the axonal supply and can change if a new nerve supply is provided.

Nerve lesions, if not too severe, have a strong tendency to recover. It is particularly important for the RLN. Several experimental studies have shown nerve regrowth through an interrupted RLN [27, 39]. However, synkinesis explains why the vocal cord remains immobile.

The position of the paralyzed vocal cord (median or lateral position with subsequent symptoms) has been the subject of a number of articles. Cricothyroid residual innervation has been thought to play a role. Residual (or recovered) laryngeal innervation is probably the main explanation [78, 79]. Consequently, the greater the residual nerve supply, the more trophic is the hemilarynx, with a vocal cord in a median position allowing effective contralateral vocal cord contact and good voice [4]. In other words, preservation (or recovery) of the viscoelasticity of the larynx is suitable for optimal voice results. This is a strong justification for laryngeal reinnervation. Moreover, no glottis scar is performed.

Some additional concepts must be understood regarding laryngeal reinnervation [17]. First, a nerve lesion stimulates axonal sprouting in the vicinity of the injured muscle. On the other hand, axon-sprouting inhibitor factor is normally found in innervated muscle. Moreover, an innervated muscle does not accept additional innervation unless the original or the supplying nerve is injured. For that reason, at the time of a reinnervation procedure, it is necessary to remove the spontaneously recovered innervation.

Biochemical properties of a reinnervated muscle are determined by the nerve transfer. For this reason, the phrenic nerve, with slow contraction fibers and firing in inspiration, is an ideal nerve graft for PCA reinnervation.

Denervation atrophy hinders reinnervation. Spontaneous reinnervation by nerves coming from the vicinity or regenerated laryngeal nerves prevent severe denervation atrophy for a long time (and might induce some synkinesis). For these reasons, reinnervation can be proposed some years after laryngeal nerve lesions if arycricoid ankylosis (a rare occurrence in our experience) has not occurred.

Surgical reinnervation of the larynx can be performed with various surgical techniques: nerve anastomosis or implantation of a nerve end or nerve muscle pedicle (NMP) into a recipient muscle to allow regenerating axons to grow and reinnervate the laryngeal muscles.

Laryngeal reinnervation can be either nonselective or selective. Nonselective reinnervation comprises anastomosis to the main stem of the RLN, leading to reinnervation of both the abductor and adductor muscle groups. It can be performed at the time of an acute nerve injury or for chronic vocal cord paralysis. It is carried out on unilateral lesions. With selective reinnervation, the abductor and/or adductor muscles are separately reinnervated, with the main goal of vocal cord mobility rehabilitation. (It is essential to enlarge the glottis in the presence of bilateral vocal cord paralysis.)

Properties of the donor nerve have to be highly similar to the original nerve, having the same function, mainly for selective functional reinnervation. Phrenic nerve and branches of the hypoglossal nerves have these properties. However, removal of the donor nerve must be well tolerated. Questions exist regarding the phrenic nerve, however. We will see later under which conditions.

Because the larynx is mobile and is elevated during swallowing, the nerve graft must be long enough to allow these movements without risk of disruption.

Nerve anastomosis is usually performed as follows: An epiperineural technique is used with interrupted sutures of 9-0 to 10-0, under amplification (an operating microscope is the most suitable). Biological glue may be used to recover the suture line, to avoid axonal escape, but mainly to secure the nerves to the muscles.

16.3 Nonselective Reinnervation (In a Unilateral Nerve Lesion)

16.3.1 Acute Lesions of the Laryngeal Nerves

A common question for the laryngologist is what to do in case of acute laryngeal nerve resection. The answer is simple: always try to fix it by nerve reconstruction during the same operating time.

At the cervical level, injury of the recurrent nerve can be induced by laryngeal trauma (cricotracheal desinsertion) or thyroid surgery. Nerve resection is sometimes performed at the time of thyroid cancer resection. Optimal rehabilitation can be obtained by nerve anastomosis. A direct anastomosis can be carried out between two stumps of the RLN using a free nerve graft if it is necessary to bridge the gap between them. If the proximal stump for the RLN cannot be found, a neighboring nerve can be used, usually the ansa hypoglossi, as described by Crumley [22].

No immediate mobility recovery is observed; nevertheless, nonselective reinnervation achieves optimal voice results after a 4- to 8-month delay. Temporary improvement can be obtained (while waiting for axonal growth) by endoscopic medialization, if possible with resorbable material (Gelfoam, fat). A contemporary external medialization is proposed based on the fact that a cervical wound gives access to the thyroid ala. The usual problem encountered is general anesthesia and the presence of the endotracheal tube, decreasing the possibility of voice adjustment.

When the RLN is injured at the thoracic level, immediate treatment can be undertaken using immediate passive medialization and/or reinnervation [80]. Medialization, associated with adapted nutrition, is useful to prevent aspiration and help cough efficacy, which are so important to pulmonary healing.

A vagus nerve lesion at the cervical or thoracic level can benefit from the same approach. Moreover, a vagus nerve lesion at the skull base or intracranial level induces vocal cord paralysis (often in a lateral position) and sensitive denervation of the homolateral hemilarynx. The risk of aspiration is high and justifies an early reconstructive method.

Laryngeal closure can be corrected by a vagus-to-vagus anastomosis, or ansa-to-RLN anastomosis.

Sensitive rehabilitation can be done, in some favorable cases, with an SLN anastomosis (directly or using a free nerve graft). A new attitude can even be proposed, adapted from our animal experiments: anastomosis to a sensitive nerve, the superficial cervical plexus [6].

In some rare cases, at the time of injury, division of the recurrent nerve can be followed inside the larynx. Selective anastomosis can be attempted, although functional results are not always achieved (H. Ganz, personal communication: 2008).

16.3.1.1 Results

Few results of acute reinnervation by RLN neurorraphy alone are reported. No return of motion is expected. Chou et al. reported significant improvement in eight patients with primarily repair of the RLN compared with four similar patients who did not undergo repair but who later required thyroplasty [11]. Other authors have shown an interest in acute neurorraphy of the RLN whatever the technique performed (direct neurorraphy, graft interposition, or ansa RLN) [52, 80]. Crumley, to avoid synkinesis, recommended the ansa RLN in these situations [20].

Time elapsed until recovery depends on the distance the axons have to travel. For instance, during cervical schwannoma surgery, vagus nerve removal reconstructed with a free interposition nerve graft can achieve reinnervation within 12 months. An ansa hypoglossi technique would have produced faster results (within 4 months).

In our department, we always recommend reconstruction of the nerve supply at the time of nerve resection if possible.

16.3.2 Reinnervation of Chronic Unilateral Vocal Cord Paralysis

16.3.2.1 Lesions of the Inferior Laryngeal Nerve (Recurrent Nerve Paralysis)

General Indications

Reinnervation is indicated:

- When the nerve lesion is severe, either by known resection, or when the time elapsed has not demonstrated any functional and electrophysiological recovery.
- When an optimal voice result is required (voice professionals).
- When delay before recovery can be expected.
- When the functional handicap is mainly *dysphonia*, with a breathy voice, or diplophonia induced by lack of adduction of the vocal cord.

Recent lesions (less than 3 years) are preferred to old lesions; however, poor residual innervation preserves trophicity and allows successful reinnervation. A recurrent nerve lesion at the entrance of the larynx is not a contraindication. An intralaryngeal retrograde dissection can easily be done. Reinnervation can be completed by passive medialization while awaiting axonal regrowth.

No recovery of the mobility is expected. However, there is improved trophicity of the ipsilateral larynx, allowing better approximation of the contralateral healthy vocal cord in phonation. Passive mobility of the arytenoid is not required.

Preoperative Assessment

The previous medical history should be carefully assessed, specifically the previous operation report with a description of the recurrent nerve lesions (severity, level) and the extent of the neck dissection (to anticipate the status of the potentially nerve grafts). Physical examination can verify the lack of vocal cord scars and the integrity of the other cranial nerves. Previous radiotherapy and/or severe neck fibrosis adds some difficulty.

Because the technique of reinnervation usually requires recurrent nerve resection, it is necessary to make sure via laryngeal electromyography (EMG) that only poor or no residual innervation remains in the intrinsic laryngeal muscles. A severe neurogenic pattern or fibrillation potentials are the most suitable traces. On the contrary, fair enrichment in phonation means good residual innervation and precludes a good functional result (reinnervation does not improve the result).

Certain preoperative voice assessments are required: questionnaires (VHI 100 or 10, or others), voice recordings for perceptual analysis and future comparisons (and medicolegal reasons), computerized analysis, and videoscopy imaging.

Surgical Technique (Including Specific Recommendations)

1. Ansa Cervicalis-to-RLN Anastomosis ("Ansa Technique") Described by Crumley

The ansa-cervicalis-to-RLN anastomosis is today the most frequently used technique [21, 23, 25, 43]. A homolateral horizontal incision is made in a skin crease at about the level of the lower edge of the cricoid cartilage. The platysma muscle is then incised followed by prudent incision of the sternocleidomastoid muscle fascia, watching for the ansa cervicalis. The ansa can usually be found traversing the jugular vein; it can also be located by careful examination of the posterior aspect of the omohyoid or sternohyoid muscles. Once identified, the nerve is dissected proximally to the lateral edge of the jugular vein and distally into the strap muscles (electrical stimulation of the nerve can be performed for confirmation). No specific branch is chosen.

The RLN is identified next. In cases of an intact cervical area (e.g., when the RLN lesion was produced by a thoracic lesion), the RLN can be identified inferior to the thyroid gland and dissected superiorly. With more frequent cases of cervical injury, a retrograde dissection can be performed. A single hook is placed around the posterior part of the thyroid cartilage, permitting its rotation. The RLN is found behind the cricothyroid joint, entering the larynx. If a scar is present in a previously dissected region, the possible site of the RLN lesion, careful section of the inferior constrictor muscle is performed, allowing dissection in an usually intact area. The RLN trunk (which must be differentiated from the Galen anastomosis) is then dissected several centimeters inferiorly.

Before either nerve is divided, it is necessary to verify that there is enough length to allow a tension-free anastomosis. Moreover, the ascending movement of the larynx during swallowing must be anticipated. The ansa is cut at the point where the diameter is similar to that RLN.

End-to-end anastomosis is performed using standard microsurgical techniques, under magnification. After frank section of the nerves, the extremities are prepared by resecting the axonal excess. The epineurium is preserved. Epiperineural anastomosis is performed using four to six sutures of 9/0. The anastomosis can be protected and stabilized by biological glue or a surrounding vein fragment. Closure is conventional.

2. XII-Recurrent Anastomosis as Described by Paniello

Paniello has reported a technique of unilateral nonselective reinnervation using the hypoglossal nerve trunk, as it is performed during facial rehabilitation with skull base surgery. The procedure is similar except that more length of the RLN is required to reach the hypoglossal nerve [56–58]. The section of the hypoglossal nerve is performed distally to ensure that the anastomosis is carried out without tension; a nerve graft to obtain adequate length can be used, but the advantage in terms of axonal supply is probably not better than that with the ansa RLN technique.

The apparent incongruence between two nerves is not a problem microscopically because much of the hypoglossal nerve diameter is constituted of nonneural material that should be removed. Neural anastomosis and closure are performed as described above.

3. Nerve-Muscle Pedicle Implantation of Tucker

Having introduced the nerve muscle pedicle (NMP) technique implantation for posterior cricoarytenoid reinnervation for bilateral vocal cord paralysis (see below), Tucker applied this technique to adductor muscle reinnervation [65, 73] (Fig. 16.1). The omohyoid muscle nerve supply is used, assuming that strap muscles contract in phonation during pitch control.

This technique can be performed in cases in which the RLN cannot be found. Nevertheless, we have observed that a retrograde dissection is always possible.

The incision is performed horizontally in regard to the cricothyroid cartilage area. A block of omohyoid muscle is dissected and mobilized with the nerve supply (a branch from the hypoglossal nerve). The strap muscles are then retracted and mobilized to expose the thyroid cartilage (as for thyroplasty). A posteriorly based perichondrial flap is created (Fig. 16.1). A block of cartilage is removed with the Striker saw (or the fissure burr) from the lower 50% of the thyroid ala so an intact posterior and inferior strut of cartilage is left intact. Having incised the internal perichondrium, the fibers of the lateral thyroarytenoid muscle are exposed. The NMP pedicle is approximated to this muscle and sutured in place with two or three 5/0 nylon sutures. The wound is closed in a normal fashion.

4. Combinations

Reinnervation techniques can be performed in addition to medialization techniques. This was proposed by Tucker, who demonstrated that the long-term results after thyroplasty were not particularly good owing to supposed muscular atrophy [71, 72].

The ansa-RLN technique can be combined with arytenoid adduction [10].

5. Reinnervation for Unilateral Vocal Cord Paralysis in Children

In children, reinnervation can be performed with ansa-RLN technique and nerve muscle adductor implantation [69]. A combination of medialization techniques and reinnervation can be performed (thyroplasty or arytenoid adduction [10]).

Recommendations for Follow-Up
(Postoperative Care)

The cervical wound is managed in a routine fashion. No antibiotic prophylaxis is required. Voice rest is unnecessary. With unilateral RLN reinnervation, the acute nerve denervation can induce some aspiration during the first few days, as does the first recurrent nerve lesion. Nasogastric feeding is recommended followed by education and thickening of the food, especially the liquids.

Even if a retrograde intralaryngeal dissection of the RLN has been carried out, no hematoma or excessive laryngeal edema has been observed in our experience.

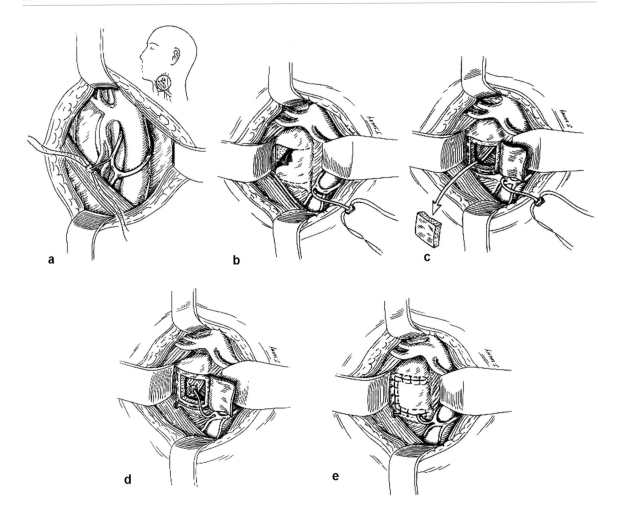

a   b   c

d   e

Fig. 16.1. Reinnervation of the adductor muscles by the nerve-muscle pedicle (NMP) technique of Tucker [65, 73] (for unilateral vocal cord paralysis). (**a**) Isolation of a branch of the ansa hypoglossi to the omohyoid muscle. (**b**) Posteriorly based thyroid cartilage perichondrial graft. (**c**) Removal of cartilage to expose adductor muscles. (**d**) Insertion of a nerve-muscle pedicle into adductor muscles. (**e**) Closure of thyroid perichondrium

Consequently, no dyspnea is observed, even if additional passive medialization is performed at the same time.

Alteration of the voice can be observed for the next few weeks, which is a consequence of removing some of the remaining innervation of the hemilarynx. Usually resection of the RLN is performed in cases of severe larynx denervation.

Voice improvement is not observed before 4 months and can be expected at 8–9 months, depending on the length of the denervation, the age of the patient, and the use of an elongation graft. The patients must be previously informed of that situation. Temporary medialization can be performed at the time of surgery, while awaiting the efficacy of reinnervation, by Gelfoam paste (or fat injection, in our experience).

Results

Ansa-RLN Technique of Crumley

Crumley has published good phonatory results based on large series [19, 22, 23, 25], and other authors have shown similar good results [36, 55]. We have had experience with this technique for more than 5 years, and the results are consistently excellent with a normal voice. Long-term results are excellent, without degradation.

The technique can be used in case of RLN resection during thyroid oncological surgery or thoracic surgery. Retrograde dissection is always possible. EMG evidence of reinnervation has been achieved in all cases [43].

Personal assessment, built on our ongoing experience, is that this technique provides optimal long-term results—better than with any other medialization technique. However, a prospective randomized evaluation is still lacking.

Hypoglossal Nerve-RLN Technique of Paniello

Paniello studied the morbidity induced by hypoglossal nerve temporarily paralysis [56, 57] and found no major problem with articulation or aspiration in this condition or in reinnervated patients. However, because the results are usually excellent with the ansa-RLN technique, the hypoglossal nerve-RLN method is a second option to be undertaken in cases where the ansa cannot be used. We think that unfavorable synkinesis is induced by such a large amount of regenerated axons [18, 24].

Nerve-Muscle Pedicle Implantation of Tucker

Among the 31 cases reported by Tucker [35, 73], some degree of adduction recovery was observed 2–18 weeks postoperatively. In 12 cases, there was synchronous adductor function and tensing of the vocal cord during phonation efforts. Voice was good in 27 cases. In four cases, additional Teflon injection was needed to achieve a better voice. No comparative evaluation of these different techniques was performed.

Combination

Combined techniques can achieve good long-term results of medialization or arytenoid adduction with immediate improvement [10, 72]. Finally, no comparison between these reinnervation techniques has been published.

16.3.2.2 Superior Laryngeal Nerve Lesions

The superior laryngeal nerve (SLN) is responsible of the sensitive innervation of the supraglottis area by the internal branch (iSLN); its external branch supplies the cricothyroid muscle. It can be injured at a high level, during skull base surgery for instance, with an associating sensitive deficit and motor paralysis of all the intrinsic laryngeal muscles in the ispsilateral side, resulting in vocal cord paralysis in an abductory position with breathy voice and aspiration (increased by a lack of pharyngeal propulsion). More often, the external branch of an SLN lesion can result as a complication of thyroid surgery or from a viral isolated disease.

Lesions of the External (Cricoid) Branch of the SLN

Often misdiagnosed is the patient who presents with mild dysphonia that becomes worse with pitch control. EMG of the cricothyroid (CT) muscle confirms the diagnosis.

Spontaneous recovery or speech therapy effects must be achieved before surgery. In addition to the framework surgery technique (cricothyroid aproximation, thyroplasty), some reinnervation can be proposed.

El-Kashlan used the muscle-nerve-muscle reinnervation technique with success [30], as described in cats by Hogikyan [33]. The principle is to implant a free nerve graft in a donor muscle (here the CT muscle) and to implant the other stump in the receptor denervated muscle. Some reinnervation can be achieved verified by electrical stimulation of the contralateral side.

Crumley used the contralateral ansa hypoglossi to reinnervate a CT muscle (combined with homolateral RLN nonselective reinnervation by the ansa) for rehabilitation of a high-level vagus lesion.

Lesions of the Internal Branch of the SLN

A lesion of the SLN internal branch may produce some aspiration, mainly if it is associated with a motor nerve, such as vagus nerve denervation. Sensory deficit can result also from stroke and can induce some severe aspiration problems. The diagnosis can be confirmed by fibroscopic sensory tests, which test the ability of the patient to feel air pressure or fibroscope tip contact. Cases of failure of swallowing reeducation can be corrected by reinnervation.

Animal experiments in dogs [5] and rabbits by our research team [6], have demonstrated the feasibility of laryngeal sensory reinnervation by direct iSLN anastomosis or other nerve transfers, primarily with the great auricular nerve (GAN). This type of neurorraphy with the GAN was reported by Aviv et al. to be successful in two patients [1].

16.3.2.3 Vagus Nerve Lesion

A vagus nerve lesion can be created at the time of schwannoma or vagus paraganglioma removal. A free nerve graft is usually required to bridge the gap between the two nerve stumps. The superficial cervical plexus (great auricular nerve) can be easily used, harvested even from the same wound, often by a separate incision placed below the external ear. A 5- to 7-cm portion can be harvested if the nerve is followed up to the parotid gland. Sensory sequelae are slight.

However, the longer the nerve graft required, the longer time is needed for recovery and probably the axonal escape. For that reason, this technique has to be performed in contrast to nonselective reinnervation, as described above.

With a high-level vagus nerve lesion (skull base or brain stem lesion), cricothyroid and sensory denervation is observed. The combination of RLN reinnervation and external and internal laryngeal nerve reinnervation can be proposed using the above-mentioned techniques. Combination with passive medialization techniques can also prevent severe aspiration while awaiting recovery of the nerve supply. Currently, we have no experience with this surgical procedure.

16.4 Selective Motor Reinnervation (Bilateral Nerve Lesion)

Selective reinnervation is defined as reinnervation of one or several groups of muscles dedicated to a function of adduction or abduction. The ultimate goal of selective reinnervation is recovery of vocal cord mobility.

In cases of bilateral RLN paralysis, or synkinesis, the vocal cords are usually immobile in a paramedian position, with dyspnea but fairly good voice. The main problem is then to recover the abductive function.

A number of animal experiments have been conducted with some success. The principle was to bring a motor supply with an inspiratory trigger to the abductor muscle—the posterior cricoarytenoid muscle (PCA)—often unilaterally but sometimes bilaterally. The motor nerve supply was either branches from the hypoglossal nerve or roots or the main trunk of the phrenic nerve.

The reinnervation was performed by one of three techniques: nerve implantation into the muscle, nerve-muscle pedicle implantation, or selective nerve anastomosis.

A combination of methods can be performed, and selective simultaneous reinnervation of both adductors and abductors can be done on one or both sides [39].

We consider here only the techniques used in humans. Indications, techniques, follow-up, and results are presented with each technique described.

16.4.1 General Indications

These techniques are usually indicated for bilateral vocal cord paralysis in an adductory position. Voice is fairly well preserved, but severe dyspnea is present. Sometimes a tracheostomy has been carried out. Reinnervation, the aim of which is to preserve an optimal voice, can be considered only if no previous laryngeal surgical treatment has been performed, and no scar alters the capacity of vocal cord mucosal vibration. Passive mobility of the arytenoid should be present. The time elapsed between onset of the paralysis and reinnervation does not appear critical if residual innervation (and usually synkinesis) can be demonstrated on EMG.

16.4.2 Specific Assessment

The usual phoniatric assessment with voice recording and videolaryngoscopy should be performed. EMG is critical for evaluating the remaining innervation of the laryngeal muscles as well as the lack of atrophy. Arytenoid palpation is also crucial for verification, at least at the time of reinnervation surgery. Temporary tracheostomy must be done, especially when bilateral vocal cord reinnervation is performed.

16.4.3 Surgical Techniques

16.4.3.1 Nerve-Muscle Pedicle with the Ansa Hypoglossi

The nerve-muscle pedicle technique described by Tucker et al. using an ansa hypoglossi nerve supply was originally intended to be used as a means for reinnervating the transplanted larynx [64, 74] (Fig. 16.2). It has since been modified and used for reinnervation of bilaterally paralyzed vocal cords in humans [67, 68, 70]. The method was thought to be able to achieve some reinnervation rapidly. Adductor reinnervation was not performed because of the tendency of the vocal cords to return to the paramedian position when not actively abducted [35]. Surgery was performed on one side alone.

Technique

A skin incision is made at the lower border of the thyroid cartilage followed by incision of the platysma and identification of the sternocleidomastoid muscle. The anterior belly of the omohyoid muscle and the jugular vein are identified. The ansa hypoglossi can usually be seen lying on or crossing the internal jugular vein. The fascia overlying the ansa hypoglossi is carefully incised, and the nerve is traced proximally and distally to the first major branch, which is usually the one to the anterior belly of the omohyoid. A 2- to 3-mm square block of muscle, just large enough to include the point of entry and arborization of the nerve, is dissected from the omohyoid. The nerve-muscle pedicle is then isolated for a sufficient length to reach the larynx. The inferior constrictor muscle is then exposed. Blunt dissection and exposure of the PCA, whose fibers pass at right angle to those of the inferior constrictor, is performed. Two or three 5-0 nylon sutures are placed in the posterior cricoarytenoid muscle

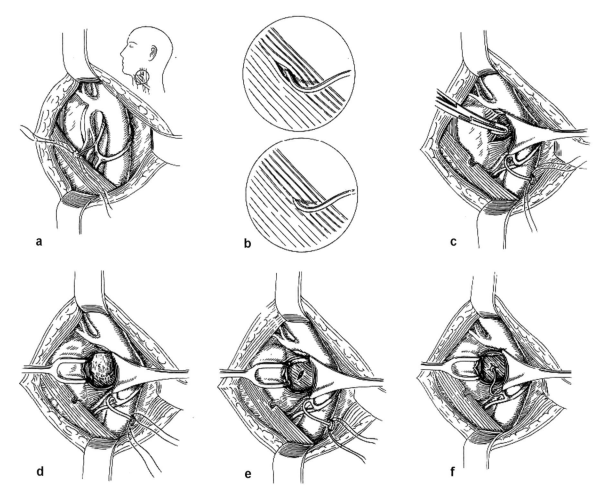

Fig. 16.2. Laryngeal reinnervation of the posterior cricoarytenoid muscle (PCA) by the NMP technique of Tucker [64, 66, 68, 74] (for bilateral vocal cord paralysis). (**a**) Isolation of a branch of the ansa hypoglossi to the omohyoid muscle. (**b**) Dissection of the ansa terminating fibers. (**c**) Separation of inferior constrictor muscle fibers and exposition of the piriform sinus. (**d**) Exposure of the PCA. (**e**) Incision of the PCA. (**f**) Insertion of a nerve-muscle pedicle into the PCA

and then sutured to the block of muscle that is part of the nerve-muscle pedicle (Fig. 16.2). The wound is closed in the usual fashion after insertion of a small Penrose drain. Postoperatively, the patient may be fed the next morning. No antibiotics are necessary.

Results

Tucker has reported a series of 214 patients with a nerve-muscle pedicle to treat bilateral vocal cord paralysis. Long-term success has been achieved in 74% of these patients. Deterioration was observed in 17% of these cases 2–5 years later (due to cricoarytenoid ankylosis) [70]. Similar success was not reported by other authors, and the technique is not done today. Main criticisms were the lack of active abduction of the arytenoid and the lack of EMG inspiratory activation. The procedure was thought to have some efficacy more by passive lateralization induced by the PCA scar than by efficient reinnervation [17]. Moreover, omohyoid and ansa activation during airway obstruction and hypoxia induces self-limitation to its action.

16.4.3.2 Selective Reinnervation Using the Phrenic Nerve

The phrenic nerve is able to produce inspiratory firing to reinnervated muscles and was considered an ideal nerve transfer for PCA reinnervation. Unilateral phrenic

nerve resection was considered to be well tolerated and was used in the past for neurorraphy of the facial nerve or brachial plexus. Some effort was exerted to preserve some nerve supply to the diaphragm.

Animal experiments and human application were performed by Crumley with the split phrenic nerve graft PCA reinnervation [14, 15, 26] (Fig. 16.3). The phrenic nerve is incised longitudinally on part of the circumference, and a free nerve graft is then anastomosed to this harvested portion. The recurrent nerve trunk is sectioned to remove the residual innervation of the larynx and stimulate the muscle to accept new innervation. The distal part of the nerve graft is anastomosed to the tiny abductor branch of the RLN inside the larynx (Fig. 16.3).

Good results were observed in animals. The first human results were presented in 1983 [15]. Some improvement in glottis diameter was observed, but there was no active arytenoid abduction.

Some variations of that technique were used in animals and were described by Rice [61], Mahieu [37], and van Lith-Bijl [75, 77]. They performed an extralaryngeal anastomosis of the phrenic nerve; and inside the larynx, they sectioned the adductor branch and implanted it inside the PCA, guiding all the axons to that muscle.

Later, Crumley [16], van Lith-Bijl [76], and Marie [40] developed some selective simultaneous reinnervation of adductor muscles (with the ansa) and abductor muscle (with the phrenic nerve graft) in animals, with some success.

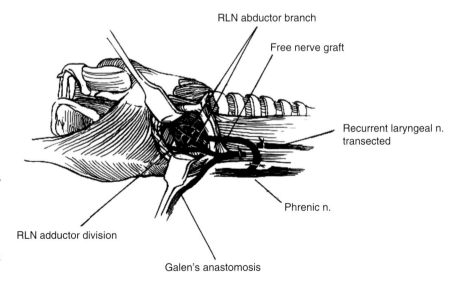

Fig. 16.3. Split phrenic nerve graft procedure of Crumley [15, 26] (for bilateral vocal cord paralysis). Inspiratory phrenic nerve fibers are connected to the abductor branch of the recurrent laryngeal nerve (RLN) (for the PCA), through a free nerve graft

RLN abductor branch

Free nerve graft

Recurrent laryngeal n. transected

Phrenic n.

RLN adductor division

Galen's anastomosis

Bilateral PCA reinnervation was performed in humans by Zheng at al. [83]: on one side by phrenic nerve neurotization (anastomosis of the RLN trunk and implantation of the proximal cut adductor branch of the RLN in the PCA; on the contralateral side by the nerve-muscle pedicle technique with the ansa. Arytenoid abduction was observed in five of six patients only on the phrenic nerve reinnervation side.

16.4.3.3 Bilateral selective motor reinnervation of adductor and abductor laryngeal muscles (total motor reinnervation)

We have previously obtained successful results in dogs with unilateral selective reinnervation of both adductor and abductor muscles using, respectively, the ansa hypoglossi and the phrenic nerve [40]. To apply this technique in humans, we first studied the effects of partial phrenic nerve resection on the respiration of rabbits and dogs and demonstrated that resection of the upper phrenic nerve root had a slight effect on respiration [45, 49–51]. Later, we studied the possibilities of bilateral PCA reinnervation to improve the glottis opening, finally performing total motor reinnervation of the larynx [39, 41] (Fig. 16.4).

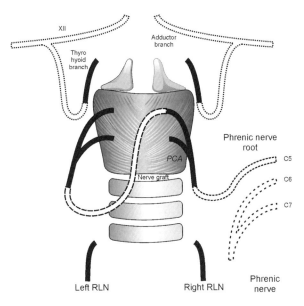

Fig. 16.4. Total motor reinnervation of the larynx. (**a**) Both posterior PCA muscles reinnervation by the upper root of one phrenic nerve. (**b**) Both adductor muscles reinnervation by thyrohyoid branches of both hypoglossal nerves [39, 41, 42, 47, 48] (for bilateral vocal cord paralysis)

We showed that the results were better with a small number of axons for both PCAs provided by just one root from one phrenic nerve [39]. Contemporary reinnervation of adductors by the thyroid branch of both hypoglossal nerves can achieve an optimal supply [46]. The technique can be used in a delayed manner, even in cases of synkinesis [42]. Therefore, we were prompted to begin a clinical prospective trial in humans. Having the Hospital's Ethical Committee approval and grants, we started the study in 2003. Today, 12 patients have undergone bilateral motor reinnervation with this technique.

Indication

The indications for this operation start with bilateral vocal cord paralysis in a paramedian position and dyspnea. Then, the delay since of the start of the paralysis is either (1) short but without signs of recovery or muscle atrophy, or (2) longer and synkinesis is present (clinical and EMG diagnosis) without cricoarytenoid ankylosis. No previous laryngeal surgery must have been done, except tracheostomy or botulinum toxin injection (no scar on the vocal cord). Intact pulmonary function must be verified. Transient tracheostomy at the time of surgery is required.

Technique

Tracheostomy is accomplished via a prior incision (usually a low neck horizontal scar after thyroidectomy). Horizontal cervicotomy is performed at the level of the cricothyroid membrane (Fig. 16.4).

Nerves Identification

Right phrenic nerve dissection (convenient for right-handed surgeons) preserves the left diaphragm in case of aspiration and right lung atelectasis. It is prudent to identify the root distribution. The upper phrenic nerve root is used. The length is variable, sometimes no more than 2 cm, and necessitates harvesting a free nerve graft to elongate it. The free nerve graft can be provided by the superficial cervical plexus—great auricular nerve (GAN). The GAN can be harvested until the point of intraparotid branching: it will be used as (1) a Y-shaped nerve graft for both PCA implantation, and (2) interposition between different transplants if necessary. Alternatively, a sural nerve graft or some branches from the ansa can be used as interposition nerve grafts.

The next step is right and left dissection of the thyrohyoid branch of the hypoglossal nerves (TH XII), which is found at the upper part of the anterior face of the thyrohyoid muscle (coming from the hypoglossal nerve, close to the hyoid bone, and anterior to the ansa).

Intralaryngeal dissection of the RLN branches is next. Hook on the posterior part of the thyroid ala, rotate the larynx, and identify the cricothyroid joint. Section the inferior constrictor just behind the joint: The RLN distribution can be immediately found. If possible, identify the RLN branch for the PCA, which is not always possible (in some cases, it originates from a common branch of the interarytenoid or from the adductor branch). A retrocricoid tunnel is then easily created between PCA muscles and pharyngeal tube, for the next part of the procedure.

Anastomosis

Two situations regarding identification of the RLN branch for the PCA and careful dissection at the lateral part of the PCA muscle are addressed.

- *If the PCA branch is found*: The anastomosis is performed between the upper phrenic nerve root and the ipsilateral RLN trunk (some interposition nerve graft should be required). Section the adductor branch of the RLN inside the larynx, and anastomose the proximal stump of the adductor branch to an interposition retrocricoid free nerve graft, going to the contralateral side (Fig. 16.4). On the contralateral side, if possible, anastomose the nerve graft to the PCA branch if the diameters of the stumps are similar; if not, section the RLN trunk and anastomose it to the interposition retrocricoid nerve graft. Then section the adductor branch the proximal end of which will be implanted inside the PCA. Ensure upper transposition of the distal part of the adductor branches of the RLN to be anastomosed with the TH XII on both sides. An interposition nerve graft is usually used to avoid tension, particularly during swallowing.
- *If the PCA branch is not found*: It is more convenient to use a Y-shaped interposition nerve graft in a retrocricoid position. Perform direct implantation inside the PCA of the distal part of one branch of the Y-shaped nerve graft (secured with thread and

biological glue). Perform retrocricoid passage of the free nerve graft to the contralateral side. Implant it inside the contralateral PCA in the same manner.

Perform low section of the RLN trunks if possible (distal to the previous RLN lesion). There should be transposition to the upper part and anastomosis to TH XII on both sides. The final step is the anastomosis between the upper phrenic nerve root and the interposition nerve graft, to bring the inspiratory axonal supply to the PCA muscles. Tunneling between the jugular vein and carotid artery can be done for shorten distances. Anastomoses are performed under an operating microscope, with epiperineural technique and 9/0 or 10/0 thread usually surrounded by biological glue.

Follow-Up

Aspiration is present for the next first days after surgery, increased by neck and laryngeal dissection. The gastric feeding tube and tracheostomy can be removed within 10 days after surgery. Resection of the RLN removes the paradoxical adduction during inspiration and usually decreases laryngeal resistance. Voice recovery and improved ventilation should start within 6 months after the procedure.

Results

Twelve patients were operated on (ten adults and two children). Ten cases were postthyroidectomy and two were of congenital origin. The results indicated decreased dyspnea in four of six evaluable patients. Three of the six have active arytenoid abduction. All are decannulated, one after arytenoidectomy. All have an improved voice [48].

16.4.4 Reinnervation of Bilateral Vocal Cord Paralysis in Children

Tucker has reported reinnervation by ansa cervicalis nerve-muscle pedicle transfer to the posterior cricoarytenoid muscle (above-mentioned procedure in adults) with some success: 50% decannulation rate in children following this procedure in 9 of 18 tracheostomized children under 5 years of age [69]. Some other teams have published the same success with that technique performed in a fewer number of children [31, 54]. Failures were attributed to alteration of the passive arytenoid mobility.

We performed bilateral selective reinnervation of abductor and adductor muscles with upper phrenic nerve roots (as described above in adults) in three young patients: two under 3 years of age and one under 17 years. Two cases were of congenital origin and associated with PCA trophicity and passive arytenoid mobility. One was secondary to cervicothoracic removal of a lymphangioma, resulting in bilateral RLN and left phrenic nerve paralysis.

The first operated patient (the 17-year-old) recovered bilateral active inspiratory abduction of the arytenoids with preservation of a normal voice. The patient was decannulated [47]. Three years later, he was able to play rugby (3 days a week) [48]. One of the younger boys has markedly improved with residual stridor during intensive efforts. We are currently waiting for the evaluation of the third patient.

16.5 Other Techniques Active on Laryngeal Innervation

We describe some other techniques that contribute to modulation of the nerve supply and are used in neurolaryngology [32].

16.5.1 Botulinum Toxin

Botulinum toxin has been extensively used for laryngeal dystonia. It can also be used to treat laryngeal paralysis and to reduce paradoxal vocal cord adduction during inspiration [12, 13, 44, 60, 62].

16.5.2 Laryngeal Denervation-Reinnervation in Laryngeal Dystonia

During the 1970s, Dedo presented the RLN unilateral resection for spastic dysphonia [29]. Berke et al. have extensive experience of adductor muscle denervation/

reinnervation in long-term, toxin-resistant laryngeal dystonia [3, 9]. Ansa hypoglossi is used to replace the adductor muscles by intralaryngeal bilateral anastomosis.

16.5.3 Laryngeal Pacing

Introduced by Bergman [2], nerve stimulation was directed to the PCA muscles by implantation [34, 82] or through nerve transfer [8]. The RLN or vagus nerve can be stimulated by a permanent system developed by Broniatowsky [7]. Some success was described by Zealer et al. in its human application [81].

16.6 Future of Nerve Reconstruction

In the future, the various techniques may be used in combination (reinnervation and pacing). Furthermore, the contribution of nerve growth factors and stem cells will help improve reconstruction of sensation and motor function of the human larynx. Functional recovery improvement, immunosuppressive and antimitotic drugs will allow to develop the concept of functional laryngeal transplantation.

16.7 Tips and Pearls

- Laryngeal reinnervation can be considered if no scar from previous surgery is present on the vocal cords and there is no severe muscular atrophy (long-term severe denervation).
- With unilateral vocal cord paralysis, the aim of reinnervation is not recovery of vocal cord mobility but correction of muscular tonus; nonselective reinnervation is mandatory.
- Ansa hypoglossi cannot be used in cases of previous extensive neck dissection. Nevertheless, a contralateral ansa can be used in some cases.
- The cricothyroid joint is the main landmark for the RLN. A healthy plane for dissection can usually be found behind the cricopharyngeal muscle, which is the starting point of the retrograde dissection.
- Nerve lengths must be adapted to the ascending movement of the larynx during swallowing.

If necessary, a free nerve graft can be harvested from the superficial cervical plexus (great auricular nerve) better than branches for the strap muscles.

- After reinnervation, voice therapy is mainly aimed at avoiding incorrect use of the larynx.
- With bilateral vocal cord paralysis, selective reinnervation of the PCA on both sides is done, if possible.
- Functional reinnervation necessitates integrity of the cricoarytenoid joints.
- The phrenic nerve is the most suitable donor nerve for inspiratory nerve supply, even if only one of it's roots can be used.
- Removal of the residual innervation is necessary to replace it by functional nerve transfers.
- Temporary degradation of the voice is usual until axonal growth is achieved (within 4–9 months).
- Aspiration is an usual temporary complication of reinnervation and must be prevented.
- Temporary tracheostomy is necessary for bilateral vocal cord reinnervation.
- In cases of failure of the reinnervation, conventional treatments can be undertaken.

References

1. Aviv JE, JP M, Blitzer A, Thompson JE, Close LG (1997) Restoration of laryngopharyngeal sensation by neural anastomosis. Arch Otolaryngol Head Neck Surg 123:154–160
2. Bergman K, Warzel H, Eckardt HU, Hopstock U, Hermann V (1988) Long-term implantation of a system of electrical stimulation of paralyzed laryngeal muscles in dogs. Laryngoscope 98:455–459
3. Berke GS, Blackwell KE, Gerratt BR, Verneil A, Jackson KS, Sercarz JA (1999) Selective laryngeal adductor denervation-reinnervation: a new surgical treatment for adductor spasmodic dysphonia. Ann Otol Rhinol Laryngol 108:227–231
4. Blitzer A, Jahn AF, Keidar A (1996) Semon's law revisited: an electromyographic analysis of laryngeal synkinesis. Ann Otol Rhinol Laryngol 105:764–769
5. Blumin JH, Ye M, Berke GS, Blackwell KE (1999) Recovery of laryngeal sensation after superior laryngeal nerve anastomosis. Laryngoscope 109:1637–1641
6. Bouchetemble P, Marcolla A, Lacoume Y, Verin E, Dehesdin D, Marie JP (2007) Laryngeal sensation recovery by reinnervation in rabbits. Laryngoscope 117:897–902
7. Broniatowski M, Dessoffy R, Shields RW, Strome M (1999) Vagal stimulation for reciprocal coupling between glottic and upper esophageal sphincter activities in the canine. Dysphagia 14:196–203
8. Broniatowski M, Kaneko S, Jacobs G, et al (1985) Laryngeal pacemaker. II: electronic pacing of reinnervated posterior cricoarytenoid muscles in the canine. Laryngoscope 95:1194–1198
9. Chhetri DK, Berke GS (2006) Treatment of adductor spasmodic dysphonia with selective laryngeal adductor denervation and reinnervation surgery. Otolaryngol Clin North Am 39:101–109
10. Chhetri DK, Gerratt BR, Kreiman J, Berke GS (1999) Combined arytenoid adduction and laryngeal reinnervation in the treatment of vocal fold paralysis. Laryngoscope 109:1928–1936
11. Chou FF, Su CY, Jeng SF, Hsu KL, Lu KY (2003) Neurorrhaphy of the recurrent laryngeal nerve. J Am Coll Surg 197:52–57
12. Cohen SR, Thompson JW (1987) Use of botulinum toxin to lateralize true vocal cords: a biochemical method to relieve bilateral abductor vocal cord paralysis. Ann Otol Rhinol Laryngol 96:534–541
13. Cohen SR, Thompson JW, Camilon FS, Jr. (1989) Botulinum toxin for relief of bilateral abductor paralysis of the larynx: histologic study in an animal model. Ann Otol Rhinol Laryngol 98:213–216
14. Crumley RL (1982) Experiments in laryngeal reinnervation. Laryngoscope 92:1–27
15. Crumley RL (1983) Phrenic nerve graft for bilateral vocal cord paralysis. Laryngoscope 93:425–428
16. Crumley RL (1984) Selective reinnervation of vocal cord adductors in unilateral vocal cord paralysis. Ann Otol Rhinol Laryngol 93:351–356
17. Crumley RL (1985) Update of laryngeal reinnervation concepts and options. In: Bailey BJ, Biller HF (eds) Surgery of the larynx. W.B. Saunders, Philadelphia, PA, pp. 135–147
18. Crumley RL (1989) Laryngeal synkinesis: its significance to the laryngologist. Ann Otol Rhinol Laryngol 98:87–92
19. Crumley RL (1990) Teflon versus thyroplasty versus nerve transfer: a comparison. Ann Otol Rhinol Laryngol 99:759–763
20. Crumley RL (1990) Repair of the recurrent laryngeal nerve. Otolaryngol Clin North Am 23:553–563
21. Crumley RL (1991) Muscle transfer for laryngeal paralysis. Restoration of inspiratory vocal cord abduction by phrenic-omohyoid transfer. Arch Otolaryngol Head Neck Surg 117:1113–1117
22. Crumley RL (1991) Update: ansa cervicalis to recurrent laryngeal nerve anastomosis for unilateral laryngeal paralysis. Laryngoscope 101:384–387; discussion 388
23. Crumley RL (1994) Unilateral recurrent laryngeal nerve paralysis. J Voice 8:79–83
24. Crumley RL (2000) Laryngeal synkinesis revisited. Ann Otol Rhinol Laryngol 109:365–371
25. Crumley RL, Izdebski K (1986) Voice quality following laryngeal reinnervation by ansa hypoglossi transfer. Laryngoscope 96:611–616
26. Crumley RL, Horn K, Clendenning D (1980) Laryngeal reinnervation using the split-phrenic nerve-graft procedure. Otolaryngol Head Neck Surg 88:159–164
27. Crumley RL, McCabe B (1982) Regeneration of the recurrent laryngeal nerve. Laryngoscope 90:442–447
28. Damrose EJ, Huang RY, Ye M, Berke GS, Sercarz JA (2003) Surgical anatomy of the recurrent laryngeal nerve: implications for laryngeal reinnervation. Ann Otol Rhinol Laryngol 112:434–438

29. Dedo HH (1976) Recurrent laryngeal nerve section for spastic dysphonia. Ann Otol Rhinol Laryngol 85:451–459
30. El-Kashlan HK, Carroll WR, Hogikyan ND, Chepeha DB, Kileny PR, Esclamado RM (2001) Selective cricothyroid muscle reinnervation by muscle-nerve-muscle neurotization. Arch Otolaryngol Head Neck Surg 127:1211–1215
31. Fayoux P, Delattre A, Delforge A (2007) Réhabilitation laryngée par transfert neuro-musculaire d'omo-hyoïdien (intervention de Tucker)chez l'enfant. In: Société de Laryngologie des Hôpitaux de Paris, Paris
32. Friedrich G, Remacle M, Birchall M, Marie JP, Arens C (2007) Defining phonosurgery: a proposal for classification and nomenclature by the Phonosurgery Committee of the European Laryngological Society (ELS). Eur Arch Otorhinolaryngol 264:1191–200
33. Hogikyan ND, Johns MM, Kileny PR, Urbanchek M, Carroll WR, Kuzon WM, Jr. (2001) Motion-specific laryngeal reinnervation using muscle-nerve-muscle neurotization. Ann Otol Rhinol Laryngol 110:801–810
34. Lacau Saint Guily J, Sebille A, Fontanges P (1989) Stimulation électrique directe du muscle cricoaryténoidien postérieur dénervé, déclenchée par la température sous-glottique chez le chat. Préliminaires au pace-maker laryngé. Ann Oto-Laryngol (Paris) 106:123–126
35. Levine H, Tucker HM (1985) Surgical management of the paralyzed larynx. In: Bailey BJ, Biller HF (eds) Surgery of the larynx. W.B. Saunders, Philadelphia, PA, pp. 117–134
36. Lorenz RR, Esclamado RM, Teker AM, Strome M, Scharpf J, Hicks D, Milstein C, Lee WT (2008) Ansa cervicalis-to-recurrent laryngeal nerve anastomosis for unilateral vocal fold paralysis: experience of a single institution. Ann Otol Rhinol Laryngol 117:40–45
37. Mahieu HF, van Lith-Bijl JT, Groenhout C, Tonnaer JA, de Wilde P (1993) Selective laryngeal abductor reinnervation in cats using a phrenic nerve transfer and ORG 2766. Arch Otolaryngol Head Neck Surg 119:772–776
38. Maranillo E, Leon X, Ibanez M, Orus C, Quer M, Sanudo JR (2003) Variability of the nerve supply patterns of the human posterior cricoarytenoid muscle. Laryngoscope 113:602–606
39. Marie JP (1999) (Contribution à l'étude de la réinnervation laryngée expérimentale; intérêt du nerf phrénique). Laryngeal reinnervation: special interest with the phrenic nerve. Rouen Ph.D. dissertation. University of Rouen, France., pp. 300
40. Marie JP, Dehesdin D, Ducastelle T, Senant J (1989) Selective reinnervation of the abductor and adductor muscles of the canine larynx after recurrent nerve paralysis. Ann Otol Rhinol Laryngol 98:530–536
41. Marie JP, Lacoume Y, Magnier P, Dehesdin D, Andrieu-Guitrancourt J (2000) Selective bilateral motor reinnervation of the canine larynx. Laryngo-Rhino-Otologie, S188–189
42. Marie JP, Choussy O, Lacoume Y, Dehesdin D, Andrieu-Guitrancourt J (2001) Delayed total motor reinnervation of the canine larynx. In: Where upper airway and digestive tract meet. Amsterdam
43. Marie JP, Navarre I, Brami P, Magnier P, Dehesdin D (2007) Réinnervation non sélective des paralysies laryngées unilatérales. Une solution optimale pour les cas difficiles. In: Société de Laryngologie des Hôpitaux de Paris, Paris
44. Marie JP, Navarre I, Lerosey Y, Magnier P, Dehesdin D, Andrieu Guitrancourt J (1998) Bilateral laryngeal movement

disorder and synkinesia: value of botulism toxin. Apropos of a case. Rev Laryngol Otol Rhinol (Bord) 119:261–264
45. Marie JP, Lerosey Y, Dehesdin D, Jin O, Tadie M, Andrieu-Guitrancourt J (1999) Experimental reinnervation of a strap muscle with a few roots of the phrenic nerve in rabbits. Ann Otol Rhinol Laryngol 108:1004–1011
46. Marie JP, Laquerriere A, Choussy O, Lacoume Y, Dehesdin D, Andrieu-Guitrancourt J (2000) Thyrohyoid branch of the hypoglossal nerve in the canine; perspectives for larynx reinnervation. In: European Laryngological Society, Paris. European Archives of Oto Rhino Laryngology, pp S1, S11
47. Marie JP, Vérin E, Woisard V, De Barros A, Choussy O, Dehesdin D (2006) Successful reinnervation of congenital bilateral vocal cord paralysis. In: IX congress of European Society of Pediatric Otorhinolaryngology, Paris
48. Marie JP, Vérin E, Woisard V, Traissac L, Lacau St Guily J, Dehesdin D (2007) Réinnervation sélective des paralysies laryngées bilatérales en fermeture. Premiers résultats. In: Société de Laryngologie des Hôpitaux de Paris, Paris
49. Marie JP, Lacoume Y, Laquerriere A, Tardif C, Fallu J, Bonmarchand G, Verin E (2006) Diaphragmatic effects of selective resection of the upper phrenic nerve root in dogs. Respir Physiol Neurobiol 154:419–430
50. Marie JP, Tardif C, Lerosey Y, Gibon JF, Hellot MF, Tadie M, Andrieu-Guitrancourt J, Dehesdin D, Pasquis P (1997) Selective resection of the phrenic nerve roots in rabbits. Part II: Respiratory effects. Respir Physiol 109:139–148
51. Marie JP, Laquerriere A, Lerosey Y, Bodenant C, Tardif C, Hemet J, Tadie, Andrieu-Guitrancourt J, Dehesdin D (1997) Selective resection of the phrenic nerve roots in rabbits. Part I: cartography of the residual innervation. Respir Physiol 109:127–138
52. Miyauchi A, Ishikawa H, Matsusaka K, Maeda M, Matsuzuka F, Hirai K, Kuma K (1993) Treatment of recurrent laryngeal nerve paralysis by several types of nerve suture. Nippon Geka Gakkai Zasshi 94:550–555
53. Nguyen M, Junien-Lavillauroy C, Faure C (1989) Anatomical intra-laryngeal anterior branch study of the recurrent (inferior) laryngeal nerve. Surg Radiol Anat 11:123–127
54. Nunez DA, Hanson DR (1993) Laryngeal reinnervation in children: the Leeds experience. Ear Nose Throat J 72:542–543
55. Olson DE, Goding GS, Michael DD (1998) Acoustic and perceptual evaluation of laryngeal reinnervation by ansa cervicalis transfer. Laryngoscope 108:1767–1772
56. Paniello RC (2000) Laryngeal reinnervation with the hypoglossal nerve: II. Clinical evaluation and early patient experience. Laryngoscope 110:739–748
57. Paniello RC (2006) Laryngeal reinnervation. In: L Sulica, A Blitzer (eds) Vocal cord paralysis. Berlin: Springer, pp. 189–202
58. Paniello RC, West SE, Lee P (2001) Laryngeal reinnervation with the hypoglossal nerve. I. Physiology, histochemistry, electromyography, and retrograde labeling in a canine model. Ann Otol Rhinol Laryngol 110:532–542
59. Prades JM, Faye MB, Timoshenko AP, Dubois MD, Dupuis-Cuny A, Martin C (2006) Microsurgical anatomy of intralaryngeal distribution of the inferior laryngeal nerve. Surg Radiol Anat 28:271–276
60. Ptok M, Schonweiler R (2001) Botulinum toxin type A-induced "rebalancing" in bilateral vocal cord paralysis?. HNO 49:548–552

61. Rice DH (1982) Laryngeal reinnervation. Laryngoscope 92: 1049–1059

62. Rontal E, Rontal M, Wald J, Rontal D (1999) Botulinum toxin injection in the treatment of vocal fold paralysis associated with multiple sclerosis: a case report. J Voice 13:274–279

63. Sunderland S, Swaney WE (1952) The intraneural topography of the recurrent laryngeal nerve in man. Anat Rec 114: 411–426

64. Tucker HM (1975) Laryngeal transplantation: current status 1974. Laryngoscope 85:787–796

65. Tucker HM (1977) Reinnervation of the unilaterally paralyzed larynx. Ann Otol Rhinol Laryngol 86:789–794

66. Tucker HM (1978) Selective reinnervation of paralyzed musculature in the head and neck: functioning autotransplantation of the canine larynx. Laryngoscope 88:162–171

67. Tucker HM (1978) Human laryngeal reinnervation: long-term experience with the nerve-muscle pedicle technique. Laryngoscope 88:598–604

68. Tucker HM (1982) Nerve-muscle pedicle reinnervation of the larynx: avoiding pitfalls and complications. Ann Otol Rhinol Laryngol 91:440–444

69. Tucker HM (1986) Vocal cord paralysis in small children: principles in management. Ann Otol Rhinol Laryngol 95: 618–621

70. Tucker HM (1989) Long-term results of nerve-muscle pedicle reinnervation for laryngeal paralysis. Ann Otol Rhinol Laryngol 98:674–676

71. Tucker HM (1997) Combined surgical medialization and nerve-muscle pedicle reinnervation for unilateral vocal fold paralysis: improved functional results and prevention of long-term deterioration of voice. J Voice 11:474–478

72. Tucker HM (1999) Long-term preservation of voice improvement following surgical medialization and reinnervation for unilateral vocal fold paralysis. J Voice 13:251–256

73. Tucker HM, Rusnov M (1981) Laryngeal reinnervation for unilateral vocal cord paralysis: long-term results. Ann Otol Rhinol Laryngol 90:457–459

74. Tucker HM, Harvey J, Ogura JH (1970) Vocal cord remobilization in the canine larynx. Arch Otolaryngol 92:530–3

75. van Lith-Bijl JT, Mahieu HF, Stolk RJ, Tonnaer JA, Groenhout C, Konings PN (1996) Laryngeal abductor function after recurrent laryngeal nerve injury in cats. Arch Otolaryngol Head Neck Surg 122:393–396

76. van Lith-Bijl JT, Stolk RJ, Tonnaer JA, Groenhout C, Konings PN, Mahieu HF (1997) Selective laryngeal reinnervation with separate phrenic and ansa cervicalis nerve transfers. Arch Otolaryngol Head Neck Surg 123:406–411

77. van Lith-Bijl JT, Stolk RJ, Tonnaer JA, Groenhout C, Konings PN, Mahieu HF (1998) Laryngeal abductor reinnervation with a phrenic nerve transfer after a 9-month delay. Arch Otolaryngol Head Neck Surg 124:393–398

78. Woodson GE (1993) Configuration of the glottis in laryngeal paralysis. II: animal experiments. Laryngoscope 103: 1235–1241

79. Woodson GE (2007) Spontaneous laryngeal reinnervation after recurrent laryngeal or vagus nerve injury. Ann Otol Rhinol Laryngol 116:57–65

80. Yumoto E, Sanuki T, Kumai Y (2006) Immediate recurrent laryngeal nerve reconstruction and vocal outcome. Laryngoscope 116:1657–1661

81. Zealear DL, Billante CR, Courey MS, Netterville JL, Paniello RC, Sanders I, Herzon GD, Goding GS, Mann W, Ejnell H, Habets AM, Testerman R, Van de Heyning P (2003) Reanimation of the paralyzed human larynx with an implantable electrical stimulation device. Laryngoscope 113:1149–1156

82. Zealear DL, Rainey CL, Netterville JL, Herzon GD, Ossoff RH (1996) Electrical pacing of the paralyzed human larynx. Ann Otol Rhinol Laryngol 105:689–693

83. Zheng H, Zhou S, Li Z, Chen S, Zhang S, Huang Y, Wen W, Shen X, Wu H, Zhou R, Cui Y, Geng L (2002) Reinnervation of the posterior cricoarytenoid muscle by the phrenic nerve for bilateral vocal cord paralysis in humans. Zhonghua Er Bi Yan Hou Ke Za Zhi 37:210–214

Helping Drugs

17

Christian Sittel

Core Messages

› Corticosteroids may prevent laryngeal edema in adults, and they facilitate extubation in the pediatric intensive care unit.

› Long-term use of corticosteroids is not a contraindication for reconstructive surgery.

› Methylprednisolone and dexamethasone are the substances of choice.

› The use of fibrin glue is heterogeneous in Europe, although there is no good evidence of potential benefits.

› During laryngotracheal reconstructive surgery, sealing the suture line has become a de facto standard.

› Most frequently recommended concentration of mitomycin C is 2 mg/ml. It is given as a topical application only, with an exposure time of 2–4 minutes.

› Mitomycin C has documented efficacy against granulation tissue and synechia formation. It is also probably effective in some cases of airway stenosis.

› Indications for mitomycin C must be carefully considered owing to its possible side effects.

› Cidofovir has shown promising results as adjuvant therapy against recurrent respiratory papillomatosis. However, there is limited evidence because controlled studies are lacking.

› Repeated treatment with cidofovir is undertaken at a high cost and possibly with significant co-morbidity.

17.1 Steroids

Corticosteroids are in wide use in laryngology throughout Europe. The main goal is to prevent or reduce postextubation stridor by suppressing mucosal inflammation, including inhibition of leukocyte migration, maintenance of cell membrane integrity, attenuation of lysosome release, and reduction of fibroblast proliferation and tissue swelling [1]. A bolus intravenous injection of dexamethasone or hydrocortisone 1 hour before extubation seems not to prevent laryngeal edema in adults [2, 3]. In contrast, a recent study suggests that a single or multiple injections of methylprednisolone 6 hours before extubation can effectively reduce the incidence of postextubation stridor in critically ill adult patients [4]. The discrepancies observed in these previous studies could be due to several factors, including age, inclusion criteria, duration of intubation, dose, timing, and length of treatment and risk levels of developing stridor.

A treatment with multiple doses of corticosteroids has been shown to reduce the incidence of postextubation airway obstruction in pediatric patients in a well designed prospective, double-blind controlled study [5]. There are no data with a similar evidence level for the adult population. It should be kept in mind that most of the studies investigating this topic are not focused on laryngological patients.

In case of reconstructive surgery for laryngotracheal stenosis, there is a widespread belief that long-term

C. Sittel
Klinik für Hals-, Nasen-, Ohrenkrankheiten, Plastische Operationen, Klinikum Stuttgart – Katharinenhospital, Kriegsbergstraße 60, 70174, Stuttgart, Germany
e-mail: c.sittel@klinikum-stuttgart.de

M. Remacle, H. E. Eckel (eds.), *Surgery of Larynx and Trachea,*
DOI: 10.1007/978-3-540-79136-2_17, © Springer-Verlag Berlin Heidelberg 2010

use of corticosteroids is associated with anastomotic complications due to impaired wound healing and increased infectious complications. Therefore, there has been a policy to attempt to wean patients from corticosteroids to very low or zero dosage prior to surgery. As a result, an operation was either deferred or canceled if a significant dosage reduction was not feasible. A retrospective study on a large cohort of patients did not support this idea [6]. Today, reduced daily corticosteroid intake, though still an aim, is not considered a prerequisite for reconstructive surgery of a stenosed airway in most centers.

For prophylaxis of postoperative swelling of the larynx, a single dose of dexamethasone (4–12 mg) or methylprednisolone (100–250 mg) seems to be the most popular choice among laryngologists and anesthiologists.

17.2 Fibrin Glue

Fibrin sealants have been commercially available for more than two decades in Europe. However, it was not until 1998 that the first fibrin sealant was approved for commercial use in the United States.

The working mechanism basically is activation of the clotting cascade. In the presence of thrombin, fibrinogen cleaves peptides A and B, leaving a soluble fibrin monomer. Factor XIII, which is also activated by thrombin, induces fibrin to crosslink covalently and form a network of fibrils. Temperature, pH, and fibronectin also have a role. The mechanical strength of the fibrin matrix is ultimately determined by the relative concentration of fibrinogen, factor XIII, and adhesive proteins in the sealant. A high thrombin concentration forms a meshwork more rapidly, whereas a higher fibrinogen concentration induces a stronger meshwork [7]. The commercially available fibrin sealants show different characteristics reflecting these differences.

There are few data on the use of fibrin glue in the human larynx. Nevertheless, many laryngologists do use fibrin sealants for a variety of indications [8]. Current indications for use and agent choice are driven mostly by surgeon preference, not by scientific evidence.

Most research has focused on hemostasis as the main indication. Across the surgical literature topical hemostats, sealants, and glues are generally considered effective for decreasing blood loss. Wide variation still exists in the reported magnitude and efficiency of hemostasis, no doubt due to the heterogeneous mixture of agents and clinical conditions among studies. In some centers, fibrin glue is routinely used after endoscopic laser resection of laryngeal carcinoma. However, there are no convincing data showing a benefit. Another motivation is to create watertight seals by the induction of tissue adhesion. Many phonosurgeons are using fibrin glue to reposition vocal fold epithelium after having raised a microflap or during surgery for Reinke's edema. Again, there are no data to support this effect.

During reconstructive surgery for airway stenosis, the use of fibrin glue has become a de facto standard. The idea is to prevent air leaks, reinforce the suture line of an anastomosis, and provide additional stability for grafts brought in to enhance the airway lumen.

In the future, there is a potential role for fibrin glue to serve as a vehicle for drug delivery. Several unique characteristics make fibrin sealants and matrix agents suitable for this role, including a predictable pattern of biodegradability due to the natural mechanism of action, site-specific application and biocompatibility of human components. In addition, drug action can potentially be lengthened or shortened as needed by modulating the antifibrinolytic agent involved. Fibrin sealant embedded with various factors, such as nerve growth factor and fibroblast growth factor, has been used for nerve regeneration, fibroblast proliferation, and angiogenesis in several animal models. Possible benefits of these innovative strategies in human laryngology are waiting to be explored.

17.3 Mitomycin C

Mitomycin C, an anthracycline antibiotic isolated from *Streptomyces caespitosus* (also used as an antineoplastic agent), has also an antiproliferative effect on fibroblasts: By bonding to DNA, it inhibits DNA-dependent RNA synthesis and reduces fibroblastic proliferation and collagen bonding. It has been proven to be effective in reducing scar formation. Therefore, it has been widely applied as a treatment option to prevent stenosis or adhesion after otolaryngological surgery. In laryngology its use is strictly topical. Complications—ulceration, necrosis, aplasia, alopecia, nausea, vomiting—are rare [9] and may be secondary to an overdosage or an inadvertent systemic injection. The risk of inducing late carcinoma is being discussed [10]. No data exist that indicate the most effective concentration, duration, or frequency of application of mitomycin C. Dosage recommendations vary surprisingly from 0.2 to 10.0 mg/ml as does the exposure time (1–10 minutes).

Diseases of the upper airway have been the main focus of investigation. Several animal studies and some clinical trials [11, 12] indicate that mitomycin C is an effective adjuvant in the prevention of restenosis after reconstruction or endoscopic dilatation of laryngotracheal stenosis. In contrast, no such effect could be shown in other investigations on the same subject [13]. There seems to be a benefit in the treatment of synechia of the anterior and, to a lesser degree, posterior commissures [14–16]. It is also being used after surgical removal of reflux-associated granulomas to decrease the risk of recurrence.

With the efficacy of mitomycin C being debatable, the potential complications of mitomycin C need to be considered thoroughly. Partial cartilage necrosis [17] and delayed wound healing through inhibition of fibrosis, especially at a laser-induced wound [18], may result from the topical use of mitomycin C.

Topical use of mitomycin C seems to be beneficial in some laryngological indications, although the evidence is weak. A concentration of 2 mg/ml and an exposure time of 2–4 minutes seems to be favored by most authors. Because of possible side effects, the application of this substance should be restricted to selected cases after careful consideration, which seems of even greater importance in the pediatric population.

17.4 Cidofovir

Cidofovir is a nucleoside analogue that has antiviral activity against the herpesvirus family. It has been shown to induce apoptosis in cells positive for the human papilloma virus. Off-label use of cidofovir has become the most commonly used adjuvant therapy to treat recurrent respiratory papillomatosis. A survey of the American Society of Pediatric Otolaryngology found that 10% of recurrent respiratory papillomatosis patients were receiving intralesional cidofovir as an adjuvant antiviral therapy [19].

A variety of antiviral therapies have been used to treat recurrent respiratory papillomatosis, including systemically administered agents (e.g., acyclovir, ribavirin) as well as others injected into the lesions (e.g., cidofovir). The mechanism of action of antiviral compounds is predominantly inhibition of viral nucleic acid synthesis. Direct action against the viruses involved in recurrent respiratory papillomatosis is the likely mechanism for antiviral therapy efficacy. Various side effects have been associated with the use of available antiviral agents. They include nausea, vomiting, abdominal pain, acute renal impairment, hepatitis, and neutropenia.

In a recent review for the Cochrane Library [20], 23 articles especially related to antivirals and recurrent respiratory papillomatosis were identified; they consisted of 8 nonsystematic review articles, 14 uncontrolled trials or case series, and 1 registered but unfinished study. It was concluded that, owing to the lack of randomized controlled trials on which to base reliable conclusions, there is insufficient evidence regarding the efficacy of antiviral agents as adjuvant therapy in the management of recurrent respiratory papillomatosis in children or adults.

However, most of the uncontrolled studies indicate a positive role for cidofovir in the treatment of recurrent respiratory papillomatosis (RRP). Most authors advocate injection of cidofovir in conjunction with mechanical debulking, usually with repeated injections at a 4- to 12-week intervals. Transoral in-office injection in the awake patient is an established alternative in some centers. In these studies, the concentrations varied from 2.5 to 7.5 mg/ml. Snoeck et al. demonstrated a complete initial clinical response in 14 of 17 adult patients with laryngeal RRP who had local injection of cidofovir, and 10 of the 14 remained disease-free. Although Pransky et al. were unable to reproduce these results in terms of a complete response, they were able to improve the airway markedly and increase the interval time between surgical procedures in 10 children severely affected by RRP without the development of significant adverse events. In a recent publication, Dikkers [21] reported similar results in a group of 18 adult patients. In this population a case of dysplasia possibly induced by cidofovir was observed, underlining a possible carcinogenic potential, which had been observed in animal studies as well. However, based on a recent review article [22] a therapy with intralesional cidofovir for patients with RRP seems not to increase the risk of laryngeal dysplasia. Systemic side effects have not been reported in patients who have received intralesional cidofovir. Treatment with intralesional cidofovir seems to be safe provided the regulations for this therapy are followed. These regulations comprehend that the intralesionally injected dose of cidofovir in adults should be < 3 mg/kg. It is recommended that the use of intralesional cidofovir be suspended during pregnancy. Pulmonary involvement of RRP seems a justified indication for intravenous administration of cidofovir.

Nevertheless, controlled studies seem mandatory before the efficacy of intralesional cidofovir can be reliably assessed as adjuvant therapy for recurrent respiratory papillomatosis.

References

1. Hawkins DB, Crockett DM, Shum TK (1983) Corticosteroids in airway management. Otolaryngol Head Neck Surg 91(6): 593–596
2. Ho LI, Harn HJ, Lien TC, Hu PY, Wang JH (1996) Postextubation laryngeal edema in adults. Risk factor evaluation and prevention by hydrocortisone. Intensive Care Med 22(9):933–936
3. Darmon JY, Rauss A, Dreyfuss D, Bleichner G, Elkharrat D, Schlemmer B et al (1992) Evaluation of risk factors for laryngeal edema after tracheal extubation in adults and its prevention by dexamethasone. A placebo-controlled, double-blind, multicenter study. Anesthesiology 77(2):245–251
4. Cheng KC, Hou CC, Huang HC, Lin SC, Zhang H (2006) Intravenous injection of methylprednisolone reduces the incidence of postextubation stridor in intensive care unit patients. Crit Care Med 34(5):1345–1350
5. Anene O, Meert KL, Uy H, Simpson P, Sarnaik AP (1996) Dexamethasone for the prevention of postextubation airway obstruction: a prospective, randomized, double-blind, placebo-controlled trial. Crit Care Med 24(10):1666–1669
6. Wright CD, Grillo HC, Wain JC, Wong DR, Donahue DM, Gaissert HA et al (2004) Anastomotic complications after tracheal resection: prognostic factors and management. J Thorac Cardiovasc Surg 128(5):731–739
7. Hong YM, Loughlin KR (2006) The use of hemostatic agents and sealants in urology. J Urol 176(6 Pt 1): 2367–2374
8. Toriumi DM, O'Grady K (1994) Surgical tissue adhesives in otolaryngology-head and neck surgery. Otolaryngol Clin North Am 27(1):203–209
9. Hueman EM, Simpson CB (2005) Airway complications from topical mitomycin C. Otolaryngol Head Neck Surg 133(6):831–835
10. Agrawal N, Morrison GA (2006) Laryngeal cancer after topical mitomycin C application. J Laryngol Otol 1–2
11. Rahbar R, Shapshay SM, Healy GB (2001) Mitomycin: effects on laryngeal and tracheal stenosis, benefits, and complications. Ann Otol Rhinol Laryngol 110(1):1–6
12. Ward RF, April MM (1998) Mitomycin-C in the treatment of tracheal cicatrix after tracheal reconstruction. Int J Pediatr Otorhinolaryngol 44(3):221–226
13. Boseley ME, Hartnick CJ (2006) Development of the human true vocal fold: depth of cell layers and quantifying cell types within the lamina propria. Ann Otol Rhinol Laryngol 115(10):784–788
14. Roh JL (2006) Application of mitomycin C after endoscopic lysis of congenital laryngeal web combined with epiglottic hypoplasia in a middle-aged man. Acta Otolaryngol 126(4): 438–441
15. Roh JL (2005) Prevention of posterior glottic stenosis by mitomycin C. Ann Otol Rhinol Laryngol 114(7):558–562
16. Roh JL, Yoon YH (2005) Prevention of anterior glottic stenosis after bilateral vocal fold stripping with mitomycin C. Arch Otolaryngol Head Neck Surg 131(8):690–695
17. Hardillo J, Vanclooster C, Delaere PR (2001) An investigation of airway wound healing using a novel in vivo model. Laryngoscope 111(7):1174–1182
18. Roh JL, Lee YW, Park CI (2006) Can mitomycin C really prevent airway stenosis? Laryngoscope 116(3):440–445
19. Schraff S, Derkay CS, Burke B, Lawson L (2004) American Society of Pediatric Otolaryngology members' experience with recurrent respiratory papillomatosis and the use of adjuvant therapy. Arch Otolaryngol Head Neck Surg 130(9): 1039–1042
20. Chadha NK, James AL (2005) Adjuvant antiviral therapy for recurrent respiratory papillomatosis. Cochrane Database Syst Rev (4):CD005053
21. Dikkers FG (2006) Treatment of recurrent respiratory papillomatosis with microsurgery in combination with intralesional cidofovir--a prospective study. Eur Arch Otorhinolaryngol 263(5):440–443
22. Broekema FI, Dikkers FG (2008) Side-effects of cidofovir in the treatment of recurrent respiratory papillomatosis. Eur Arch Otorhinolaryngol. Aug; 265(8):871–9
23. Bouchayer M, Cornut G (1992) Microsurgical treatment of benign vocal fold lesions: Indications, technique, results. Folia Phoniatr 44:55–84
24. Van Gogh CDL, Verdonck-de Leeuw IA, Boon-Kamma BA, Rinkel RNPM et al (2006) The efficacy of voice therapy in patients after treatment for early glottic carcinoma. Cancer 106:95–105
25. Dejonckere PH, Bradley P, Clemente P, Cornut G et al (2001) A basic protocol for functional assessment of voice pathology, especially for investigating the efficacy of (phonosurgical) treatments and evaluating new assessment techniques. Guideline elaborated by the committee on phoniatrics of the European Laryngological Society (ELS). Eur Arch Otorhinolaryngol 258:77–82
26. Speyer R, Wieneke GH, Dejonckere PH (2004) Documentation of progress in voice therapy: perceptual, acoustic, and laryngostroboscopic findings pretherapy and posttherapy. J Voice 18(3):325–340

Preoperative and Postoperative Speech Therapy

18

Niels Rasmussen and Frederik G. Dikkers

Core Messages

> Evidence based medicine has not quite reached the field of pre- and post-operative speech therapy.

> Spontaneous healing of the vocal folds after surgery using standardized microphonosurgical techniques is the key to voice restoration.

> Pre- and post-operative speech therapy should be tailored to the nature of the vocal fold pathology.

> Precise, truly objective measures of the quality of speech are warranted.

> Better definitions of and precise goals for speech therapy are desirable.

This chapter on preoperative and postoperative speech therapy builds on European experience and pertinent international literature. The organization and application of speech therapy for patients undergoing phonosurgery varies widely across Europe. The aim of the present section is to describe these variations, their background, the arguments, and the causes for this diversity. Areas needing further research are identified. A proposal is provided based on this information to guide phonosurgeons to the most efficient use of speech therapy in relation to phonosurgery.

N. Rasmussen (✉)
Department of Otolaryngology,
2100 Copenhagen, Rigshospitalet, Denmark
e-mail: niels.rasmussen@rh.regionh.dk

18.1 History of Preoperative and Postoperative Speech Therapy

The classic article of Bouchayer and Cornut in 1992 [1] simply stated that pre- and postoperative speech therapy for all laryngeal conditions was indispensable. However, until recently there have been no randomized controlled studies to support this contention.

18.2 Organization of Speech Therapy

The organization of health care varies considerably across Europe. In some countries or areas of the same country, speech therapists are employed by the national health care system and work intimately with the phonosurgeon in the examination and treatment of the patients. In other countries or areas of the same country, speech therapists are employed by the Ministry of Education and are only involved in the examination and treatment on the demand of the phonosurgeon. This also applies for countries where speech therapists work exclusively in private practice.

18.3 Educational Programs

There are several schools of speech therapy. The effect of these various treatments for the same entity has not been validated. A major reason for this is that the personality and personal skills of the speech therapist appear to be important. For details concerning specific methods of speech therapy, one is advised to read specific literature.

M. Remacle, H. E. Eckel (eds.), *Surgery of Larynx and Trachea*,
DOI: 10.1007/978-3-540-79136-2_18, © Springer-Verlag Berlin Heidelberg 2010

18.4 Evidence for the Effect of Speech Therapy Preoperatively and Postoperatively

Evidence for the effect of speech therapy pre- and postoperatively is sparse. In 2006, van Gogh and colleagues [2] showed that there is a beneficial effect of voice therapy in patients treated for early glottic carcinoma, but only 11 and 12 patients were included in the two arms of the study.

A major reason for the lack of evidence of a beneficial effect of speech therapy has been that quantification of this effect is difficult. This, again, is intimately linked to the proposed mechanism of speech therapy. If one takes the holistic point of view, any professional care to comfort the patient in relation to his or her fear of the surgery and the uncertainty of the postoperative result is of benefit. This effect must be ascertained by psychological measures. However, if the mechanism of improvement of speech is thought to be based on a specific training of the entire mechanism of speech focusing on correct use of the laryngeal muscles, the accessory muscles of the neck and thorax, and the remaining muscles of the body involved in speech, other measures such as glottic closure, phonation time, and breathing parameters are relevant.

The evaluation of the voice quality also remains a problem. Attempts at standardizing the auditive as well as the acoustical analysis of speech have been made by the European Laryngological Society (ELS) [3]. Despite this standardization, it is still difficult to establish reproducible measures of the quality of the voice [4] even though it appears simple to conclude whether the voice of the individual patient has improved.

18.5 Relevance of Speech Therapy Related to Diagnosis

The presumed causative mechanisms for the conditions requiring phonosurgery are multiple. It is therefore necessary to look at the individual conditions.

18.5.1 Edema of the Vocal Fold Edge (Acute Type of Vocal Cord Nodules)

Edema of the vocal fold edge is frequently found in rhythmic singers and is localized at the site of vocal cord nodules. These bilateral slight edematous lesions best seen on stroboscopy, may wax and wane depending on the use of the voice. They can be reduced by local steroid inhalation but reappear when treatment is stopped. Such edemas are presumed to be due to inappropriate technique while singing. It is therefore assumed that speech therapy is the treatment of choice. In a number of cases, however, such edemas are consistent, and removal by surgery is indicated. The evaluation of the effect of surgery or speech therapy in these cases is hampered by the fact that most patients are professionals and do not agree to being in a randomized study.

18.5.2 Vocal Cord Nodules (Chronic Type)

Chronic vocal cord nodules are believed to be caused by inappropriate use of the voice. They are most often observed in children with hyperfunctional voices. It is therefore tempting to speculate that speech therapy pre- and postoperatively is indicated for these conditions. However, vocal cord nodules in children often disappear during adolescence, more frequently for boys than for girls, irrespective of speech therapy. The right time for surgery has therefore been a subject of discussion. At present, speech therapy has been used prior to surgery as a rule, but this approach has not been validated. This also accounts for "sandwich therapy," in which speech therapy is offered before and after surgery.

18.5.3 Reinke Edema

Patients suffering from Reinke edema are frequently women around the menopause with heavy smoking habits and who have complained of increasing dysphonia over many years. The causative mechanism is unknown. The only known factor of importance for recurrence after surgery for edema is tobacco smoking, indicating that this is an important causative mechanism. Inhaled steroids are not effective.

Speech therapy preoperatively is used by some to prepare the patient for operation. It aims at treating the hyperfunctionality, which is presumed to represent a compensatory mechanism for inadequate glottic closure. As the dysphonia is primarily due to the organic condition, speech therapy usually does not change the quality of the voice preoperatively. This makes evaluation of the effect of treatment difficult.

As the patients experience a large benefit from surgery [5], they are frequently less motivated to undergo speech therapy postoperatively. Postoperative speech therapy has not been shown to influence the rate of recurrence of the edema, but treatment of the hyperfunctionality is believed to be of benefit. This has not been validated.

18.5.4 Cysts and Polyps

Cysts and polyps are thought to be due to local trauma as they frequently appear in relation to a specific situation with abnormal and/or forceful use of the voice. In such cases, speech therapy seems of little importance, as the patient is usually painfully aware of the offense. No validated evidence exists.

18.5.5 Vocal Cord Palsy

Speech therapy may be applied prior to medialization of the paralyzed vocal cord. However, a significant number of patients spontaneously compensate for insufficient glottic closure without speech therapy, and others do not make any progress with speech therapy. Depending on the school of speech therapy, an attempt is made at increasing the compensatory movement of the contralateral vocal cord and/or increase blood flow to the nerve to speed healing. Other schools simply teach the patients to have patience and use short sentences. A role for postoperative training does not seem evident.

18.5.6 Laryngeal Papillomas

Laryngeal papillomas are treated primarily with surgery, which frequently has to be performed repeatedly (up to several times a year) after the primary episode—possibly for the rest of their lives. The quality of voice appears to depend entirely on the scarring after surgery. Speech therapy seems of little importance.

18.5.7 Precancerous and Cancerous Lesions

Precancerous and cancerous conditions may cause physical changes in the vocal cords due to surgery and/or irradiation. Preoperative speech therapy does not influence the decision on further treatment and is therefore of little

importance unless one takes the holistic point of view into consideration. Postoperative speech therapy is limited by the natural cause of the repair process after surgery and/or irradiation. Speech therapy appears to be of value in certain cases with phonastenia because of the disease course. It may also be useful with regard to the psychological impact of treatment of a life-threatening disease and in some cases with undesired counterproductive compensations such as using the false vocal cords. These factors may explain the effect of speech therapy shown by van Gogh and colleagues [2].

18.6 Timing of Speech Therapy in Relation to Surgery

Preoperative speech therapy (if indicated) should be started so it can have an effect before surgery. This depends entirely on the nature of the lesion, of course, as discussed above.

Postoperative speech therapy may be started immediately after surgery if the holistic point of view is applied. Some argue that patients may start vocal abuse immediately after surgery owing to the change of the voice after surgery, and therefore speech therapy should be started immediately to prevent this. Others find that the natural healing process must take place before onset of speech therapy and that the previously mentioned risk is negligible. This has not been validated.

18.7 Voice Restrictions

In the treatment of acute (soft) as well as chronic (hard) vocal cord nodules, speech rest may be recommended. Its effect does not appear lasting and is frequently negligible (especially regarding the chronic nodules).

Postoperatively, it is frequently recommended that the patients keep absolutely silent to let the epithelium and subepithelial tissue heal. However, others recommend only that patients speak as little as possible using their normal voice but refrain from shouting or using their voice professionally. The time period for such restraints also appears to vary. Some use days and others a week, as the integrity of the vocal fold epithelium is usually reestablished by then. Even voice rest up to 3–4 weeks may be prescribed as phonosurgeons await reestablishment of the epithelial wave using laryngostroboscopy. The combination of voice restrictions and speech therapy also seems to vary widely.

References

1. Bouchayer M, Cornut G (1992) Microsurgical treatment of benign vocal fold lesions: Indications, technique, results. Folia Phoniatr 44:55–84
2. Van Gogh CDL, Verdonck-de Leeuw IA, Boon-Kamma BA, Rinkel RNPM et al (2006) The efficacy of voice therapy in patients after treatment for early glottic carcinoma. Cancer 106:95–105
3. Dejonckere PH, Bradley P, Clemente P, Cornut G et al (2001) A basic protocol for functional assessment of voice pathology, especially for investigating the efficacy of (phonosurgical) treatments and evaluating new assessment techniques. Guideline elaborated by the committee on phoniatrics of the European Laryngological Society (ELS). Eur Arch Otorhinolaryngol 258:77–82
4. Speyer R, Wieneke GH, Dejonckere PH (2004) Documentation of progress in voice therapy: Perceptual, acouastic, and laryngostroboscopic findings pretherapy and posttherapy. J Voice 18(3):325–340
5. Bouwers F, Dikkers FG (2009) A retrospective study concerning the psychosocial impact of voice disorders: Voice Handicap Index change in patients with benign voice disorders following treatment (measured with the Dutch version of the VHI). J Voice 23(2):218–224

Subject Index

Printing and Binding: Stürtz GmbH, Würzburg